k library

Medical Ethics and Sociology

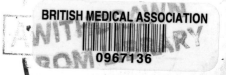

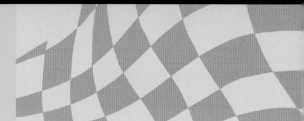

First edition authors

Keith Amarakone
Sukhmeet S. Panesar

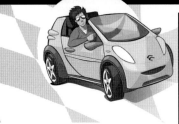

2nd Edition
CRASH COURSE

SERIES EDITOR
Dan Horton-Szar
BSc (Hons) MBBS (Hons)
Northgate Medical Practice
Canterbury

FACULTY ADVISORS
Carolyn Johnston
LLB LLM MA PhD
Adviser in Medical Law & Ethics
King's College London, School of Medicine
London

David Armstrong
CBE MB MSc PhD FFPH FRCGP
Professor of Medicine and Sociology
King's College London
London

Medical Ethics and Sociology

Andrew Papanikitas
BSc (Hons) MA MBBS DCH MRCGP DPMSA
Portfolio GP, London and Buckinghamshire
Sessional Tutor/Facilitator in Ethics
King's College London, London

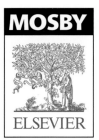

MOSBY

ELSEVIER

Edinburgh London New York Oxford Philadelphia St Louis Sydney Toronto 2013

Content Strategist: Jeremy Bowes
Senior Content Development Specialist: Ailsa Laing
Project Manager: Andrew Riley
Designer: Christian Bilbow

First edition 2006

Second edition 2013

ISBN   978-0-7234-3634-8

British Library Cataloguing in Publication Data
A catalogue record for this book is available from the British Library

Library of Congress Cataloging in Publication Data
A catalog record for this book is available from the Library of Congress

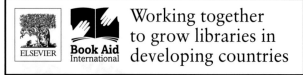

Series editor foreword

The *Crash Course* series was first published in 1997 and now, 16 years on, we are still going strong. Medicine never stands still, and the work of keeping this series relevant for today's students is an ongoing process. These new editions build on the success of the previous titles and incorporate new and revised material, to keep the series up-to-date with current guidelines for best practice, and recent developments in medical research and pharmacology.

We always listen to feedback from our readers, through focus groups and student reviews of the *Crash Course* titles. For the new editions, we have completely re-written our self-assessment material to keep up with today's 'single-best answer' and 'extended-matching question' formats. The artwork and layout of the titles has also been largely re-worked to make it easier on the eye during long sessions of revision.

Despite fully revising the books with each edition, we hold fast to the principles on which we first developed the series. *Crash Course* will always bring you all the information you need to revise in compact, manageable volumes that integrate basic medical science and clinical practice. The books still maintain the balance between clarity and conciseness, and provide sufficient depth for those aiming at distinction. The authors are medical students and junior doctors who have recent experience of the exams you are now facing, and the accuracy of the material is checked by a team of faculty advisors from across the UK.

I wish you all the best for your future careers!

Dr Dan Horton-Szar

Author

Ethics and sociology as applied to medicine can sometimes appear isolated and unimportant in a crowded curriculum. These subjects, however, *are* important, not just because they contribute towards qualification as a doctor (they are tested in exams), but because they influence the practice of medicine itself. Medical students cannot hope to experience every dilemma first hand, or to spend time with every single kind of clinician or every single kind of patient. But medical students and junior doctors are expected to deal with new and problematic clinical situations in a reasoned and professional way, whether this is in a clinical examination or a clinic.

There are several ways that medical students (in the UK at least) can experience ethics and sociology. Lectures, self-selected components and intercalated degrees provide opportunities to learn. There has to be a point to learning, however, and as a medical student, a doctor and more recently, as a teacher and OSCE examiner, I have seen the concepts in this book are often tested, whether in extended-matching questions and OSCEs, or out in the real world of clinical practice.

This second edition has been extensively revised. Not only have many of the sections been updated, but the book also contains a complete set of practice questions. The ethics and law sections take into account the revised core curriculum in Medical Ethics and Law. The book is written to be used as a revision guide and a springboard to further reading and discussion. Every chapter contains suggestions for further reading. There is a 'health warning' that comes with this book, however. While every effort has been made to bring the book up-to-date, laws will change, and like all other disciplines, ethics and sociology are always updating their ideas. If something does not appear to make sense, then do look it up in the most current text you can find, or search online.

In the meantime, I hope this book will be your passport to exam success!

Andrew Papanikitas

Faculty Advisor

Why should medical students open a book on ethics, law and sociology? Practising good medicine requires more than knowledge and application of science and technical skills. An understanding of the principles of medical ethics and law is crucially important in order that doctors know how to identify and deal with ethical dilemmas arising in clinical practice. In 2005 the Royal College of Physicians Working Party report on *Ethics in Practice* noted that, 'medical practitioners are encountering ethical uncertainties and even dilemmas in their daily practice with increasing frequency' (Executive summary, page ix, paragraph 1), so preparedness through study and understanding of ethical concepts is a necessary pre-requisite to the practice of medicine.

In the UK, the General Medical Council (GMC) requires that medical graduates behave according to ethical and legal principles and must know about and comply with the GMC's ethical guidance and standards. In 2010 an updated consensus statement was published outlining core learning outcomes in medical ethics and law for medical students and foundation year doctors (Stirrat et al. 2010 Medical ethics and law for doctors of tomorrow: the 1998 Consensus Statement updated. *Journal of Medical Ethics* 36: 55–60.

Crash Course; Medical Ethics and Sociology builds upon these core learning outcomes and provides accessible and relevant information for students, whether revising for an examination, studying for an assignment, and for those who just want to develop their understanding. I hope you will find the book useful and thought-provoking.

Carolyn Johnston

Acknowledgements

I would like to thank Dr Carolyn Johnston and Professor David Armstrong for their invaluable guidance and constructive criticism, as well as Elizabeth Morrow (PhD student, Dept of Political Economy, King's College, London) for her co-revision of Chapter 9. I would like to thank all the people who have commented on sections of the book, especially Dr Catherine Quarini, Dr Catherine Marshall and Dr Nawal Bahal. I would like to thank my PhD Supervisors, Professors Alan Cribb and Sharon Gewirtz, and my family for tolerating my distractedness around the time of manuscript submission, and especially Dr Emma McKenzie-Edwards for providing much needed moral support and inspiration at the finish-line. This edition would not have taken shape as it did without the hard work of Alison Taylor, Ailsa Laing, Andrew Riley, Jeremy Bowes, Barbara McAviney and the team at Elsevier, and editorial comment from Dr Dan Horton-Szar.

Dedication

For my family, my friends and my teachers ...
but also for my students, who make it all worthwhile.

Andrew Papanikitas

Contents

Contents

Foundations of medical ethics and law ① 1

WHAT IS 'MEDICAL ETHICS' AND WHY IS IT IMPORTANT?

'Ethics' or 'moral philosophy' is the study of morals in human conduct. Like all branches of philosophy, it deals with the critical evaluation of assumptions and arguments. Within the field of philosophy, 'Medical ethics' is the study of morals in the medical arena (Fig. 1.1). In practice this means that medical ethics plays a role wherever the question, 'What ought to be done?' is raised in the medical context. Campbell and Higgs (1982) describe three concepts of 'ethics' held by doctors:

1. Professional etiquette: the accepted conventions of a social role
2. Synonymous with 'morals or morality'
3. Moral philosophy: the critical study of morality.

In the past, many medical schools did not formally teach ethics. It was thought that the student would be able to learn what was considered right and wrong by observation of senior doctors, *and by doing as they did.*

The explicit teaching of ethics aims to help to foster *an ability to make rational, moral decisions* – rather than to simply do things as they have been done before.

The importance of this for the medical student, in real life and in exams, is that it is not just the conclusion you reach that is important. Rather, it is also the strength and coherence of the arguments that lead you to your conclusion, which are important.

Ethics deals with:

- what is right and wrong
- what is good and bad
- what ought and ought not to be done.

Medical ethics, therefore, critically examines the reasons that underlie any medical decision that involves these concepts. Medical ethics aims to produce and emphasize a rational, coherent and consistent approach to making moral decisions in medicine.

It is sometimes helpful to distinguish philosophical medical ethics from:

- law and professional codes of practice, which rely on the interpretation of pre-existing legal and professional rules
- religious teaching or theological arguments, which derive from one or more sources of religious scripture
- sociological or psychological explanations for why we behave in certain ways do not necessarily indicate if the behaviour is good or bad
- the discussion of moral decision-making within medicine, in a historical or anthropological light. This does not necessarily answer the question, 'what is the right thing to do?'

However, all of the above disciplines may contribute to the study of medical ethics.

THE CORE CURRICULUM IN MEDICAL ETHICS AND LAW

The core curriculum in medical ethics and law was updated in 2010 (Stirrat et al 2010) and sets out a core content of learning for medical ethics and law in the UK. It has been endorsed by the General Medical Council (GMC), which means it will form a basis for the standards expected from medical schools and hence of medical students.

In Years 1 and 2 medical students are expected to:

- recognize and understand core ethical and legal topics
- apply common ethical arguments using constructed case scenarios
- be able to understand and discuss differing viewpoints
- be aware of the requirements of GMC on student fitness to practice.

In Years 3 and 4 medical students are expected to:

- be familiar with the GMC's professional codes of conduct
- recognize ethical and legal issues and be able to apply common ethical arguments to actual clinical encounters in different specialties and public health interventions
- recognize and conform with professional and legal obligations in practice

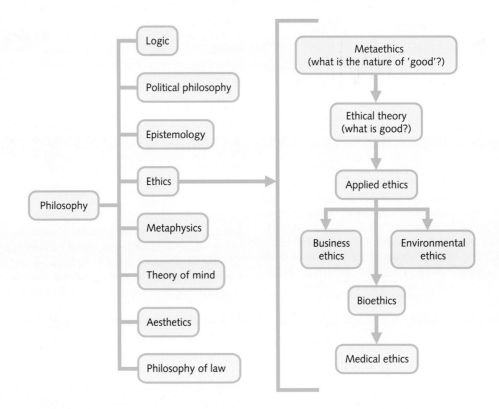

Fig. 1.1 Branches of philosophy and the position of medical ethics.

- demonstrate the ability to reflect on ethical practice of self, peers and teachers.

In Year 5 (and 6 where applicable) medical students are expected to be able to:

- integrate ethical analysis of actual clinical encounters with clinical knowledge and skills and legal obligations
- elaborate on common ethical arguments
- propose action/decision based on this synthesis
- display professional attitudes and behaviours consistent with Good Medical Practice
- be aware of their own values.

In the foundation years and their subsequent careers, doctors should be able to demonstrate increasing competence in how to identify, acknowledge and deal with ethical, legal and professional issues on which good medical practice is based. Teaching and learning should be relevant to both their particular stage of training and relevant specialty-specific ethical issues.

The updated curriculum also specifies a core content of learning for medical ethics and law:

- Foundations of medical ethics and law (see Ch. 1)

- Professionalism: 'good medical practice' (see Ch. 2)
- Patients: their values, narratives, rights and responsibilities (see Ch. 3)
- Informed decision-making and valid consent or refusal (see Ch. 3)
- Capacity and incapacity (see Ch. 3)
- Confidentiality (see Ch. 2)
- Justice and public health (see Ch. 5)
- Children and young people (see Ch. 3)
- Mental health (see Ch. 3)
- Beginning of life (see Ch. 4)
- Towards the end of life (see Ch. 4)
- Medical research and audit (see Chs 2 and 11).

ETHICAL ARGUMENTS

Medical students and indeed qualified doctors often find it disheartening that medical ethics asks questions more often than it provides answers. You *could* argue that abortion (or euthanasia, cloning, dating patients and so on) is right or wrong – there seem to be arguments either way.

Fig. 1.2   How to write an ethics essay:

Make an outline/plan of the essay before writing a first draft

Answer the question: Work out what the question is asking and make sure that everything you say is relevant to the essay title. Ways to help you to do this include:
    Define how you interpret any unclear terms at the beginning of your essay
    State in your own words what the problem is and the issues you plan to address in your essay
    Briefly state the scope of the question.

When making your arguments in the body of the essay, try and develop points in a logical way by:
    Stating your perspective and reasons for holding it
    Looking at opposing arguments: you must use other people's ideas as well as your own to show that you are aware of the major arguments in a certain area. Don't forget to reference ideas you have read (especially important in coursework essays)
    Saying why your arguments are better/more convincing.

When you re-read your first draft, decide what the 'purpose' of each paragraph is, and whether what you have written is achieving that purpose.
When concluding, sum-up the reasons for your argument that you have already outlined: don't include new arguments in the conclusion.
No-one expects a definitive right answer: ethical debates have raged for millennia without resolution. Conclude your essay, however. You should say why you believe one argument is better than another, while still acknowledging that both have their merits.

However, it is important to use arguments that are valid or justifiable (Fig. 1.2). Having a structure can help to make an argument logical and relevant. Ethical theory can provide this structure.

ETHICAL THEORIES

Ethical theories attempt to provide an over-arching theoretical framework for addressing the problem of how human beings should behave with one another in the world. There are three key theories which have historically dominated medical ethics teaching: *Utilitarianism, Deontology and Virtue Ethics*. More recent frameworks attempt to reconcile different theories and values. The widely taught four principles of biomedical ethics attributed to Beauchamp and Childress is one such attempt. 'Values-Based Practice' or 'Values in Medicine' has recently gained prominence in psychiatry and general practice, and is taught on some undergraduate medical degrees (these theories are considered below).

Rights-based approaches to ethics are often used in public debates, and particularly around the availability of healthcare services.

Why should we bother with these theories? Can we not rely on some 'Golden principle' such as 'Do unto others as you would have them do unto you?' Perhaps such a principle is sufficient to help to guide our moral decisions on a day-to-day basis, but often it falters on the ethical dilemmas where there is no obvious path to take. In addition, we need to provide reasons why any such golden principle is right and why others might be wrong. The purpose of ethical theory is to help us to think more clearly about ethical problems.

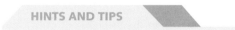

HINTS AND TIPS

There are three key theories which have dominated medical ethics: Utilitarianism, Deontology and Virtue Ethics. You must have a basic idea of what these theories say.

Utilitarianism

Utilitarianism is founded on the work of Jeremy Bentham (1748–1832) and John Stuart Mill (1806–1873). It is based on a single principle of what is good: the principle of utility. The morally correct decision or course of action is often summed up as that which promotes *'the greatest good for the greatest number'*. The principle of good holds that we ought to produce the maximum amount of good. It is a *consequentialist* theory, as it holds that the predicted outcomes (i.e. the consequences) of an action are the most morally important component of that action.

What then is 'utility'? Bentham and Mill thought that utility was pleasure or happiness. Others have considered utility to include values such as friendship, knowledge, health and beauty. Still others believe that the concept of utility is best applied to the satisfaction of preferences rather than any intrinsic values.

Bentham believed that law and morality could be made rational by a scientific study of human nature. He thought that humans were governed by two factors: 'pleasure and pain', and that it was in their nature to seek pleasure and avoid pain. For Bentham, laws were only 'good' if they maximized pleasure and minimized pain for the majority of people. The 'scientific' foundation of utilitarianism comes from the requirement to do 'happiness sums'. Bentham thought it was possible to classify how good an action is by measuring how much pleasure or pain was brought about by that action. He called this process 'felicific calculus'.

Mill differed from Bentham in two important ways:

1. He thought that cultural and spiritual pleasures should be sought in preference to physical pleasures.
2. He thought that people should ordinarily stick to moral rules rather than calculate the balance of utility for each ethical problem.

Even though Mill advocated moral rules, he is still a utilitarian, because he held that these moral rules should be calculated using the principle of utility. This is what is known as *rule utilitarianism*. For example, lying in general might produce less utility than telling the truth. Therefore, there is a rule that says 'Do not lie!' However, we could imagine a scenario where telling a particular lie might produce more utility than telling the truth would. The rule utilitarian would still tell the truth. Other utilitarians, known as *act utilitarians*, would appeal directly to the principle of utility and lie (Fig. 1.3).

The advantages of utilitarianism are that:

- it fits with two strong intuitions, i.e.
  - morality is about promotion of well-being
  - we should maximize well-being
- it is a single principle that tries to deal with appropriateness of other principles, such as a principle of *always* telling the truth or of *always* acting to prevent suffering
- it incorporates a principle of equality: each person's happiness is equal
- it can be extended to the animal kingdom: some utilitarians have argued that the capacity to suffer (and feel pain) means our treatment of animals also ought to be subject to moral scrutiny.

The disadvantages of utilitarianism are that:

- there are problems dealing with intuitively immoral actions: is it right to kill one patient in order to harvest their organs and perhaps save five lives?
- utilitarianism demands too much: in always asking us to do the *best* action, everyone is expected to be both heroic and saintly. For example, it could be argued that 'maximizing utility' demands that not only should we donate blood and bone marrow as often as we can, but also that we may well be morally obliged to donate one of our kidneys as well
- the equality principle is overly impersonal in demanding that we treat the well-being of our friends and family as equivalent to that of strangers
- in principle, a small increase in pleasure for the majority will override a vast degree of pain for a minority.

Deontology

Deontology covers those theories that emphasize moral *duties* and *rules*, rather than consequences (from the Greek *deon*, meaning 'duty'). Perhaps the best *known* deontological principles are those set down in the *Ten Commandments*.

Deontology is associated with Immanuel Kant (1724–1804). He believed that morality was not dependent on how much happiness resulted from particular actions. Rather, he thought morality was something humans imposed upon themselves because they are rational beings. Although Christian, Kant did not believe that God was necessary for moral law.

Kant argued that we can find out which moral rules to obey by using our powers of reason. He said that by seeing whether our desires can be applied universally, we can tell whether or not they follow rational moral principles. This 'universalizability' test is called the 'categorical imperative'. It states:

> Act only on that maxim through which you can at the same time will that it should become a universal law.

This means that we should behave in such a way that we can imagine everyone can behave. For example, if our 'maxim' or 'desire' is to 'steal other people's things when we want them', we need to consider whether or not this maxim could be held for everyone. Kant said that if everyone stole things whenever they wanted, the whole notion of theft and personal property would collapse; if this happens, the concept of 'stealing' becomes illogical. The same holds for the idea of lying. Telling a lie only 'works' if people generally tell the truth. If everyone lied whenever it might benefit them, then this general belief in truth-telling would collapse and lying would itself become pointless. Therefore, Kant said that the moral law obliges us not to steal and not to lie.

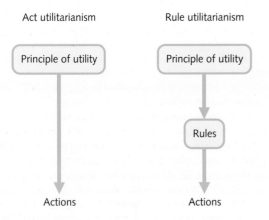

Fig. 1.3 Act vs rule utilitarianism. In 'act utilitarianism', the principle of utility is directly used to guide actions. In 'rule utilitarianism', the principle of utility is used to formulate general rules which in turn are used to guide actions.

Kant also said that because humans are rational beings, we should never treat people *simply as a means but always at the same time as an end*. The emphasis here is on the fact that all people are equal (because they are rational) and deserve equal respect.

The advantages of Kantian deontology are that:

- it has a simplicity of structure: moral rules must pass the 'categorical imperative'
- it places a special responsibility upon individuals for their actions
- it addresses factors other than consequences, such as motives, which intuitively seem important in moral decision-making
- it allows a certain degree of choice; if more than one option is morally acceptable, then the individual can choose which to carry out (unlike utilitarianism where the *best* option *must* be selected).

The disadvantages of Kantianism are that:

- it depends on freedom of will and rationality: are we perfectly free and rational?
- it seems to be absolutist in nature: the imperative 'do not lie' is intractable – it means 'do not lie . . . EVER', even if it prevents great harm from occurring
- the moral rules can seem quite abstract and unable to deal with the complexities of real-life ethical dilemmas
- two duties (imperatives) may conflict, so what happens then?

Duties often go hand-in-hand with rights. When someone has a 'right', this usually implies that someone else has a 'duty' to respect that right (this may entail a duty to do something, or to refrain from doing something). Ronald Dworkin (1977) suggests that rights are special kinds of fact – moral facts – which carry more influence in moral disputes. This way of thinking sees moral rights as 'insistent normative demands' that take precedence over other types of moral argument.

Rights can be positive or negative:

- A negative right: generally confers a freedom from interference, e.g. the 'right to life' involves a freedom from being killed.
- A positive right: confers a duty on someone else to provide for the right holder, e.g. the 'right to health care' imposes a duty on the government to provide hospitals, nurses and doctors for its citizens.

Virtue theory

Virtue theory does not focus on either moral rules or consequences; rather, it concentrates on character and motivation. It originates in the philosophical writings of the ancient Greeks. Socrates (469–399 BC) asked, 'How should a man live, in order to achieve *eudaimonia* (happiness or flourishing)?' His answer was that the good life was the one lived in accordance with *arête* (virtue). Ancient virtues included wisdom, justice, courage, moderation and piety.

Aristotle (384–322 BC) claimed a more practical approach. He believed that people were preprogrammed with the virtues, but were responsible for the degree to which they implemented them. 'Good' people choose a 'golden mean', an 'average' between extremes and so do everything in moderation. So the virtuous man would be neither reckless (too courageous) nor timid (not courageous enough).

According to virtue theory, it is the cultivation of virtue within one's character that is the function of morality. Philosophers such as Alisdair MacIntyre (b. 1929) have advocated that the study of ethics should be directed towards how we ought to live our lives, and advised which ethical characteristics we should try and develop. In a sense, virtue theory tries to concentrate on what it is that makes some people 'good' or 'virtuous' and how they are different from those who are not. The right thing to do in a given dilemma is that which a 'virtuous' person would do. Virtue theory emphasizes:

- the *interpretation* of certain facts of a dilemma, within a specific *context*. That is by looking at the values pertinent to those involved in a dilemma rather than abstract hypothesizing
- *reasoning by analogy* rather than reasoning by deduction or from principles.

The advantages of the virtue theory:

- It is more personal than either utilitarianism or Kantianism: it supports those actions done out of benevolence, friendship, honesty and love in and of themselves, rather than because they are 'maximizing positive value' or are carried out in accordance with 'moral duty'
- It is more adaptive to the particular context of a dilemma, rather than being bound by rules or applying a 'calculation' to a dilemma.

The disadvantages of the virtue theory:

- A list of virtues is insufficient to justify why we should promote them
- It is unhelpful in *resolving* moral conflicts
- There is no universally agreed-upon list of virtues to promote. Some writers, however, have attempted to come up with a set of medical virtues (Pellegrino & Thomasma 1993). Pellegrino and Thomasma's list of virtues includes trust, compassion, prudence, justice, fortitude, temperance, integrity and self-effacement. The key virtue in a physician's character is phronesis, or prudence, which is 'both a moral and an intellectual virtue that disposes one habitually to choose the right thing to do in a concrete moral situation'.

Values-based medicine

Consideration for individual values, particularly those of the patient, can be difficult within the context of modern health care, where complex and conflicting values are often in play. This is particularly so when a patient's values seem to be at odds with evidence-based practice or widely shared ethical principles, or when a health professional's personal values may affect the care provided.

Values-based practice, a framework developed originally in the domain of mental health, maintains that values are pervasive and powerful influences in healthcare decisions and research, and that their impact is often underestimated. It suggests that our current approaches lead us to ignore some important manifestations of values at both the general level, as relevant in legal, policy and research contexts, as well as at the individual level, as relevant in clinical practice. All students and trainees are continually exposed to areas of ethical difficulty throughout their training; the important thing is to try to be aware of them. Fulford (2004) calls this the 'squeaky wheel principle' of values-based medicine. This metaphor means that we tend to notice values only when they are diverse or in conflict. Learners may have difficulty doing this on their own. Discussion with others is essential to bring out a proper range of responses to ethical problems or value conflicts and to challenge individual views.

Values-based practice expands on the ideas that may be regarded as value-laden. It suggests that one of the reasons for overlooking values is that they are presumed to be shared when not obviously in conflict. Fulford and others (Fulford 2004, Fulford et al 2002) have suggested that since primary care is an area of significant diversity of values, values-based practice may have particular relevance there.

THE FOUR PRINCIPLES

In the late 1970s, two Americans, Tom Beauchamp and James Childress, introduced the idea of the 'four principles' or 'principlism'. Historically, principlism represents the most widely taught ethical framework in UK medical schools and probably the most widely used ethical framework by clinicians in English-speaking countries.

The four principles are:

- autonomy: the principle of respecting the decisions made by those capable of making decisions. Autonomy also includes respecting (as far as is possible) the autonomy of people whose ability to make decisions is limited, e.g. by senility or illness
- beneficence: the principle of doing good or providing benefit

- non-maleficence: the principle that a person should avoid doing harm, or minimize harm as much as possible if it is unavoidable
- justice: the principle of ensuring fairness and equity in the distribution of risks and benefits. This includes the idea of treating equals equally and recognizing relevant inequalities.

HINTS AND TIPS

The four principles do not constitute an 'ethical theory' as such, rather they are guidelines: a framework around which an ethical discussion can be based, regardless of the favourite ethical theory held by the participants.

Respect for autonomy

Autonomy literally means 'self-rule'. In essence, it refers to an ability: (1) to reason and think about one's own choices; (2) to decide how to act and (3) to act on that decision, all without hindrance from other people. Autonomy is more than simply being free to do what one wants to do. It implies that rational thought is involved in a decision. While many animals are free to do what they want, they are not autonomous because they do not critically evaluate the benefits and risks to themselves, or others, involved in their decisions.

In respecting a person's autonomy, we recognize that they are entitled to make decisions that affect their own lives. Justification for this principle is most obviously found in Kantian theory: the idea that people should be treated not simply as means, but as ends in themselves. However, support for autonomy can also be found in those versions of *rule-utilitarianism* which hold that the best outcomes arise when autonomy is respected.

Often, depending on how young or old, sick or insane, people may be more or less autonomous. We may judge that they have the capacity to make all decisions, some decisions or no decisions. The degree to which a person is autonomous is central to the concepts of consent and capacity in medical ethics and law. This is discussed in Chapter 3.

Beneficence and non-maleficence

Beneficence is the principle of doing 'good'. In the medical context, this generally means improving the welfare of patients. Non-maleficence involves 'not harming patients'. It is associated with the Latin phrase *primum non nocere* or 'above all, do no harm'. As 'doing good' and 'not doing harm' seem to fall on a continuum, there is often confusion about where non-maleficence ends and beneficence begins. One way of looking at the two, is to think of non-maleficence as a duty towards all people, whereas beneficence, as we cannot help everyone, is a duty we choose to discharge on specific people. Medical staff, by accepting a patient, have chosen to act beneficently towards that person. The principles of beneficence and non-maleficence are broadly similar to the utilitarian principle of maximizing benefit and minimizing harm.

Justice

The principle of justice within the medical context refers to the allocation or distribution of resources among the population. Basically, this principle demands the fair treatment of 'equals' within the healthcare system. There is, however, no single answer as to what constitutes fair and equal distribution. The following are possible answers:

1. *Equality* – Each person receives an equal share of the resources available
2. *Need* – Each person receives resources appropriate to how much that person needs
3. *Desert* – Each person receives resources according to how much they deserve them (in terms of contribution, effort or merit)
4. *Desire* – Each person gets what they want. Desire forms the basis of a utilitarian outlook: utilitarianism is important as it forms the basis for cost-effective analysis and quality-adjusted life years.

Justice is considered more fully in Chapter 5, which deals with commissioning and resource allocation in health care (Fig. 1.4).

EMPIRICAL BIOETHICS

Just as medicine has become more evidence-based in the twentieth century, medical ethics research has also taken an 'empirical' or 'scientific-evidence'-based turn.

At the simplest level, ethicists will argue, 'If x is true, then y should happen'. Thus, research is needed to find out if x is true and whether y indeed has the effect ethicists want it to. At a more complicated level, social scientists ask, 'What does ethics mean to people?' and 'How does ethics come about in a particular context?' Some of this interaction has resulted in the theoretical critique of bioethics by sociologists (Hoeyer 2006) on the following grounds:

- Social sciences instil the sense of context that philosophical ethics lacks – philosophers by contrast come up with unrealistic scenarios on which to test reasoning.
- Social scientists do ethics in a better way than philosophers – are better suited to spot injustice and understand the imperfections of the real world (as opposed to solving the dilemma in a hypothetical thought experiment).
- Ethics is just another way of having power over what other people do – ethical rules are written by the people in charge.

WHY IS ALL THIS IMPORTANT IN MEDICINE?

Medical practice may be influenced by various ethical approaches. The General Medical Council's code of conduct, *Good Medical Practice*, is essentially deontological, founded on the duties of a doctor, and can be seen as a rulebook. The use of evidence-based medicine to produce guidelines on cost-effectiveness by organizations such as the National Institute for Health and Clinical Excellence (NICE) is utilitarian, based on ideas of what promotes the greatest good for the greatest number. Undergraduate and specialty training is still rooted in the concepts of professional growth and development,

Fig. 1.4 A comparison of the four principles and ethical theories.

Principle	Utilitarianism	Deontology	Virtue theory
Respect for autonomy	This generally brings about best consequences but can be overridden	An essential component of why we should be moral – a respect for all rational (autonomous) beings	Respectfulness is consistent with virtuous behaviour
Beneficence	Maximizing good (beneficence) is the central concept	Not central – the 'right' action is the one that is one's moral duty – benevolence is not important	The principle of beneficence can be seen as equivalent to a virtue of benevolence
Non-maleficence	Can also be seen as a very utilitarian goal – minimizing harm	As above	The principle of non-maleficence is equivalent a the virtue of non-malevolence
Justice	Not necessarily concerned with the distribution of utility – simply the maximization of it	The universalizability criterion ensures a type of justice where all people are equal by virtue of their rationality	Corresponds to virtues of justice or fairness

aimed at producing life-long learners who aspire to excellence – and this is arguably virtue-based. Some medical schools and the Royal College of General Practitioners have taken up 'Values-based medicine' as a way to promote ethical behaviour in a multicultural society. Most importantly, society increasingly expects doctors to be able to justify their decisions in ethical as well as scientific terms.

AN INTRODUCTION TO MEDICAL LAW

The role of the law

Like everyone else in society, doctors and medical students are subject to the laws of society.

The law has a number of functions, including the following:

- To promote civil order
- To resolve disputes without resorting to use of force
- To establish and define standards of acceptable behaviour
- To maintain those standards and punish 'offences'
- To provide rules enabling trade and business
- To provide fair recompense for injury
- To do justice and put right wrongs.

The UK legal system has two *sources* of law: parliament and the courts:

- Parliament-made law consists of Acts/Statutes
- Court-made law is described as 'Common Law' or 'Case Law'.

Case law

The courts are able to interpret statutes, but not overturn them. In contrast, parliament can overrule judge-made decisions. Parliament can 'change' the law, especially on controversial matters.

English Common Law is built on case law – the body of decided judgements, from which legal principles have been established. These principles are applied in subsequent cases, unless the facts of the case are different or a compelling case for change can be made. 'Precedent' is the term describing the binding power of previous decisions on subsequent similar cases. However, decisions in 'higher' courts are binding on 'lower' courts: decisions in the High Court are binding on Magistrate's and Coroner's Courts, and usually followed in High Court decisions. Judgements from the Court of

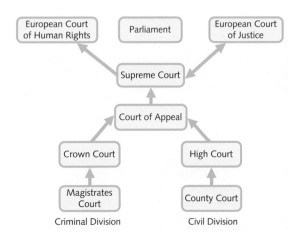

Fig. 1.5 Hierarchy of the UK justice system.

Judgements in the Supreme Court are binding on the Court of Appeal, and judgments from both are binding on all lower courts. The Supreme Court of England and Wales was formerly known as The House of Lords. The Supreme Court may very rarely reverse a decision of its own. Since the Human Rights Act 1998, cases founded on the European Convention of Human Rights may (rarely) have a final appeal to the European Court of Human Rights (ECtHR). Several recent cases of relevance to UK medical law and ethics have found their way to the ECtHR. The European Court of Justice is only concerned with questions which relate to European Union laws or institutions (Fig. 1.5 shows the division and hierarchy of the Court System in England and Wales).

Court cases are either heard in the civil, or in the criminal division of the justice system. A civil case arises from a conflict between two or more people and aims to fairly compensate the injured person or people. A criminal case examines whether someone has broken the law of the state and whether they should receive punishment, such as the unlawful killing of a patient. A major difference between the two is that in criminal cases, the prosecution must demonstrate beyond all reasonable doubt (i.e. be certain) that the accused has broken the law in order to secure a conviction. To be decisive in a civil case, the burden of proof is 'the balance of probabilities', i.e. one side needs to demonstrate that their facts are more likely and arguments are more persuasive than the other's. Most medical law cases are brought within the civil-justice system (rather than the criminal). Most of these cases are brought under the tort (or wrong) of negligence. However healthcare professionals can be, and are, charged with criminal offences, including battery and assault.

Statute law

Statutes are laws created by Acts of Parliament. Acts are still subject to interpretation by the courts. Only parliament may reverse or amend an Act of Parliament, by passing another Act to do this. Many Acts delegate the detail of how they are implemented to minister, local authority or other official. When there are concerns that these powers have been used unreasonably, an application may be made in the courts for a judicial review. However, a successful challenge needs to demonstrate that, e.g. a ministerial decision is clearly unreasonable or in conflict with other laws (judicial review in the context of healthcare resource allocation is explored in Chapter 5).

Health legislation is a complex area that has required frequent amendments in order to keep policies in-line with evolving circumstances. Specific Acts of Parliament relating to different aspects of medical law will be discussed in relevant sections. However, most health legislation made since 1977 has recently been summarized within three Acts of Parliament:

- The National Health Service Act 2006
- The National Health Service (Wales) Act 2006
- The National Health Service (Consequential Provisions) Act 2006
- The Health and Social Care Act 2012.

This is relevant because the legal duty of care owed by doctors to NHS patients is statutory (i.e. enshrined in the NHS Act 2006) and not contractual.

Legal rights and the Human Rights Act

In the UK, legal rights are created either by Acts of Parliament or by judges in case-law. The most important piece of legislation that deals with rights is the Human Rights Act 1998. This makes rights from the 1950 European Convention on Human Rights (ECHR) enforceable against public authorities, which includes hospitals, in England and Wales. Some of the rights are absolute and signatories to the convention are obliged to protect them. Others are 'qualified' and may be superceded by other duties a state has, e.g. to protect the health of its citizens and promote law and order (for a recent example of an important medico-legal case considered by the ECtHR, see the discussion of *Pretty v. UK* [2001], in Chapter 4).

Some of the Articles that are important in medicine are:

Article 2: Right to life (Absolute Right)

Everyone's right to life shall be protected by law:

- This Article might be used to challenge a 'Do not attempt resuscitation' order placed against a patient's wishes.

- This might be used to challenge the withholding or withdrawal of life-saving or life sustaining treatment.

However, this is not always a breach of Article 2.

Article 3: Prohibition of torture, inhuman and degrading treatment (Absolute Right)

No-one shall be subjected to torture or inhuman or degrading treatment or punishment:

- This could be used to challenge poor-quality treatment or failure to provide treatment within a certain time. Consider – Does waiting 18 months for a hip replacement constitute degrading treatment? Does waiting for 24 hours on a trolley in A&E constitute degrading treatment?
- It has been argued (unsuccessfully so far in the UK) that laws prohibiting the assisted suicide/euthanasia of terminally ill patients constitute inhuman or degrading treatment.

Article 8: Right to respect for private and family Life (Qualified Right)

Everyone has the right to respect for his private and family life, his home and his correspondence:

- How might this affect issues of confidentiality? For example, where a teenager does not want parents to know she is taking contraception? The teenager could claim that her right to privacy is supported by Article 8.

Article 9: Freedom of thought, conscience and religion (Qualified Right)

Everyone has the right to their religious and cultural beliefs:

- How might this affect the rights of others? For example, where a doctor or nurse does not wish to provide information about or take part in contraception services because they believe that this is morally wrong?

Article 12: Right to marry and found a family (Qualified Right)

Men and women of marriageable age have the right to marry and found a family according to the national laws governing the exercise of that right:

- This Article could be used to challenge limitations on access to fertility treatment.

Article 14: Right to protection from discrimination (Qualified Right)

- This Article could be used to challenge limitations on access to fertility treatment on the basis of, e.g. race or sexual orientation.

Think about how you might encounter the Articles of the European Convention on Human Rights and fundamental freedoms in medical practice. In this book, see how absolute and qualified human rights have been discussed in the courts and think about how the Human Rights Act might apply to those cases which have not.

Medical negligence

Doctors may sometimes fall foul of the criminal law (this is discussed in relevant sections over the next four chapters) but the majority of cases against doctors are heard in the civil courts. Civil law cases involving doctors are usually actions in medical negligence. There are some basic components of a medical negligence action.

A duty of care: it must be shown that the defendant (that is the person or authority accused of negligence) owed the claimant (that is the injured party or the person accusing the defendant of negligence) a duty of care:

- The duty of care of a GP crystallizes when the patient registers with that GP and then consults with the GP on the occasion in question.
- The duty of care of a hospital doctor crystallizes when the patient is formally accepted into hospital.

English law does not oblige doctors to give emergency treatment outside of the above situations except when:

- a patient presents to an A&E department
- when a GP is requested to provide emergency treatment to a person in his practice area.

By contrast in France, 'Good Samaritan' laws oblige doctors to stop and assist anyone who is taken ill or injured.

Breach of the duty of care

There must be a standard of care that could be expected from the defendant – this is normally the standard of reasonable care – that is the level of care that could be expected from an ordinary member of that branch of medicine.

The standard of care doctors are expected to reach was asserted by the case *Bolam v. Friern Hospital Management Committee* [1957]. The standard of care was set as that of 'the ordinary skilled man exercising and professing to have that special skill'. This standard has become known as the Bolam Test – it is applicable to all aspects of treatment, diagnosis, the disclosure of information or risks to patients.

This standard was possibly modified in *Bolitho v. City and Hackney Health Authority* [1998], where it held that a court must find the medical opinion to be 'reasonable'

and 'responsible'. The claimant must show that the defendant did not reach a reasonable standard of care.

Causation: the claimant must then show that that breach of the duty of care caused the damage they claim to have suffered: the test used to prove causation is often referred to as the '*but for*' test. It says the claimant must demonstrate that *but for* the defendant's negligence, he would not have suffered the harm in respect of which he seeks damages. For example in *Barnett v. Chelsea and Kensington HMC* [1969], a casualty officer refused to attend three night watchmen who were vomiting after drinking tea. One later died from arsenic poisoning. Though there was a breach of duty, the claim failed because, even if he had received treatment, the man would have died anyway and there was therefore no causation.

Damages: some level of damage must have occurred to the claimant for compensation to be awarded. The purpose of bringing an action is to usually gain compensation for damages; if no damages have occurred, there is little point in bringing an action.

Remember: To succeed, a medical negligence case must demonstrate that there was a duty of care, there was a breach of that duty, and the breach caused harm to the patient.

As well as being subject to the requirements of the law, doctors are also subject to the requirements of professional regulation. In the UK, the General Medical Council (GMC) issues guidance on what it considers to be the ethical duties of British doctors. It publishes this in *Duties of a Doctor*, which covers truth-telling, confidentiality and good medical practice in general. The professional duties set down by the GMC have been described as quasi-legal (Fulford et al 2002). This is because the duties set down by the GMC are *enforced*. Failure to adhere to the GMC code of practice can mean removal from the register of licenced doctors. Being 'struck off' means you can no longer work as a doctor in the UK, and are unlikely to find work as a doctor in Europe or elsewhere in the world. (Professionalism and professional regulation are discussed in the next chapter.)

Key questions

- What is the purpose of medical ethics?
- What does the 2010 Core Curriculum in Medical Ethics and Law expect from students and medical schools?
- What is the difference between act utilitarianism and rule utilitarianism?

- What is virtue ethics?
- What are the two central ideas associated with Kantianism and the categorical imperative?
- What are the four principles of bioethics?
- How might deontology, utilitarianism, virtues and values influence UK medicine?
- Name a positive right and negative right – can you justify them?
- What is the role of the law?
- How do the Articles of the European Convention on Human Rights as stated in the Human Rights Act 1998, affect the provision of medical treatment in England and Wales?
- What are the components of a negligence case?
- Why might professional regulation be considered 'quasi-legal'?

References

Barnett v. Chelsea and Kensington HMC, 1969 1QB 428; 2 WLR 422.

Bolam v. Friern HMC, 1957 1WLR 583.

Bolitho v. City and Hackney HA, 1998 AC 232 and [1998] Lloyds Rep Med 26.

Campbell, A.V., Higgs, R., 1982. In That Case: Medical Ethics in Everyday Practice. Darton, Longman and Todd, London.

Dworkin, R., 1977. Taking rights seriously. Duckworth, London.

Fulford, K., 2004. Ten principles of values-based medicine. In: Radden, J. (Ed.), The Philosophy of Psychiatry: A Companion. Oxford University Press, New York, pp. 205–234.

Fulford, K., Dickenson, D., Murray, T., 2002. Healthcare Ethics and Human Values: an Introductory Text with Readings and Case Studies. Blackwell, Oxford.

Hoeyer, K., 2006. 'Ethics wars': reflections on the antagonism between bioethicists and social science observers of biomedicine. Human Studies 29, 203–227.

Pellegrino, E., Thomasma, D., 1993. The Virtues in Medical Practice. Oxford University Press, New York.

Stirrat, G.M., Johnston, C., Gillon, R., et al., Medical Education Working Group of Institute of Medical Ethics and associated signatories, 2010. Medical ethics and law for doctors of tomorrow: the 1998 Consensus Statement updated. J. Med. Ethics 36, 55–60.

Further reading

Garside, 2006. Law for Doctors, Principles and Practicalities, third ed. RSM Press, London.

Garside, J.P., 2006. Structure and sources of English law. In: Law for Doctors: Principles and Practicalities, third ed. RSM Press, London, pp. 1–10.

Gillon, R., 1986. Philosophical Medical Ethics. John Wiley & Sons, Chichester.

The 2nd edition, by Gillon R and Sokol D, is expected in 2013–2014.

Hope, T., 2004. Medical Ethics. A very short introduction. Oxford University Press, Oxford.

Hope, T., Savulescu, J., Kendrick, J., 2008. Medical Ethics and Law: The Core Curriculum, second ed. Elsevier, London.

Petrova, M., Dale, J., Fulford, K.W.M., 2006. Values-based practice in primary care: easing the tensions between individual values, ethical principles, and best evidence. Br. J. Gen. Pract. 56, 703–709.

Raphael, D.D., 1981. Moral Philosophy. Oxford University Press, Oxford.

Professionalism and medical ethics

2

This chapter outlines the role of the key professional bodies involved in regulating and providing ethical guidance for doctors. Truth-telling, confidentiality and conscientious objection are considered here because they are issues particularly identified with professional behaviour. Professional boundaries and their relevance to medical students are discussed. The chapter concludes with a practical overview of research ethics and publication ethics.

PROFESSIONALISM, OATHS AND DECLARATIONS

Oaths and declarations are a way in which professions promise to the public that they will uphold a publically accepted set of values, enabling that profession to be trusted and have a certain status within society. They also represent a way in which a profession can remind its members of those core values.

The Hippocratic Oath (~425 BC) has historically been seen as part of the Western medical tradition. It encourages a number of concepts that are still relevant today: the teaching of medicine; the consideration of the patient's best interests; confidentiality and the abstinence from 'whatever is deleterious and mischievous'. However, it does not mention concepts such as autonomy or justice, and forbids performing surgery. The original Hippocratic Oath is now rarely taken in UK medical schools, though some have written modern versions.

The Declaration of Geneva (1948, amended 1968 and most recently revised in 2006) is a modern-day Hippocratic Oath, requiring doctors to make the health of their patients their 'first consideration'.

The Declaration of Helsinki (1964, revised in 2008) deals with biomedical research. It states that 'the interests of the subject must always prevail over the interests of science and society'.

Both declarations arose from the general concern by the world medical community at how the medical profession in Germany became complicit in the activities of the Nazi party in the time leading up to and during the Second World War.

Since the nineteenth century, in the UK there has been professional regulation of doctors. Initially, this was to prevent unqualified practitioners from claiming the title. Today, professional regulation is far more extensive. This is discussed further later in this chapter.

Professional regulation

In the UK, doctors are obliged to register with the General Medical Council (GMC) *and* to take membership of a Royal College relevant to their area of practice. At present, membership of the British Medical Association (BMA) is optional. Each of these bodies has an important, if sometimes overlapping, role.

HINTS AND TIPS

You should know what the GMC, the BMA, the Royal Medical Colleges and the indemnity bodies do – each plays an important role for doctors.

The General Medical Council

The role of the GMC (established 1868) is broadly:

- to set professional standards of practice
- to ensure that those allowed to practise medicine (registered medical practitioners) are fit to do so, in terms of knowledge, skills and their behaviour
- to maintain a register of doctors who are licensed to practise medicine in the UK. It is illegal to practise medicine without a licence in the UK
- to supervise standards of undergraduate and postgraduate education – the GMC sets out a syllabus for medical schools to follow, and since 2008, now also works with the Royal Colleges to ensure appropriate standards for specialist training and continuing medical education. (The GMC has taken over this role from the Postgraduate Medical Education and Training Board.) This latter role includes supervising revalidation (see below), supervision of doctors' fitness to practise after qualification as a general practitioner (GP) or specialist
- to enforce professional discipline – the ultimate sanction is to 'strike a doctor off the register', either temporarily or permanently. More often, however, the GMC will issue a warning or recommend remedial action, such as a supervised period of practise, or additional training in the area of deficiency.

The GMC also administers the Professional and Linguistic Assessment Board (PLAB) test, which doctors from outside the European Union have to pass before being allowed to practise in the UK.

The GMC sets out guidelines on what it deems to be *Good Medical Practice* (Fig. 2.1). These guidelines are important because any doctor who violates them may be subject to disciplinary procedures and possible erasure from the register – effectively losing the ability to practise as a doctor in the UK. Moreover, other countries often require a certificate of 'good standing' from doctors who emigrate, and therefore a doctor who is 'struck off' in the UK may also have difficulty finding work abroad. Because *Good Medical Practice* represents a set of rules with possible sanctions against those who break

them, some authors (Fulford et al. 2002) talk of them being quasi-legal. Others (Gillies 2004) would hold the GMC duties to be an example of a deontological framework (see Ch. 1) because they represent rules that should not be broken.

DUTIES FOR MEDICAL STUDENTS

The GMC also sets out duties for medical students. Medical students have legal restrictions on the clinical work they can do, but must be aware that they are often doing things that a qualified doctor might do (such as 'taking a history') and that their activities will affect patients. Patients may see students as knowledgeable, and may consider them to have the same responsibilities and duties as a doctor. Students must be aware that their behaviour outside the clinical environment, including in their personal lives, may have an impact on their fitness to practise (professional boundaries are discussed later in this chapter).

Therefore:

- students have a duty to make sure that patients know that they are students and not doctors. For example: should medical undergraduates introduce themselves as medical students or as student doctors? The title 'Student doctor' could mislead a patient that the person seeing them is medically qualified
- students have a duty to behave in a professional way in the clinical and educational environment, and are subject to the same ethical duties as doctors, such as maintaining confidentiality or not performing a procedure unless competent to do so
- students have a duty to avoid behaving in an antisocial or criminal manner outside the clinical setting (e.g. this could include taking recreational drugs, drunken driving or disorderly behaviour in public).

COMMUNICATION

Remember: Students have a professional duty to make sure that patients know that they are medical *students* and not doctors.

For full guidance, see *Medical Students: Professional values and fitness to practice, Medical Schools Council and General Medical Council, November 2009*. Online. Available at: http://www.gmc-uk.org/static/documents/content/GMC_Medical_Students.pdf

Students whose behaviour falls below an acceptable standard may not be allowed to qualify and/or register with the GMC. Currently, there is talk of introducing student GMC registration.

Fig. 2.1 The duties of a doctor registered with the General Medical Council.
Patients must be able to trust doctors with their lives and health. To justify that trust you must show respect for human life and you must:
Make the care of your patient your first concern
Protect and promote the health of patients and the public
Provide a good standard of practice and care
Keep your professional knowledge and skills up-to-date
Recognize and work within the limits of your competence
Work with colleagues in the ways that best serve patients' interests
Treat patients as individuals and respect their dignity
Treat patients politely and considerately
Respect patients' right to confidentiality
Work in partnership with patients
Listen to patients and respond to their concerns and preferences
Give patients the information they want or need in a way they can understand
Respect patients' right to reach decisions with you about their treatment and care
Support patients in caring for themselves to improve and maintain their health
Be honest and open and act with integrity
Act without delay if you have good reason to believe that you or a colleague may be putting patients at risk
Never discriminate unfairly against patients or colleagues
Never abuse your patients' trust in you or the public's trust in the profession.
Summarized from GMC 2006 'Good Medical Practice'. General Medical Council.

The Royal Medical Colleges

The chief role of the Royal Medical Colleges is to set educational, professional and clinical standards for their specialty. Trainees in a given specialty must now generally pass a membership examination from the relevant college before obtaining a certificate of completion of specialist training. Some newer specialties have their standards set by a faculty of a Royal Medical College. For example, forensic medical examiners have their standards set by the Faculty of Forensic Medical Examiners at the Royal College of Physicians. Now that doctors will have to supply evidence of fitness to practise after specialization (a process called revalidation), the Royal Colleges will set specialty-specific standards on behalf of the GMC. The colleges also pass comment on issues relating to their specialty and the health service. The colleges support research (e.g. with financial grants and opportunities to showcase research at conferences and in college journals) and will have a committee which produces specialty-specific ethical guidance. For example, the Royal college of General Practitioners has an ethics committee, which produces educational material on ethics for GPs and reports to the RCGP council.

The British Medical Association

The main function of the BMA (established 1832) is to protect the interests of its members; it is the trade union for doctors in the UK. It is involved in the negotiations on behalf of doctors at national level as well as representing members at a local level in employment-related disputes (English et al. 2004). Membership of the BMA is optional. A doctor who is a 'paid-up' BMA member has to raise a problem locally for industrial relations officers to become involved in a local dispute over work conditions (otherwise there would be no point in paying to be a member of a trade union). As well as representing members' interests, it also passes comment on behalf of the profession on matters related to health such as banning tobacco advertising, and on global issues such as the role of doctors in executions and torture. The BMA also has a research unit and an ethics department, which provides guidance on contentious issues (see below). BMA members can seek personal advice from the ethics department, and it also collects data on the ethical issues of concern to doctors.

The top 10 issues for which doctors sought advice from the BMA medical ethics department in 2010 (on the BMA website each of these is hyperlinked to guidance from the Ethics department) were the following:

1. Under what circumstances can confidential health information be disclosed?
2. Who can apply for access to a patient's health records?
3. What should a doctor do when they have child protection concerns about a patient?
4. How much information should patients be given in order for consent to treatment to be valid?
5. What should a doctor do if they are asked by a terminally ill patient to write a medical report to use abroad for assisted dying?
6. Does a patient have a right to see a medical report written about them?
7. Under the Mental Capacity Act 2005, when is a person judged to lack capacity?
8. How and when, can a doctor broach the subject of private treatment with NHS patients?
9. Are GPs able to register asylum seekers and refuse asylum seekers?
10. What is the BMA's position on organ donation?

Ethical issues faced by medical students

The BMA medical ethics committee has also asked the BMA medical students' committee to make a list of common 'ethical dilemmas' faced by medical students (list adapted from the BMA Handbook of Ethics and Law, 2004). The list they supplied comprised:

- The proper form by which students should be introduced (e.g. see above)
- Patients' consent to student involvements in consultations and treatments
- The sharing of confidential information with clinical firms
- Inexperience in carrying out procedures
- Carrying out intimate examinations on patients while under anaesthetic
- Conflicts between medical education and patient care
- Witnessing poor practice
- How to respond when senior colleagues have impaired judgement
- Physical or verbal assault from patients
- Disclosure from patients that they have been subjected to abuse
- Concealment of mistakes by senior colleagues
- Responding to admissions of criminal behaviour from patients
- Providing medical treatment to family or friends
- When questions arise about the competence or behaviour of fellow students
- Students being recruited to take part in the research projects of their teachers.

Many of the above issues repeat the concerns of qualified doctors, but not all. Some relate to the specific duties of medical students (see above). Many of the sources of support for medical students are the same as for doctors – medical students are entitled to use their medical indemnity body (see below) and the BMA ethics department. As well as clinical advisors and other responsible staff, some medical schools have student clinical ethics discussion groups and medical ethics societies. Think about what is available to you – if there is no easy source of ethics support – consider setting something up!

Medical indemnity

Doctors working in a clinical setting in the UK are obliged to have medical indemnity (in other countries, they may be obliged to have malpractice insurance). Indemnity bodies have two key roles:

1. To safeguard doctors' reputations from unwarranted accusations
2. To compensate patients who have suffered as a result of medical negligence.

Medical students may also join medical indemnity organizations – at present, this is free for students and a very small sum for Foundation Year doctors, but gets much more expensive as doctors acquire responsibility and experience. Indemnity organizations are an excellent source of confidential advice on professional and medico-legal issues for their members. If you are not sure about the legality or the ethics of a clinical or professional decision, all such organizations have a helpline and will give advice to their members 24 hours a day, 7 days a week in emergencies.

Trust, honesty and truth-telling

From ancient times until comparatively recently, lying to patients was not necessarily disapproved of, or even discouraged, provided it was for the patient's own good.

Current professional opinion is rather different; the document *Good Medical Practice* and the *Good Medical Practice: Framework for Appraisal and Revalidation* (GMC 2011) states that doctors have a duty to be honest and trustworthy. Dishonesty in general is viewed in a particularly harsh light. Some of the behaviours below have parallels at undergraduate level, e.g. allowing patients to think you are a junior doctor or cheating in exams.

Dishonest behaviours include (list adapted from Whitehouse 2011):

- misleading patients into receiving treatment which they do not need
- omitting or lying about information which would affect the choice a patient makes
- claiming a qualification or expertise which is not possessed
- making untrue statements in mortgage or job applications, passport or visa applications
- making fraudulent applications on claims forms in relation to insurance companies, and other third-party funding organizations

- altering an entry in healthcare records which has been made on a previous occasion
- cheating in professional examinations.

Telling the truth

The concept of 'telling the truth' has two facets:

1. The 'telling' part, which deals with the *communication* of information
2. The 'truth' part, which holds that the information given has to be *true*.

From an ethical perspective, truthful information is important for a number of reasons: even if the information does not lead to a treatment decision, the patient may still wish to know information about their health, because their health is intricately linked with their sense of self.

It is generally accepted that truth-telling promotes a sense of trust between both the doctor and their patient, and in general between doctors and the public.

Medical schools spend a huge amount of time and money teaching communication skills (the telling part, above) so that doctors can break bad news and help patients make difficult decisions, rather than be tempted to avoid such encounters or even mislead patients.

It thus seems that, in general, truth-telling is a necessary duty. However, is it an absolute one? Are there any circumstances in which it might be right to lie to patients? What about not telling the *whole* truth? Is there a difference between avoiding answering a direct question, and telling a lie? The following scenarios illustrate the general principles at stake.

COMMUNICATION

The concept of 'telling the truth' has two facets: the 'telling' part, or communication of information, and the 'truth' part, which holds that the information given has to be true.

Scenario 1

A patient, Mrs X, is brought to the emergency department after being caught in a house fire with her two children, who have both died. Mrs X herself has sustained burns which will be fatal in the next few hours. Mrs X asks you, the doctor treating her, how her children are.

You fear that knowing the truth will distress her. Do you deceive her, for the short period of time she has left to live, and tell her that her children are alive?

If we use the four principles (see earlier) to look at this case, we have a conflict of ethical principles:

1. Respect for autonomy holds we should not lie to patients.
2. Beneficence holds that lying may be crucial in easing the patient's distress.

The conflict in principles is mirrored by a conflict in different ethical theories as well. Utilitarianism might suggest we should lie, because telling a lie is more likely to make the patient happy (or ease her distress). Deontology would oblige us to tell the truth because if people lie, no-one can trust that what anyone says is true. How can a compromise be reached? Virtue ethics might see a conflict between honesty and kindness. Using the four principles: beneficience and non-maleficence could (if hope is good and distress is a harm) appear at first glance to outweigh patient autonomy and right to know the truth. However, we do not know, for example if Mrs X wants in her final lucid moments to make sure that her money and property are appropriately inherited.

It has been suggested that lying to patients is justified only 'if a person, acting rationally, were presented with the alternatives, he or she would always choose being lied to' (Gert & Culver 1979). But how can you know that someone would choose to be lied to?

Scenario 2

Mr Y has a poor (but not end-stage) prognosis due to cancer. You are treating Mr Y, and are about to tell him his diagnosis and prognosis.

Before you do so, his son, a local GP, who has guessed the diagnosis, urges you not to tell his father the truth, either that this is a cancer or that it has a poor prognosis. The son explains that his mother, Mr Y's wife, died a mere 2 months ago of a very aggressive cancer, and he fears that if his father knows the truth, he will 'give in' because the father thinks that *any* diagnosis of cancer is one without hope of recovery.

The deception which the son requests is not a short-term one. The conflict of principles (if you believe the son) is similar: If you respect Mr Y's *autonomy* and tell him the truth, he may 'give in', become depressed and refuse all treatment. He might also elect to have appropriate treatment and have a better opportunity to manage what remains of his life, given the prognosis. If you truly respect Mr Y's *autonomy*, you may consider that he has a right to 'give in' and refuse all subsequent help if he chooses to.

If you do as the son suggests, following a *beneficent* aim of allowing him to live his remaining days free from despair, this may deny him the opportunity to have appropriate treatment for any chance of cure or management of symptoms. After all – why see a cancer specialist if he does not have cancer? It may also produce more distress if he ever finds out the truth. If doctors routinely lied about serious illnesses, then reassurance might provide no comfort anyway.

You may consider that each of the above scenarios has an obvious answer. However, a short-answer or essay question in an exam should examine both sides of an argument before deciding which decision to support.

In both cases above, actively deceiving a patient is clearly problematic but telling the truth may also be difficult.

Telling the whole truth and the law: therapeutic privilege

Therapeutic privilege is where a clinician withholds information (usually during the consent process) from a competent patient in the belief that disclosure of this information would cause harm to the patient. Information that a patient would ordinarily be told is deliberately withheld for the patient's benefit, as perceived by the healthcare professional. Therapeutic privilege is recognized and discouraged by medical indemnity organizations (Whitehouse 2011), as it would otherwise suggest the erroneous belief that any form of dishonesty (or incomplete honesty) can be condoned if the patient benefits from not receiving the full truth. Johnston and Holt (2006) argue that although clinicians should have discretion as to how sensitive or distressing information is disclosed, they are neither qualified nor justified to make a judgement to deliberately withhold information or deceive patients, because:

- in considering patient welfare, the clinician must consider the patient's overall best interests (not just the medical best interests)
- the law recognizes that a competent patient determines his or her own best interests
- therefore it is unlikely that any clinician will know the patient well enough to make such a judgement
- withholding information about risks prevents the patient from making an effective decision in his or her own interests.

Informed consent, autonomy and disclosure of risks is discussed in Chapter 3.

CONFIDENTIALITY

> Whatever, in connection with my professional practice . . . I see or hear, in the life of men, which ought not to be spoken of abroad, I will not divulge, as reckoning that all such should be kept secret.
>
> Hippocratic Oath ∼425 BC

The duty of confidentiality is a cornerstone of the therapeutic relationship between patients and doctors. It has been included in professional oaths and declarations from Hippocrates to the present day. A duty of confidentiality can be explicitly invoked by the patient requesting that information provided be kept confidential, but more usually in clinical practice, there is an implicit obligation on the part of doctors, and expectation on the part of patients, that information will not be disclosed to third parties (Slowther 2010). The most common reason in 2009/2010 for doctors telephoning the BMA for advice concerned whether to disclose confidential patient details. It is important to note that even the Hippocratic Oath has a 'get out' clause, however. 'Which ought not to be spoken', implies that some things ought to be!

The right to confidentiality derives ultimately from a right to autonomy, in that self-determination includes deciding who knows what about oneself. Medical consultations consist of a disclosure of information to a healthcare professional. The purpose of such information is to treat the patient – it has not been given for any other reason. That information in a sense 'belongs' to the person who disclosed it and ought not to be broadcast to third parties without specific consent. If a healthcare professional does not treat patients as autonomous, she is not treating them as equals – in the sense of being rational beings in control of their own lives.

When thinking about or discussing confidentiality, it is helpful to think in terms of three categories:

- A theoretical basis for confidentiality – which can be justified in terms of deontology (we have a duty to respect autonomy by not disclosing information without consent), consequentialism (if doctors keep confidences, patients trust doctors and disclose more relevant details), virtue ethics (sensitive and respectful doctors keep their patients' private details confidential), as well as other ethical theories.
- A professional basis for confidentiality – quasi-legal codes of practice set down by the GMC, and advice from the Royal Colleges and indemnity organizations serve as a reminder of what the medical profession and the public expect of doctors. The GMC asserts that 'Patients have a right to expect that information about them will be held in confidence by their doctors' and 'Confidentiality is central to trust between doctors and patients. Without assurances about confidentiality, patients may be reluctant to give doctors the information they need in order to provide good care' (GMC 2009).
- A legal basis, which asserts a duty to maintain confidentiality exists and states where exceptions are made (e.g. in the case of *X v. Y (UK)* [1988]; a newspaper that obtained confidential medical records identifying two doctors with HIV was restrained from publishing the information. The court held that the confidentiality of the medical records was more important than protecting the public from the theoretical risk the doctors might pose and the freedom of the press.).

COMMUNICATION

Remember: The duty of confidentiality is a cornerstone of the doctor–patient relationship.

Legal regulation of confidentiality and disclosure

This duty of confidentiality in law arises when a person gains information in circumstances where there is an assumption, or a specific agreement, that the information is confidential. Such a duty is held to apply to doctors. The Medical Protection Society describes three general conditions that establish a duty of confidentiality and what constitutes a breach of that duty (adapted from MPS Guide to Ethics: a map for the moral maze, 2011):

1. Information must have an inherent quality of confidentiality, e.g. obtained during a medical history or a treatment carried out
2. Information must be disclosed in circumstances implying an obligation of confidence. If information given to a doctor in a medical practice, hospital or in a clinical area (including at the bedside or in a patient's home), then those circumstances imply an obligation of confidentiality
3. Unauthorized disclosure would cause some harm to the provider. This is more likely to be psychological other than physical harm. This could include financial losses. Consider the criteria for a successful claim in negligence (breach of duty, causation, loss; see Ch. 1).

Case discussion (adapted from Hope et al. 2003):

Dr B is a GP in a small town. Three days ago, she saw Miss X in her surgery. Miss X is a 20-year-old student who had been feeling unusually tired for over a month. Dr B had sent off a number of blood tests. Dr B is shopping in the local supermarket when she bumps into Miss X's mother, who asks what is happening with her daughter. What should Dr B reply?

It is potentially a breach of confidentiality for Dr B to even confirm that Miss X, an adult patient has been to see her, let alone tell her mother the test results. Dr B does not know what Miss X would wish her mother to know, and might reply that she does not discuss patients outside the surgery.

Later in the day, Dr B is back at work. While Dr B is conducting a review of another patient, Mr R's blood pressure medication, he says, 'While I'm here doctor can I pick up my wife's prescription?' How should Dr B respond?

Again Dr B needs to be sure that Mrs R is happy for her prescription to be collected by her husband and/or that her husband knows its contents.

Statutory basis of confidentiality and patients' access to healthcare records

The Data Protection Act (DPA) 1998 is extremely relevant to doctors and medical students. This is because it sets down and describes the statutory duty to maintain the confidentiality of medical records (as well as all other personal information which might be stored about a person). It applies to both computer records and paper records. There are eight principles of the Act. (Think about how these might relate to patient health-care records.):

- Information is processed fairly and lawfully
- Information is obtained for specified and lawful purposes
- Information is adequate, relevant and not excessive in relation to the purpose for which obtained
- Information is accurate and, where necessary, kept up-to-date
- Information is not kept for longer than necessary
- Information is not used in ways contrary to the rights of the data subject (the patient in the medical records)
- Appropriate measures are taken to prevent un-authorized disclosure of information
- Information is not transferred to areas that cannot provide the above assurances.

The Data Protection Act 1998 gives the patient a certain number of rights with respect to their medical records. These include:

- *The right to be informed* about what information is being held, and why
- *The right of access to personal data.* Patients have a right to a copy of their medical records. They also have the right to have this information communicated to them in a way they can understand it. However, in order to obtain this information, the patient must make a written request, and may be required to pay a fee
- *The right to correct information that is inaccurate.* If a patient feels that the information about them is misleading, they can ask for it to be changed
- *The right to seek damages as a result of misleading information.*

HINTS AND TIPS

The Data Protection Act 1998 is extremely relevant to healthcare professionals. You should know what rights it gives to patients and what duties it creates for doctors.

When should confidential information be disclosed?

Sokol (2008) considers that, if we want patients to be really informed about confidentiality, hospital doctors and GPs might tell patients at the outset that there are limits to this. Otherwise, some patients may believe that doctors are committed to absolute confidentiality.

Hence, a GP might start the consultation: 'Hello, I'm Dr Jones. I don't yet know the reason for your visit, but I must tell you something first. I shall respect your confidences, but if doing so is likely to put others at risk of serious harm, then I might need to violate your confidentiality, even if you object'.

Sokol's statement above sounds a bit silly (this is intentional), but think about these two statements, frequently used by medical students:

'You can tell me anything, nothing you tell me will leave this room' *and*

'I have an obligation to keep anything you tell me confidential, everything you tell me will stay within the healthcare team'.

The first statement is obviously misleading. The second statement still omits the idea that confidentiality is not absolute.

The GMC has outlined that confidential information about a patient can be disclosed:

- with the patient's consent (or the consent of a person properly authorized to act on the patient's behalf, e.g. the parent of a young child)
- within healthcare teams: This is in order to provide the best care possible, and the patient should be informed so as to understand why and when information may be shared between team members
- when disclosure is required for a procedure that has been agreed to, *explicit* consent would not be required, e.g. giving relevant clinical information to the radiologist when sending a patient for an X-ray
- in an emergency, if a patient is unable to give consent, disclosure of confidential information to members of the healthcare team can be in the patient's best interests.

It must be noted, however, that if a patient does not wish you to share particular information with team members, you must respect those wishes (provided that this does not endanger the safety of others). It is the responsibility of *all* members of the team to ensure that other team members understand and observe confidentiality:

- Confidential information should be disclosed to employers and insurance companies, only with the patient's *written* consent. The purpose of the consultation (if on behalf of a third party) should be made clear from the outset.
- *For the purpose of education, audit or research*: inform the patient of the purpose of disclosure and that the person given access to the records will be under a duty of confidentiality. Seek their consent and as far as possible, anonymize the data and keep the disclosures to the minimum required. Where research projects are using identifying information, and it is

not practical to inform patients, then this needs to be brought to the attention of the research ethics committee. Expressed consent should be obtained before publishing case histories and photographs (many journals now require written consent from the patient).

- *In the patient's best interest*: if a patient is unable to give consent owing to immaturity, illness or mental incapacity. However, the patient should, as far as possible, be informed of your intention. If a patient is a victim of neglect, physical or sexual abuse *and* unable to give valid consent *and* you believe disclosure will prevent further harm, you *must* disclose information to the *appropriate* responsible person or statutory agency.
- *In the interests of others*: if not doing so will lead to a risk of serious harm or death (e.g. contact tracing in HIV). However, you should inform the patient of your intention to make the disclosure.
- If a colleague, who is also a patient, is placing patients at risk.
- If disclosure is required for the prevention or detection of a serious crime.
- *When it is required by statute or the courts*: for example there is a requirement by statute to give information under the Public Health (Infectious Diseases) Regulations SI 1988/1546 about certain 'notifiable' diseases (HIV is *not* a notifiable disease), if ordered to disclose by a judge or the coroner. Doctors are allowed to object to disclosure if an attempt is made to obtain information about those not involved in a particular proceeding or if irrelevant details are requested.
- *After a patient's death*: the obligation of confidentiality in general persists after the patient's death. There are some instances when disclosure is appropriate. For example, in order to assist a coroner, as part of National Confidential enquiries or other clinical audits, on death certificates or to obtain information relating to public health surveillance.
- *To the Driver and Vehicle Licensing Agency (DVLA)*: the DVLA is responsible for deciding if a person is medically unfit to drive. If a patient has a condition that impairs their ability to drive, you should explain to them that they have a legal duty to inform the DVLA. If the patient cannot understand this advice, e.g. owing to dementia, you should inform the DVLA. If patients refuse to accept your diagnosis, you should advise them to seek a second opinion and refrain from driving until that time. If a patient continues to drive when they are not fit to do so, you should make every effort to persuade them to stop; this can include telling their next of kin. If they cannot be persuaded, you should inform the medical advisor at the DVLA. Inform the patient that this is your intention and write to confirm that a disclosure has been made.

Laws which permit or require disclosure of confidential information

There are a number of Acts of Parliament which either permit or require that confidential information be disclosed in particular circumstances. These include:

1. *Disclosure in court*, e.g. when a doctor is brought to give evidence on the extent or cause of an injury
2. *If the police request access to records* in accordance with the Police and Criminal Evidence Act 1984
3. *'Notifiable' disease must be reported to the authorities* in accordance with the Public Health (Infectious Diseases) Regulations 1988 (SI1988, No. 1546). These include, among others: cholera, meningitis, anthrax, diphtheria, measles, mumps, rubella and tuberculosis (neither HIV nor AIDS is a notifiable disease)
4. *In accordance with the Terrorism Act 2000*. All individuals have a legal obligation to disclose to the police, as soon as reasonably practicable, any information that they know or believe might be of material assistance in preventing the commission of an act of terrorism anywhere in the world. It is a criminal offence not to disclose such information, punishable by up to 5 years in prison
5. *The Children Act 1989/2004* holds that information pertaining to child abuse must be given if requested by the local authority – it does not oblige doctors to report suspected abuse, although both the GMC and the BMA advise there is a duty to report
6. *The Health and Social Care Act 2012* deals with the regulation of patient information. It allows the Secretary of State to make provision for the disclosure of information in the interests of improving patient care or in the public interest. In particular, this allows for the disclosure of patient records to the patient or a prescribed individual on behalf of the patient.

Case discussion: Mr S

You are a GP at a university student health centre. One of your patients, Mr S, reveals in the course of a consultation that he has thoughts about harming another student, Ms L, who has rejected his romantic advances. You are aware that Mr S has been under the care of mental health services as a teenager, and has been before the university's disciplinary board for disorderly conduct while under the influence of drugs and alcohol. Mr S says he expects you to keep the consultation confidential as he wishes to remain on his university course and feels that disclosure of the consultation could result in his being suspended or expelled. He agrees to be referred for counselling. Should you warn the university authorities, or Ms L?

Reasons for keeping Mr S's consultation confidential:

1. Without the assurance of confidentiality, Mr S may be deterred from seeking assistance

2. Confidentiality is essential in eliciting the full disclosure necessary for effective treatment, and an integral part of the trust between patient and physician or therapist.

Reasons for breaking confidentiality:

1. The clinician–patient relationship – where there is a relationship with someone whose conduct needs to be controlled or the foreseeable victim of that conduct, the clinician has the discretion to break confidentiality
2. Autonomy of the person at risk – given that the duty of confidentiality is based on respect for autonomy, we should also consider the loss of autonomy of the victim and weigh that against the loss of autonomy (to the patient) caused by disclosure, even if unwarranted
3. Public interest in disclosure – there is a public interest in the maintenance of confidence, but this could be outweighed by a public interest in safety.

Case discussion: Mr L

Mr L, an HIV-positive patient demands you tell no-one else of his diagnosis, including others of the healthcare team. Key points include confidentiality and preventing risk to third parties.

What makes HIV/AIDS different from other diseases is that there is still no cure for the disease, that patients can live apparently unaffected for a long period of time (but still be infective) and that there is a degree of stigma associated with the disease.

The ethical thinking behind maintaining confidentiality and not disclosing includes:

1. The right to privacy, based on a respect for autonomy
2. The fact that the erosion of confidence in the medical consultation will lead to worse consequences (e.g. fewer people with HIV seeking treatment).

Factors that might persuade us in this case to break confidentiality would include:

1. Not disclosing the patient's HIV status to the patient's sexual partner could put the partner at risk of infection if sex is unprotected
2. Other healthcare professionals might be unaware of their risk of infection, and some procedures, such as dentistry and surgery may involve accidental contact with blood
3. Not telling other members of the healthcare team may lead to the provision of inappropriate treatment for Mr L or someone infected with HIV after sexual or blood-borne contact.

In practice, a reasonable course of action would start with explaining to the patient why you think it is necessary that the healthcare team knows about his HIV status. The patient should also be informed that all healthcare staff (and students) are under a duty of confidentiality and, in particular, a GP is not well placed to manage the patient's condition unless informed about the patient's HIV status. However, with regard to informing a GP, if the patient continues to refuse a disclosure, his wishes ought to be respected. If he has communicated an intention to engage in risky unprotected sex, there may be a duty to warn the patient's partner. Contact-tracing for non-notifiable diseases (see above) is at the discretion of the patient. Rarely, e.g. if the patient is violent or severely mentally disturbed, disclosure to the GP without consent may be appropriate.

What then of disclosing information to the patient's partner?

1. The harm in the breach of confidentiality lies in distress caused by ignoring the patient's wishes, and the loss of trust that follows. The loss of trust may deter the patient from seeking help in the future. There may be additional consequential harms such as break-up of the patient's relationship, and stigma, as a result of the diagnosis becoming known.
2. The main benefit is the potential avoidance of a serious risk to the patient's partner's health. It seems reasonable that preventing infection with HIV is a good enough reason to breach confidentiality. The view that doctors have a duty of care only towards patients and as such, do not need to look out for the interests of their partners or other relevant third parties, is not generally accepted. The GMC advises that you should disclose information in order to protect a person from risk of death or serious harm (even with significant improvements in the management of the disease, contracting HIV is arguably a serious harm). However, you must not disclose information to relatives or others who have not been, and are not, at risk of infection. The approach of the courts has been to consider the public interest in maintaining confidentiality (confidentiality encourages patients to seek treatment) against the public interest in disclosure (protection of people at risk).
3. For a discussion of legal issues linked to HIV, see Yeoman 2007.

CONSCIENCE AND PERSONAL BELIEFS

Doctors may hold personal beliefs or values which may conflict with those of their patients and colleagues. There is for example a conscientious objection clause in the Abortion Act 1967 (amended 1990), which allows a doctor to opt out of providing abortions (see Ch. 4). Savulescu argues (2006) that where a service is provided legally in the UK, doctors should be obliged facilitate it, irrespective of their personal beliefs. Otherwise, some people are unfairly denied a service they are entitled to, purely because of their doctor's beliefs. Seale (2010) has suggested that the medical profession is often not representative of the general population in terms of ethnicity and religion, in his study for example specialists in geriatrics were more likely to be Asian, Hindu and Muslim, and specialists in palliative care were more likely to be white and Christian. The GMC guidelines (2008) state:

- you must not unfairly discriminate against patients allowing your personal views to affect adversely the professional relationship with patients
- if carrying out a particular procedure or giving advice about it conflicts with your religious or moral beliefs, and this conflict might affect the treatment or advice you provide, you must explain this to the patient and tell them they have the right to see another doctor. You must be satisfied that the patient has sufficient information to enable them to exercise that right. If it is not practical for a patient to arrange to see another doctor, you must ensure that arrangements are made for another suitably qualified colleague to take over your role
- you must not express to your patients your personal beliefs, including political, religious or moral beliefs, in ways that exploit their vulnerability or that are likely to cause them distress.

Medical schools usually make some allowances for conscientious objection. For example students are not currently obliged to assist in abortions if they have a conscientious objection. However, there is controversy around whether a student stating a conscientious objection in an objective structured clinical examination (OSCE) could pass or obtain full marks. Students who have difficulty even offering simulated advice, which conflicts with their beliefs or ethical position should think about what other skills are being tested (e.g. there may be as many marks for taking an adequate sexual history as for offering contraceptive advice in an OSCE station). They should also discuss this issue with a clinical advisor and/or find out what the position the medical school takes on this issue. Attempting to evangelise patients, whether real or simulated, is considered to be an inappropriate use of a doctor's influence over a potentially vulnerable patient (personal boundaries and power imbalance in the doctor–patient relationship are considered below).

DISCLOSURE OF MISTAKES AND MISCONDUCT

Mistakes happen in all workplaces; however, given that medicine does literally deal with matters of life and death, the results of mistakes may be considerably more grave than those made in other walks of life. The Bristol Royal Infirmary Inquiry addressed the question of how to learn from mistakes. This inquiry identified a 'culture of blame and stigma' within the NHS. How then should students and doctors react when they realize they have made a mistake? How should they react if they become aware that one of their colleagues is making mistakes or behaving in an unprofessional way?

If you make a mistake, a reasonable course of action may be to:

- inform your clinical supervisor and rectify the mistake
- with the agreement of your supervisor, apologize to the patient and explain why the mistake was made – also explain the consequences of the mistake. The patient may wish to speak to a more senior doctor, and depending on the gravity of the mistake, this may be appropriate. Inform the patient what steps are being taken to rectify the mistake.

It is difficult to ethically justify *not* telling the patient that a mistake has been made.

If you believe that a colleague is behaving in a way which calls into question his or her fitness to practise there are a number of options:

- Consider whether or not patients are at risk: The GMC guidance is that 'You must protect patients from risk of harm posed by another colleague's conduct . . . The safety of patients must come first at all times'
- If you feel able to, you could approach your colleague directly and voice your concerns. You may be able to reach an agreement whereby your colleague takes time off work and seeks professional help
- If you are uncomfortable approaching your colleague directly, or your colleague denies there is a problem, you should voice your concerns to an appropriate person from the employing authority, e.g. your colleague's educational supervisor, the educational sub-Dean (if in a hospital) or the medical director. If the concern is about a medical problem such as drug/alcohol addiction, psychiatric illness or a serious infectious disease, you may wish to speak to a consultant in occupational health
- Remember that you still have obligations of confidentiality towards your colleague and any patients involved (see above)
- You may wish to discuss your options with your defence organization or the GMC.

The Public Interest Disclosure Act 1998, which is sometimes called the 'Whistle-Blowing Act', aims to protect those employees who report their concerns about the performance of colleagues (to the appropriate authorities). Employees who claim they have been dismissed or passed over for promotion as a result of such a disclosure, may bring the case before an employment tribunal. It does not protect the 'whistleblower' from libel proceedings if an allegation of misconduct turns out to be false. The Act does not cover volunteers and self-employed individuals.

Ethics and occupational health

It is important to determine whether or not patients are at risk because of the behaviour or illness of a health professional. What are the sorts of professional issues which might arise from illness in clinicians? The GMC is not completely specific, rather it talks about any condition that leads to a colleague 'placing patients at risk as a result of illness or another medical condition'. One envisages that this could include the following:

- Serious communicable diseases: particularly HIV, tuberculosis, hepatitis B and C. The GMC recommends that if you believe a medical colleague has a serious communicable disease and is continuing to practise *in a way which places patients at risk*, you must inform an appropriate person in the healthcare worker's employing authority, such as an occupational health physician. Of course, doctors with disease are allowed to continue to practise; however, they may be restricted in the invasive procedures they perform
- Psychiatric disorders, including depression (that hinders the ability of the doctor to properly care for his or her patients), personality disorders and psychotic disorders
- Alcohol and drug addiction.

Occupational health staff may have conflicting responsibilities. The well-being and confidentiality of the worker may conflict with the needs of the employer and protection of patients. Doctors have an ethical duty to prioritize patient safety.

PROFESSIONAL BOUNDARIES

The GMC and indemnity organizations tell us that it is always the doctor's responsibility to maintain appropriate professional boundaries. Sheather (2011) argues that, ordinarily, the primary obligation of a doctor is to promote the best medical interests of their patients. To an extent, therefore, the requirement to respect the integrity of professional boundaries is allied to the ethical requirement to avoid, as far as reasonably possible, those circumstances in which conflicts of interest are likely to arise.

Power relationships

The doctor–patient relationship may involve an imbalance of power between the doctor and the patient. This could arise, e.g. from the doctor having access to expertise and healthcare resources which the patient needs, or the possible vulnerability – emotional or physical – of a patient seeking health care. This may be particularly acute in some specialties such as psychiatry but can arise in any relationship between doctor and patient. GMC guidance (Maintaining Boundaries, 2006) states that in successful doctor–patient relationships, a professional boundary exists between the doctor and patient. If this boundary is breached, this can undermine the patient's trust in their doctor, as well as public trust in the medical profession.

Boundary violations

Much literature about professional boundaries concerns 'improper' sexual behaviour. However, professional boundary issues can include:

- Doctors as patients
- Doctors treating their friends and relatives
- Dealing with poorly performing colleagues or misconduct by colleagues (see above)
- Accepting gifts from patients and colleagues.

Blurred professional boundaries and the use of social media

The popularity of internet-based social media has grown rapidly in recent years. There is widespread use of internet sites such as Facebook and Twitter among medical students and doctors and there are a growing number of well-established blogs and internet forums that are aimed specifically at medical professionals, such as doctors.net.uk and the BMJ's doc2doc. The BMA's ethical advice is summarized below:

Key points:
- Social media can blur the boundary between an individual's public and professional lives
- Doctors and medical students should consider adopting conservative privacy settings where these are available but they should be aware it is hard to protect online information
- The ethical and legal duty to protect patient confidentiality applies equally on the internet as to other media
- It is inappropriate to post informal, personal or derogatory comments about patients or colleagues on public internet fora
- Doctors and medical students who post online have an ethical obligation to declare any conflicts of interest

- The BMA recommends that doctors and medical students should not accept Facebook friend requests from current or former patients
- Defamation law can apply to any comments posted on the web made in either a personal or professional capacity
- Doctors and medical students should be conscious of their online image and how it may impact on their professional standing.

Sexualized behaviour

The GMC, in its 2006 guidance 'Maintaining Boundaries', draws a number of distinctions regarding intimate relationships.

With current patients they are prohibited: 'You must not pursue a sexual or improper emotional relationship with a patient'. The ban on sexual relationships with current patients is absolute (Sheather 2011). Sheather explains that this is because illness can still render even the most self-assured person, temporarily vulnerable to exploitation. Nor is it just a question of authority. During medical consultations, patients may need to reveal the most intimate details. A relationship predicated on such one-sided disclosure must raise questions about the balance of power.

Sexualized behaviour has been defined as acts, words or behaviour designed or intended to arouse or gratify sexual impulses and desires. If a patient displays sexualized behaviour, wherever possible, doctors are encouraged to try and re-establish a professional boundary. Where this is not possible, sometimes doctors have to end the professional relationship.

But what if I practise in a remote location and everyone in the local community is my patient?

The GMC does not really answer this question. It states that 'If circumstances arise in which social contact with a former patient leads to the possibility of a sexual relationship beginning, you must use your professional judgement and give careful consideration to the nature and circumstances of the relationship . . .'. Take into account the following:

- When the professional relationship ended and how long it lasted
- The nature of the previous professional relationship
- Whether the patient was particularly vulnerable at the time of the professional relationship, and whether they are still vulnerable

- Whether the doctor will be caring for other members of the patient's family.

If you are not sure whether you are – or could be seen to be – abusing your professional position, it may help to discuss your situation with an impartial colleague, an indemnity organization, the BMA or (confidentially) with a member of the GMC Standards and Ethics team.

Chaperones

One of the ways in which professional boundaries are managed is with effective use of chaperones, where an intimate examination is to be performed. In the medical context, a chaperone is a person (who should be trained for the role) who witnesses a doctor's conduct during circumstances where either a patient is vulnerable (mainly during intimate examinations) or to protect the doctor against allegations of indecent assault. The use of chaperones has been particularly encouraged since 2000, when GP Clifford Ayling was convicted of 12 counts of indecent assault and accused of 23 others. The case resulted in a Department of Health (2004) investigation.

What is an intimate examination?

1. Examination of the breasts, genitalia and rectum are generally assumed to be intimate examinations.
2. Any examination where it is necessary to touch or be close to the patient, can be considered intimate, such as eye examinations in dimmed lighting, palpating the abdomen or looking for an apex beat.
3. Cultural and religious factors may play a role in whether an examination is intimate and whether a chaperone is needed.
4. Patients may consider themselves, or could be considered, vulnerable – this is regardless of whether the examining clinician considers them to be sexually attractive.

The presence of a chaperone protects the doctor. It is unlikely that a doctor will be accused of sexual assault if a chaperone is present. A chaperone also may protect potentially vulnerable patients and may be practically useful: e.g. assistance might be needed with the examination, with undressing and dressing and the chaperone may act as an interpreter or help answer questions.

However, there may not be an appropriate (or indeed any) chaperone available. Also, the patient may have cultural objections to another person being present and has the right to decline a chaperone. The patient may have concerns about confidentiality.

In the consultation

Caution is advisable:

- Offer a chaperone if you think that there is a need for an intimate examination.
- Obtain and record informed consent for the examination and the presence of a chaperone. Record the name *and* role of the chaperone.
- If the patient declines but you would prefer a chaperone to be present, explain why this is the case and try and get agreement from the patient. Record this in the notes.
- Be sensitive to cultural differences – these may have a bearing on the patient's decision.
- It is good practice to give the patient privacy to undress and dress; use curtains if needed to maintain a patient's modesty while they are being examined.
- Explain to the patient what you are doing, throughout the examination. Avoid making irrelevant or personal comments.
- The chaperone should be present for the minimum appropriate period. They do not necessarily need to remain for the whole consultation.
- Record any concerns you or the patient have about the examination.

Be especially wary of:

- vulnerable patients, e.g. with mental health problems
- patients who have made previous allegations of indecent assault
- if the patient suggests explicitly or implicitly that they find you sexually attractive
- if you find the patient sexually attractive, this can be more obvious and threatening than you think
- patients of the same sex as the doctor may also require a chaperone
- some examinations can be deferred (e.g. a non-urgent presentation in general practice) if you are concerned about a particular patient making allegations or exhibiting sexualized behaviour.

Intimate examinations under anaesthetic

Coldicott et al (2003) suggest that, 'The teaching of vaginal and rectal examinations poses ethical problems for students and educators, and guidelines exist to protect patients from unethical practice'. The findings of their exploratory survey suggested that best practice is not always followed and that in many cases, consent has not been given for procedures. The GMC guidance is clear:

- Prior consent is needed, usually in writing, for the intimate examination of anesthetized patients.
- Doctors supervising a student should ensure that valid consent has been obtained before they carry out any intimate examination under anaesthesia.
- Students are also under an obligation to make sure that consent is obtained.

Students in Coldicott's survey were still reluctant to speak out if they found something inappropriate or were experiencing ethical discomfort, fearing repercussions. Intimate examinations performed with anaesthetic had a much higher anecdotal reportage of no consent being gained (Coldicott et al. 2003). The GMC guidance is that 'You must protect patients from risk of harm posed by another colleague's conduct . . . The safety of patients must come first at all times'. In this instance, conducting an intimate examination on someone without their consent is considered legally to be causing harm to that person.

Financial dealings and gifts

Another area where potential boundary problems can arise, is in relation to financial dealings involving patients. These can include gifts from grateful patients, patients telling doctors that they have been made the future beneficiaries of their wills and doctors having financial interests in care homes or other healthcare providers to which they wish to refer their patients.

Consider whether it would be appropriate for a doctor to accept any of the following:

- A box of chocolates from a patient to Emergency Department staff, just before she asks for a 2-week supply of sleeping tablets
- A case containing six bottles of Champagne, from a grateful patient after his GP spots a skin cancer in time for it to be removed with clear margins
- Free educational meetings at a local private hospital, led by consultants at that hospital
- A limited edition luxury car, from an elderly lady to her favourite geriatrician
- A cheque for £300 towards a new piece of equipment for a GP health centre from a patient who has just been diagnosed with a terminal illness
- An all-expenses-paid trip to a dermatology conference in the South of France, courtesy of a leading brand of topical steroids.

Although, on the face of it, a gift from a grateful patient may be harmless enough, professional bodies urge caution. As the BMA says in *Medical Ethics Today*, 'doctors need to be aware that in some rare cases gifts or loans may be offered by patients as a means of establishing an improper sense of closeness'.

Doctors also need to be sensitive to potential issues arising where they are made beneficiaries to a patient's will. They need to avoid, e.g. any involvement in assessing the patient's capacity to make legal and financial decisions, and be sensitive to the possibility that financial interests might be seen to have an impact on clinical decision-making. Where such conflicts of interests cannot be avoided, they should be disclosed to those with a relevant interest.

Treating friends and family and doctors as patients

Scenario

You have come to work early at a busy suburban GP surgery. Two of you colleagues are sick and there is a backlog of paperwork. As you are about to read the first letter, there is a knock on your office door. The receptionist tells you that one of the local hospital consultants, whom you know to be a good friend of the senior GP partner, has popped in early on the 'off chance' of seeing a GP before work. Would you make special allowances for a colleague? Why might you and why might you not do this?

Would you be more likely to see him before morning surgery if:

- he is a relative?
- he is a personal friend?
- he used to be your boss?
- he used to be your teacher?
- he is a local celebrity?
- he is a local politician?
- he is a local religious leader?
- None of the above?

Why would any of these influence your decision? If there are good reasons which you might give preferential treatment to any of the above types of person, then consider where you might set your limits. Doctors can be put under pressure by those seeking to blur boundaries for their own interests. Friends and family members short on time, or medical colleagues doubtful about confidentiality or the impact of disclosures on their careers can seek informal consultations. Sheather (2011) suggests that the requirement to respect clinical boundaries can therefore insulate doctors from pressures that might otherwise be coercive.

A PROFESSIONAL APPROACH TO RESEARCH ETHICS

The argument that research of some sort is necessary runs as follows:

- Research can improve the human condition and/or aims to reduce human suffering
- Research can contribute to the sum of human knowledge
- Medical research can increase the length and quality of life.

Medical research has been regarded as a particularly worthy activity. However, previous abuses, particularly under the auspices of medical research, require us to remain vigilant in order that the rights of the individual are not ignored. Thus, there exists a tension between reducing future suffering and the rights of the individual.

There is an ethical difference between research and audit. Research ethics committees are generally reluctant to give opinions on audits. Medical research is the systematic acquisition and pursuit of medical knowledge. A medical audit specifically assesses how well an established standard is met in practice. (Research and audit are covered in more detail in Chapter 11.) As such, this is an essential part of ensuring quality in healthcare delivery. Even so, UK hospitals have personnel dedicated to approving formal audits, both to ensure the quality of the audit and to safeguard patient information. The ethical boundary between audit and research may sometimes be blurred, especially with regard to the use of patient information.

A brief history of ethics guidelines in medical research

The current regulations around medical research have largely arisen as a result of public outrage at human-rights abuses conducted in the name of medical research during the twentieth century.

1932–1970

The US Public Health Service undertook an experiment to study the progression of syphilis. This took place in Tuskegee, where up to 400 black men with syphilis were studied. They were denied effective treatment (penicillin) even after it became available.

1940–1945

Medical experiments were carried out in Nazi Germany under the direction of Dr Josef Mengele. Human subjects were treated like, or indeed worse than, animals in medical research.

1949

The Nuremburg Court specified 10 points – known as the 'Nuremburg Code' – as a result of the case *United States v. Brandt*. (Brandt was Hitler's personal physician – although the case also heard 19 other Third Reich doctors and three biomedical scientists; and the trial was conducted under US military patronage.) The key points of the Code are:

1. An *absolute* need for *voluntary* consent
2. A justification in terms of potential 'fruitful results'
3. Proper design and previous animal experiments
4. The avoidance of 'unnecessary physical and mental suffering and injury'
5. The conduct of the experiment by 'scientifically qualified persons'

6. The termination of the experiment if it becomes clear that harm will result or if the human subject wishes to bring it to an end.

1954

The World Medical Association (WMA) adopted a Code for Research and Experimentation that allowed proxy consent; effectively a weakening of the position of the Nuremburg Code.

1964

The WMA's Declaration of Helsinki allowed for some experimentation on human subjects, including the very young, the unconscious and those who lacked legal capacity such as the mentally ill. More popular with the medical profession, as the Nuremburg Code is more restrictive.

1968

Informal research ethics committees (RECs) established in the UK after a report by the Royal College of Physicians; these are non-statutory bodies composed of members drawn predominantly from the health professions (although there are some lay members) to consider proposals for clinical trials. The role of RECs is considered below.

1984 and 1990

Principal guidelines covering research in the UK issued by the Royal College of Physicians require that experimentation be subject to ethical review prior to being carried out. The guidelines make a number of recommendations about the review process. Key points:

- It is ethical for a controlled trial to be undertaken only if, at the outset, the investigator does not know whether the trial treatment is more effective or less effective than the standard treatment with which it is to be compared (or than no treatment at all in the case of a placebo controlled study).
- Withholding effective treatment for a short time can sometimes be acceptable but patient consent is necessary and the patient may agree that he need not know precisely when this will take place.
- If a patient expresses a strong preference for a particular treatment, he is probably ineligible as a participant.
- Randomization of treatment without the consent of the patient is unethical.

1991–2001

Department of Health issued guidelines (HSG(91)5) to local research ethics committees and (HSG(97)23) to established multi-centre research ethics committees. The document, 'Governance arrangements for NHS research ethics committees' (2001) provided a framework for the ethical review of proposals for research in the NHS and social care.

2001

International Conference on Harmonization – Guidelines for Good Clinical Practice. This sets out an international ethical and scientific standard for research on human subjects. It is consistent with the principles of the Declaration of Helsinki and it aims to provide a unified standard for the European Union, Japan and the USA.

2004

The Medications for Use (Clinical Trials) Regulations aim to standardize the regulation of medical research throughout the EU, including the factors that a research ethics committee must consider before approving a clinical trial. Responsibility for not breaking the law remains with the researcher and the research institution.

2009

The Integrated Research Application System (IRAS) is a single online system for applying for permissions and approvals for health and social care/community research in the UK. In theory, the system allows all the information relating to an NHS research project in one site, from which other relevant forms such as Site Specific Information forms for local approval in multi-centre studies, can be generated.

The ethical issues at stake in medical research

Medical research in the UK is subject to ethical review by an NHS research ethics committee. In 1991, The Department of Health required that every health district set up a local research ethics committee to scrutinize the ethical justification for local medical research. These committees require a multidisciplinary approach and commonly consist of lay members, clinicians and often a philosopher/theologian and/or a statistician/scientist. The main remit of NHS RECs is clinical trials such as trials of new medications in the UK. What then do these committees look for in research proposals? How do they weigh potential public benefit against potential harm to individuals?

1. *The position of equipoise*: In order to carry out medical research, you must be in a position of equipoise – this means that it isn't *known* whether the experimental

treatment is any more effective than current treatments. You should have reason to believe that, e.g. it has been demonstrated to be more effective in animal studies, but have no actual evidence. This means there is a responsibility to ensure that the research proposed has not already been carried out.

2. *A clear purpose*: You must establish a need for doing the proposed experiment – it is important not only that there is a position of equipoise before the experiment, but that when the experiment is completed, the results will in some way be important. If the experiment is not scientifically valid, then it is unlikely that it will be ethically justifiable.

3. *The principle of least harm*: You should ensure that the experiment's design allows only the minimal amount of harm to befall the individual. This usually means that experiments should compare a new treatment against the current standard treatment, rather than against a placebo. You must demonstrate that the potential benefits are greater than the potential risks of the treatment.

4. *Consent*: Before commencing research, the participants should give their fully informed consent to take part. You must inform patients of the potential risks and benefits, and, if appropriate, whether or not they will randomly be allocated to a treatment or control group. Patients should be informed that they can refuse to participate – and their refusal will not affect their level of care. Patients should also be aware that they can withdraw from the experiment at any time – and that their withdrawal will not affect their subsequent level of care. Valid consent needs to be informed, voluntary and from a competent patient.

5. *The difference between therapeutic and non-therapeutic research*: Therapeutic research involves giving patients an experimental treatment in order to see how effective it is. Non-therapeutic research involves doing something to healthy individuals. That is, therapeutic research has potential benefits for the patient, whereas non-therapeutic research does not. Many people believe that non-therapeutic research should involve lower levels of risk – because there is little area for benefit. This distinction has been dropped from the 2000 Helsinki Revision, but still has legal force with respect to children and those decisions to include individuals in a trial in their *best interests*.

6. The philosophical approach (see Ch. 1) one uses can affect whether one considers medical research to be ethical or unethical (Fig. 2.2).

7. Adults lacking capacity and other vulnerable groups are considered below.

HINTS AND TIPS

Research ethics committees have to ask: 'Is the research needed? Is the research sufficiently well designed? Is the use of animals justified or is there adequate consent for people? What is the possibility of benefit or risk of harm to participants?'

Research on vulnerable groups

In ethical terms, a vulnerable group is any group that lacks the ability to make informed choices about themselves. Thus, vulnerable individuals include children, the incapacitated, the mentally ill and groups that may be easily exploited (e.g. prisoners or those in the developing countries).

Research in children

The basic problem posed by the involvement of children in research is that they are not always able to give valid consent. They may be competent to make some decisions, but not others. Children over 16 are presumed to have competence to consent to medical treatment

---

Fig. 2.2 A comparison of three different ethical approaches to research.

	High-risk research where participants are *not* fully informed	High-risk research where participants *are* fully informed	Low-risk research where participants are *not* fully informed	Low-risk research where participants *are* fully informed	Poor-quality research: *low risks* but patients *are* fully informed
Libertarian (rights-based)	No	Yes	No	Yes	Yes
Paternalistic (duty-based)	No	No	Yes	Yes	?No
Utilitarian (consequentialist)	?No	Yes	Yes	Yes	No

Source: *Adapted from Hope T, Savulescu J, Hendrick J 2003 Medical Ethics and Law: the core curriculum. Edinburgh: Churchill Livingstone.*

and, therefore, possibly consent to therapeutic research. Children under 16 *may* be sufficiently competent to give such consent as well. However, if a child is incompetent, consent to participate in research should be obtained from an individual with parental responsibility. Furthermore, the risks of the research must be sufficiently low to say that participating in the research is still in the best interests of the child. Whether or not a child can take part in non-therapeutic research is contentious. However, if the research involves something relatively low-risk, e.g. taking a blood sample, then it may be ethically defensible to allow such research (assuming the other criteria above were met). If at all possible, it would be better to seek the child's assent to the procedure, even if fully informed consent cannot be obtained.

Research in incapacitated adults and adults with mental disabilities

Research in this group has some parallels with that in children, but unlike the situation with children, in UK law, no-one can consent on behalf of adults. All treatment, which includes being entered for a trial, is made on the basis of the patient's best interests. However, it is hard to justify proceeding with experimental treatment on incapacitated adults (e.g. stroke victims) without consulting relatives first, simply because this shows a willingness to communicate and a desire to find out what the patient's wishes would have been if they were able to express them.

Research on adults lacking capacity is covered by sections 30–34 of the Mental Capacity Act (MCA) 2005, in addition to the Clinical Trial Regulations 2004, The Data Protection Act 1998 and the Human Tissue Act 2004.

In summary the MCA 2005 states that:

- the research must be connected with an impairing condition affecting the mind or brain of an adult with incapacity
- the research must be approved by a REC
- if the research is therapeutic, the benefits must clearly outweigh the risks and the REC must have reasonable grounds to believe that the research cannot be carried out as effectively with people capable of giving consent
- if the research is non-therapeutic, the risks must be minimal and not unduly invasive, restrictive or interfere with a participant's freedom or privacy
- the research cannot do anything contrary to a valid advance decision by a participant
- the research cannot proceed if the participant appears to be unwilling or objects.

Animal research

A range of animals are used in research and it is not obvious that standards appropriate for treating mice are necessarily the same as the standards we think ought to exist for experiments on primates. Furthermore, there are good and bad experiments; some with the potential to provide significant benefits to science and health and some without. As a result, it seems simplistic to either say that animal experiments should be allowed or that they should not. Rather more debate should be centred on what sort of potential benefit justifies experimenting on animals.

A useful list of points to consider when deciding whether a particular experiment justifies the use of animals might be as follows:

1. Is the experiment well designed, and will it produce significant results?
2. Could the experiment be done without using laboratory animals?
3. Can animal suffering be reduced, e.g. if the experiment involves new surgical techniques, will the animals used be given anaesthesia as well as agents for anaesthesia and muscle paralysis?
4. When using primates for research, consider the following question, 'Is this the sort of research we would be happy doing to humans with a mental capacity that is equivalent to that of the animals being used? If not, why are we happy to do it on primates but not the mentally ill?'

A Select Committee on Animals in Scientific Procedures reported in 2002 that:

- it is morally acceptable for human beings to use other animals for research, but it is morally wrong to cause them unnecessary or avoidable suffering
- there is a continued need for animal experiments both in applied research and in research aimed purely at extending knowledge
- there is scope for the pursuit of the three Rs of animal research.

HINTS AND TIPS

The three Rs of animal research:

*R*eplacement of conscious, living animals by non-sentient alternatives

*R*eduction in number of animals used to obtain information of a given amount and precision

*R*efinement of procedures to produce a minimal amount or severity of suffering experienced by the animals used.

Researching healthcare staff and students

Invitations to take part in research are an almost daily part of university life in the UK. Certain types of university research (e.g. when doing social science research for an intercalated BSc, MSc or MD) do not strictly involve conducting studies in the healthcare setting. This may include sociological, psychological and educational research. These studies, however are also required to go through an approval process by the university (or other relevant) ethics committee. The same considerations set down in the declaration of Helsinki will apply. Students undertaking these kinds of projects may need to consider additional factors:

1. What other kinds of harm can be caused by research? Harm may include the distressing nature of certain topics of conversation in social science research. It may also include the duty of the researcher to report unethical or illegal conduct disclosed by research participants.
2. Are there issues of safety for the researcher? Travelling alone to interview people in their own homes may involve risk if it involves travel to locations of social deprivation, or where research participants have the potential and opportunity to be violent.
3. How will the personal information of participants be protected? This includes how the identity of participants is anonymized in publications.

Publication ethics

Publication ethics is an important part of ensuring that we trust findings published in academic journals. Issues considered include:

1. Falsifying results, e.g. in order to support a theory or minimize dangers of a new procedure – journals have statisticians who advise if results are 'too perfect'. This can result in an article being retracted, as well as loss of registration and possible legal proceedings against authors
2. Not disclosing financial interests – has the research funding shaped the direction of research?
3. Authors (and reviewers) not disclosing other sources of major bias, such as being a shareholder in a company (financial); on the board of a charity or other campaigning organization linked to the area of interest (personal). In recent times there has been debate about whether political or religious views should be considered as major bias
4. Gift authorship – putting someone's name on the paper who did not contribute to any of the work
5. Plagiarism – using someone else's work as if it is your own and claiming credit for it
6. Submitting the same piece of work to multiple journals
7. Where research does not have appropriate REC approval.

The Committee on Publication Ethics (COPE, at: www.publicationethics.org) was established in 1997 by a small group of medical journal editors in the UK but now has over 6000 members worldwide from all academic fields. Many of the leading medical journals are members of COPE.

> **Key questions**
> - What are the respective roles of the GMC, the BMA, the Royal Colleges and Medical Indemnity organizations?
> - What are the duties of medical students as envisaged by the GMC?
> - What kinds of ethical issues are faced by medical students?
> - Outline why truth telling is important and describe a situation where medical information might be withheld.
> - Outline the main ethical justifications for maintaining patient confidentiality.
> - Discuss the statutes which provide exceptions to confidentiality in the medical context.
> - Give an example of conscientious objection in medicine – what are the arguments for and against?
> - What is the key difference between audit and research?
> - What are the main ethical considerations when conducting research on animals?
> - What are the key requirements of the Mental Capacity Act 2005 for research involving adults with incapacity?
> - What kinds of issues might concern publication ethics?

References

Coldicott, Y., Pope, C., Roberts, C., 2003. Education and debate: the ethics of intimate examinations. Teaching tomorrow's doctors. BMJ 326, 97–101.

Department of Health, 2004. Independent Investigation into How the NHS Handled Allegations about the Conduct of Clifford Ayling. HMSO, London. Online. Available at: http://www.dh.gov.uk/prod_consum_dh/groups/dh_digitalassets/@dh/@en/documents/digitalasset/dh_4089065.pdf.

English, V., Romano-Critchley, G., Sheather, J., et al., 2004. Medical Ethics Today. The BMA's Handbook of Ethics and Law, second ed. BMJ Books, London.

Fulford, K.W.M., Dickenson, D.L., Murray, T.H. (Eds.), 2002. Many voices: human values in healthcare ethics. In: Healthcare Ethics and Human Values. An Introductory Text with Readings and Case Studies. Blackwell, Oxford, pp. 1–19.

General Medical Council, 2006. Maintaining Boundaries. Online. Available at: http://www.gmc-uk.org/guidance/ethical_guidance/maintaining_boundaries.asp.

General Medical Council, 2008. Supplementary Guidance: Personal Beliefs and Medical Practice. Online. Available at: http://www.gmc-uk.org/static/documents/content/Personal_Beliefs.pdf.

General Medical Council, 2009. Confidentiality: Supplementary Guidance. GMC, London.

General Medical Council (GMC), 2011. Good Medical Practice and the Good Medical Practice: Framework for Appraisal and Revalidation. Online. Available at: http://www.gmc-uk.org/doctors/revalidation/revalidation_gmp_framework.asp.

Gert, B., Culver, C.M., 1979. The justification of paternalism. Ethics 2 (199–210), 204.

Gillies, J., 2004. Practical ethics for general practice (book review). Br. J. Gen. Pract. 54, 884.

Hope, T., Savulescu, J., Hendrick, J., 2003. Medical Ethics and Law: the core curriculum. Churchill Livingstone, Edinburgh.

Johnston, C., Holt, G., 2006. The legal and ethical implications of therapeutic privilege – is it ever justified to withhold treatment information from a competent patient? Clinical Ethics 1 (3), 146–152.

Savulescu, J., 2006. Conscientious objection in medicine. BMJ 332, 294–297.

Seale, C., 2010. The role of doctors' religious faith and ethnicity in taking ethically controversial decisions during end of life cases. J. Med. Ethics 36, 677–682.

Sheather, J., 2011. Improper relationships. Student BMJ 19, d3857.

Slowther, A., 2010. Confidentiality in primary care, ethical and legal considerations. InnovAiT 3 (12), 753–759.

Sokol, D., 2008. A crisis of confidence. BMJ 336, 639.

Whitehouse, S. (Ed.), 2011. MPS Guide to Ethics: A map for the moral maze. Medical Protection Society, Leeds. Online. Available at: www.medicalprotection.org/uk/booklets/MPS-guide-to-ethics-a-map-for-the-moral-maze.

X v. Y, 1988 2 All ER 648.

Yeoman, E., 2007. HIV and the law. Student BMJ 15, 293–336.

Further reading

Biggs, H., 2011. Children and health-care research; best treatment, best interests and best practice. Clin. Ethics 6, 15–19.

BMA, 2011. Using Social Media: Practical and Ethical Guidance for Doctors and Medical Students. BMA Medical Ethics Department, London. Online. Available at: http://www.bma.org.uk/images/socialmediaguidancemay2011_tcm41–206859.pdf.

Sidaway v. Board of Governors of the Bethlem Royal Hospital and the Maudsley Hospital, 1985 AC 871, 889, per Lord Scarman.

The doctor, the patient and society (3)

This chapter discusses two key themes in medical ethics and law, namely consent and the ability to make autonomous choices (capacity). The discussion focusses on areas where consent may be problematic in medicine, including the treatment (sometimes without consent) of children and patients without capacity. As well as liberty and consent, the other key issue discussed in this chapter is the vulnerability of those who are very young, very old or less capacitous for other reasons. The chapter concludes with a discussion of ethics and mental health problems. Just as the ethical treatment of a person depends on what we consider to be the criteria of personhood (see Ch. 4), the ethical treatment of mental disorders depends on what we consider to be a mental disorder.

CONSENT

Consent is arguably the most important concept in medical law. In Chapter 1, we discussed the central concept of autonomy and self-determination – this is reflected in law through the concept of consent. Usually, medical treatment may only be lawfully undertaken with a patient's consent. The provision of consent prevents the doctor from being held liable for trespass to the person (i.e. assault and battery). A doctor who gives treatment without consent risks criminal prosecution for assault, if consent is not valid, or may be sued for damages, if consent is valid but not adequately informed.

The law does not always require consent to be in writing:

- *Expressed verbal consent*: where the patient explicitly agrees to what the doctor proposes.
- *Implied consent*: where the patient's behaviour suggests that she agrees. For example where the doctor tells a patient she needs to have a blood test and the patient holds out her arm to have this done.
- *Written consent*: this is likelier for more invasive treatment such as any form of surgery. The patient explicitly agrees to the proposed treatment and then signs a consent form to state that they have understood and agree with what is proposed. A signed consent form is only evidence (and not conclusive proof) that valid consent has taken place.

A legally valid consent (or refusal) for treatment has three elements:

1. The patient must be competent to consent to (or refuse) treatment
2. The consent (or refusal) must be based on adequate information
3. The consent (or refusal) must be given voluntarily.

> ### HINTS AND TIPS
>
> *Remember*: The law does not always require that patient consent must be in writing. Also, a signed consent form may not be valid if consent has not been obtained properly.

COMPETENCE

Competence is the patient's ability to understand, deliberate, make choices and communicate them to the doctor. A patient is competent to consent or refuse treatment if they have 'capacity'. A patient has capacity if he or she can:

1. comprehend and retain the relevant information
2. weigh the relevant information in the balance to make a choice
3. communicate that choice.

This test is enshrined in the Mental Capacity Act (MCA) 2005. It is sometimes referred to as the 'Re C Test'. It was outlined in a case where a schizophrenic patient, C, who was detained in a psychiatric hospital, successfully brought a legal injunction to prevent the proposed amputation of his gangrenous leg without his express written consent (Re C [1994]). Despite having a number of clearly delusional beliefs, C was able to comprehend and retain, believe and weigh up the relevant information in order to make the choice to refuse a potentially life-saving amputation. The key difference between the 'Re C Test' and the test of capacity in the MCA is that patients are not required to *believe* that medical information is true in the MCA test. The MCA is an important piece of legislation which affects many aspects of health care. It is considered in a separate section below.

All adults of age 18 and over are presumed to have the capacity to consent or refuse. A patient may have the capacity to consent to or refuse a particular treatment, while not having the capacity to make other decisions. Mental illness does not necessarily diminish capacity to consent or refuse (see below). Capacity may be diminished by the undue influence of others. A patient's capacity may also be diminished by exhaustion or pain, as in the case of *NHS Trust v. T* [2004].

A patient must understand in broad terms, the basic nature and purpose of medical treatment. Doctors have a legal duty to provide enough information so that a patient understands what will be done, why it will be done and what the likely consequences will be. Consent is invalid if it is obtained though fraud or misrepresentation as to the nature of the medical procedure.

Clinical scenario

Just as she is about to receive a general anaesthetic for a hysterectomy, a woman tells the anaesthetist that she plans to start trying for children as soon as her gynaecological problem 'has been sorted'. She has a signed consent form for the procedure. Should the operation go ahead?

HINTS AND TIPS

Remember: A signed consent form is not proof of informed consent. If it is obvious that a patient does not understand the nature of the procedure – the nature of a hysterectomy is that it will render a woman incapable of bearing children – then this casts the patient's consent into doubt. The operation should be postponed until the patient understands what it involves.

HINTS AND TIPS

Remember: Mental illness does not necessarily diminish a person's ability to consent to or refuse treatment.

SOME LEGAL CASES ILLUSTRATING THE BROAD NATURE AND PURPOSE OF TREATMENT

In the case of *Appleton and Others v. Garrett* [1997], a dentist performed unnecessary treatments for the purpose of making money. Because he misrepresented the purpose of the treatment by telling patients they needed the dental work (when in fact he knew they did not), the claimants succeeded in an action for 'trespass to the person' (a charge which includes 'battery'), and were awarded aggravated damages.

The attributes (including the qualifications) of the clinician are also relevant to consent. In the case of *R v. Tabassum* [2000] a man was prosecuted for conducting breast examinations while falsely claiming to be medically qualified – both the nature of the person conducting the examination and its purpose were misrepresented (Herring 2010).

Appleton and Others v. Garrett [1997] contrasts with the case of *Chatterton v. Gerson* [1987], where a patient developed neurological damage after a phenol nerve block and argued that battery had taken place because of inadequate informed consent. Because the patient had been informed in broad terms of the nature of the procedure, consent was held to be valid.

VOLUNTARINESS

Consent (or refusal) must be given voluntarily. Capacity to consent or refuse may be compromised if the patient is subject to coercion or undue influence. In the case of *Re T* [1992], a mother persuaded her daughter to forego a blood transfusion on religious grounds. The court overruled the patient's refusal on the grounds of undue influence.

SUFFICIENT INFORMATION

While only the 'broad terms' are needed for consent to avoid a charge of assault and battery, doctors also have a duty to make the patient aware of the inherent risks and side-effects of treatment, but only as far as is reasonable. But who decides what is reasonable? In the leading case of *Sidaway v. Board of Governors of the Bethlem Royal Hospital and the Maudsley Hospital* [1985], the majority of the House of Lords held that the degree of disclosure was an issue to be judged primarily on the basis of what a responsible body of medical opinion accepted as proper practice. However, regardless of the professional standard, the court considered that disclosure of a particular risk may be so obviously necessary to an informed choice on the part of the patient that no reasonably prudent clinician would fail to make it. By contrast, in *Pearce v. United Bristol Healthcare NHS Trust* [1999], it appeared that the Court of Appeal was moving towards the idea that whether a risk is significant, and therefore should be disclosed, should be measured from the perspective of a 'reasonable patient' (Johnston & Holt 2006).

If reasonable risks are not disclosed, the doctor may be liable in negligence on the basis that they have breached a duty to disclose reasonable risks. It is not necessary to discuss every risk and possible side-effect (however rare), but doctors need to keep three ideas in mind when discussing risks and side-effects (Garside 2006):

- How likely is the risk or side-effect? A side-effect which is likely should be disclosed. In *Sidaway* [1985], Lord Bridge gave the example of an inherent 10% risk of a stroke from an operation. A 1–2% chance of paraplegia was deemed significant in *Chester v. Afshar* [2004]. However, the statistical risk of 0.1–0.2% of stillbirth was not considered *by the court* to be 'significant' in *Pearce* [1999].
- How severe might the side-effect be? A risk of severe disability of death should be mentioned.
- Is there any particular concern a patient might have? For example a person who only has sight in one eye might be particularly concerned with the side-effects of any treatment on that eye. An opera singer might be particularly keen to know of any treatment side-effect that might damage his voice.

In order to sue a doctor for negligence with regard to sufficient information (in the context of consent), a patient has to prove that it was more likely than not that: the information given was inadequate by accepted standards; the patient would have withheld consent at the time, had adequate information been given; harm resulted from the procedure for which informed consent was inadequate.

The legal case often referred to in discussions about sufficient information is *Chester v. Afshar* [2004], which was ultimately heard in the House of Lords: A patient developed cauda equina syndrome following spinal surgery. The House of Lords held that it was sufficient for her to prove that she would have postponed her decision and surgery, even if she might have consented to undergo the procedure at a later date.

THE MENTAL CAPACITY ACT 2005 (MCA 2005)

This provides a statutory framework to empower and protect vulnerable people who are not able to make their own decisions. It makes clear who can take decisions, in which situations, and how they should go about this. It enables people to plan ahead for a time when they may lose capacity. The MCA 2005 *only* concerns adults who are legally incapable (*Note*: In England and Wales the Mental Capacity Act applies from the age of 16).

Capacity is not present if a person is unable to do any of the following: (1) understand relevant information; (2) retain the relevant information; (3) use the information to come to a decision; (4) communicate the decision (whether by talking, using sign language or any other means).

The MCA 2005 is underpinned by five key principles:

1. Presumption of capacity – every competent adult has the right to make his or her own decisions and must be assumed to have capacity to do so unless it is proved otherwise
2. The right for individuals to be supported in making their own decisions – people must be given all appropriate help before anyone concludes that they are incapable of making their own decisions
3. Individuals retain the right to make what might be seen as eccentric or unwise decisions
4. Best interests – anything done for or on behalf of people without capacity must be in their best interests
5. Least restrictive intervention – anything done for or on behalf of people without capacity should be the least restrictive of their basic rights and freedoms.

The MCA 2005 also makes a number of provisions about decisions taken in advance of the loss of capacity:

- It allows people to choose a person to whom they give 'lasting power of attorney' or LPA. LPA allows decisions to be made about health, wealth and social care; however, the person who is choosing the LPA decides what decisions the LPA can make. This must be done in advance of a person becoming incapacitated, e.g. a patient in the early stages of Alzheimer's may decide who should be able to make decisions on their behalf when they are no longer capable and specify what decisions the LPA relates to. However, a person with LPA must still consider the incapacitated person's best interests.
- The Court of Protection makes decisions on behalf of those without capacity. Decisions on financial and social care as well as medical care can be made.
- The Court of Protection delegates to the 'Office of the Public Guardian' (OPG) the power to assign a court-appointed deputy to make decisions on the incapacitated person's behalf: this will usually be a relative or friend.
- Those who have not appointed someone with LPA and do not have a suitable carer are appointed an Independent Mental Capacity Advocate (IMCA).
- It makes 'advance' directives legally enforceable:
  - An 'advance decision' means a decision made by a person of 18 years or over, while that person has capacity, which refuses a specified treatment for a time when that person is no longer capable of making such treatment decisions.
  - Advance decisions must be 'valid' and 'applicable': Advance decisions are *invalid* if the person has withdrawn the decision at a time while capable of doing so, has given an LPA permission to make decisions about the advance decision, or behaved inconsistently with the advance decision being a fixed decision. Advance decisions

are *not applicable* if the treatment proposed is not the one specified by the advance decision, or if any circumstances specified in the advance decision are absent, or if circumstances that the person did not envisage and that may have affected that person's decision are present.

- Advance decisions are not applicable to a life-sustaining treatment unless explicitly specified in the advance directive.

Medical treatment without capacity

Clinical scenario

An unconscious adult is brought into the emergency department. He is bleeding from a stab wound to his abdomen. The on-call surgeon says that he needs urgent surgery if he is to survive. Is consent from the next of kin needed before he is taken to the operating theatre?

In the UK, urgent treatment may be given to an adult who is incapable of giving consent. Similarly, in an emergency, children may also receive treatment without parental consent. This is referred to as the 'doctrine of necessity' and prior to the MCA 2005 would have been the sole legal basis on which, e.g. an unconscious adult might be treated in the emergency department. Treatment must be in the patient's best interests. It is considered best practice, where this is possible, to consult relatives and next of kin as to what the patient would want, and what would be in the patient's best interests. Only someone who holds a Lasting Power of Attorney (LPA) for medical decisions or has been appointed as an IMCA may consent or refuse treatment on behalf of an adult. They may only make decisions in-line with the patient's best interests and enduring prior wishes. Procedures which are of debatable benefit (such as sterilization) or withdrawal of life-sustaining treatment should involve someone who is legally responsible for making decisions on the patient's behalf – where there is disagreement, a court declaration may be required as to the lawfulness of the proposed treatment.

Deprivation of liberty

One of the ways in which institutional healthcare settings can interfere with the autonomy of a patient is by deprivation of liberty (Fig. 3.1). Specific safeguards against the deprivation of liberty were introduced into the Mental Capacity Act by the Mental Health Act 2007 (remember that an Act of Parliament may only be amended or repealed by another Act of Parliament, see Chapter 1). There are a number of situations which should raise the possibility that there is a deprivation of liberty in the care environment (adapted from Brindle & Branton 2010):

- Restraint is used, including sedation, to admit a person to an institution where that person is resisting admission
- Staff exercise complete and effective control over the care and movement of a person for a significant period
- Staff exercise control over assessments, treatment, contacts and residence
- A decision has been taken by the institution that the person will not be released into the care of others, or permitted to live elsewhere, unless the staff in the institution consider it is appropriate
- A request by carers for a person to be discharged to their care is refused
- The person is unable to maintain social contacts because of restrictions placed on their access to other people
- The person loses autonomy because they are under continuous supervision and control.

The use of sedation in an emergency situation to manage an individual's disturbed behaviour would probably not in itself constitute a deprivation of their liberty. However, it may be, if: it is used to prevent a patient's persistent attempts at leaving a hospital or care home; it is used in a non-emergency situation; or the purpose of the sedation is to protect people other than the individual concerned.

CHILDREN

Why does the clinical care of children raise ethical issues?

Children can be seen to be vulnerable:

- On account of physical and mental immaturity as well as social (e.g. financial) inadequacy, children may be unable to look after their own interests and needs.
- The consequences of events in childhood (whether physical or psychological) can last a lifetime.

Although children in general are considered to have less autonomy than adults, this is transient. Children mature into adults who have their own interests and preferences. In order to preserve their 'open future', there is an argument that parents have a duty, as far as possible, to ensure that children reach adulthood with all their options intact (Rogers & Braunack-Mayer 2010: 154–155).

Example: male circumcision

An argument against the routine circumcision of male children is that this removes the option for personal choice when the child reaches adulthood. The operation

Fig. 3.1 Requirements for a deprivation of liberty (DOL) authorization.

Assessment	Purpose	Who can carry this out
Age	Is the relevant person over 18?	Anyone who the supervisory body is satisfied is eligible to be a best interests assessor (approved mental health practitioner or other suitably trained professional)
No refusals	Would a DOL authorization conflict with another existing decision-making authority, e.g. is there a valid advance decision applicable to some or all of the treatment in question? Is there conflict with the valid decision of a donee or court-appointed deputy?	Anyone who the supervisory body is satisfied is eligible to be a best interests assessor (approved mental health practitioner or other suitably trained professional)
Mental capacity	Does the relevant person lack the appropriate decision-making capacity on whether they should be accommodated in the hospital or care home or receive the recommended treatment?	Registered medical practitioner approved under Section 12 of the Mental Health Act or with appropriate training and experience in diagnosis or treatment of mental disorder. Or best interests assessor (approved mental health practitioner or other appropriately trained professional)
Mental health	Does the relevant person have a mental disorder within the meaning of the Mental Health Act 1983? How will the mental health of the person being assessed likely be affected by being deprived of their liberty? Must report their conclusions to the best interests assessor	Registered medical practitioner approved under Section 12 of the Mental Health Act or with special experience in diagnosis or treatment of mental disorder, e.g. GP with special interest. Must have completed appropriate training
Eligibility	Is the relevant person not eligible for DOL authorization because: they are detained under the Mental Health Act 1983 or the authorization would be inconsistent with an obligation placed on them under that Act. If proposed authorization relates to treatment of mental disorder then whether they meet criteria for detention needs to be considered	Approved mental health practitioner or registered medical practitioner approved under Section 12 of the Mental Health Act
Best interests	To establish whether deprivation of liberty is occurring or going to occur and if it is in the best interests of the relevant person. Is it necessary to prevent harm and is it a proportionate response to the likelihood and seriousness of that harm?	Approved mental health practitioner or other professional such as social worker, nurse, occupational therapist or psychologist with appropriate level of experience and competencies

Adapted from Brindle & Branton 2010.

is not reversible and carries immediate risks such as pain, bleeding and infection. The counter argument is that this may allow a child to more fully engage in a particular communities, and their options in this regard may be increased.

It often assumed that young children are incapable of deciding the best course of action. So parents usually make decisions for their children, and this is supported by the law in most countries. This is because:

- society expects that parents will act in their children's best interests as part of the parenting role – granting parents power ensures that children's interests are protected
- there may be some shared values in families and that children's values and beliefs may be similar to those of their parents. Decisions made by

parents are likely to take account of these values and beliefs

- parents are the ones (apart from the children themselves) most affected by decisions made about their children – and this gives them a moral stake in those decisions.

Children and the Law

From the late 1960s to the early 1990s, the rights of children have been made more explicit both in the UK and internationally. The 1989 United Nations Convention on the Rights of the Child, ratified by the UK in 1991, creates positive obligations on states to ensure that resources and services are made available to serve children's needs and interests. It mandates every child's right to dignity, respect and the opportunity to participate in decision-making (De Zulueta 2010).

The Children Act 1989 (amended 2004)

This Act is relevant in a number of ways:

1. It asserts that the welfare of the child is of *paramount importance* in court decisions about the future of the child.
2. It outlines who has parental responsibility for a child and how to make decisions where those with parental responsibility disagree.
3. It outlines the arrangements that can be made in order to protect a child from harm or to provide care in the event of those with parental responsibility being unable to.
4. The Act provides a 'child welfare checklist' in order to guide the decisions made by the courts. In making decisions, courts need to consider:
   - the wishes and feelings of the child concerned (dependent on age and understanding)
   - the physical, emotional and educational needs of the child
   - the likely effect of any change on the child
   - the age, sex, background and any other relevant characteristic of the child
   - any harm this child has suffered or is at risk of suffering
   - the capability of each parent in meeting the needs of the child.

Children and consent

The *Children Act 1989* (*s.105*) defines a child as any person under 18 years old. Under Section 8 of the Family Law Reform Act 1969, minors of 16 and 17 years are presumed to be able to consent to their own treatment. Those with parental responsibility can consent to medical treatment on behalf of a child – regardless of the child's consent. The ability of children to consent to their own treatment is discussed below. For young children and older children who are unable to consent to treatment, consent is usually provided by someone with parental responsibility (Fig. 3.2).

Knowing who has parental responsibility is important for healthcare professionals, as it is only these individuals who can consent to *non-urgent* medical assessment and treatment if the child is unable to do so. Although a number of people may have parental responsibility, a doctor requires consent from only one individual (Fig. 3.3).

Fig. 3.2 Consent and developing competence.

Explanation: appropriate for use with children of *any* age – talking in a soothing manner may help to reassure any child regardless of their verbal ability

Assent: should be sought from any child that can understand the purpose of treatment:
  6–7-year-olds may view treatment as punishment
  7–10-year-olds may begin to understand the need for treatment, but not necessarily why it may be painful
  10–12-year-olds may start to take a more mature approach to treatment–understanding that investigations may be painful, but beneficial in the long run
  12–14-year-olds may be able to satisfy *Gillick* competence

Consent:
  14–16-year-olds is the age group to which *Gillick* competence is most likely to apply
  16+ capacity to consent is presumed

Note: *Where there is fluctuating capacity in a child, the child is assessed with respect to their capacity when they are at the least lucid, i.e. on bad days. This is inconsistent with the approach to adults where it is the capacity at the time of the act that is relevant.*

Gillick competence and the Fraser guidelines

The authoritative case in relation the ability of children to consent to medical advice and treatment is the *Gillick* case. This case clarified two important points of law, which are often confused:

1. It clarified the idea that children under the age of 16 who demonstrate sufficient maturity can consent to medical advice and treatment, and have their confidentiality respected. This is what is referred to as 'Gillick competence'.
2. It clarified the idea that in the specific circumstance of contraceptive and sexual health advice doctors who provided treatment or advice to Gillick-competent child would not be found guilty of being an accessory to a sexual offence on the basis that the legal age of consent for sexual intercourse in the UK is 16. The Gillick judgement has been incorporated into the 2003 Sexual Offences Act.

In the Gillick case, Lord Fraser produced guidelines for clinicians who provide contraceptive advice or

Fig. 3.3 Who has parental responsibility?

The following individuals have parental responsibility:

The mother
The father – if currently married to the mother or was married to the mother at the time of insemination or at birth

If not married to the mother at the time of insemination or birth, the father can acquire parental responsibility by:
    marrying the mother
    a written agreement with the mother (if not married to her)
    a court order
    being appointed the child's guardian after the mother's death
    by registering as the father (with the mother) on the birth certificate

Adoptive parents – in this case, the original parents cease to have parental responsibility
Guardians – parents may appoint a person(s) to be responsible for their children after their death
A person obtaining a residence order (by which a child is placed in their care – often with grandparents or other relatives) will also usually obtain parental responsibility. The original parents do not lose parental responsibility
A local authority named in a care order – again the original parents do not lose parental responsibility
An applicant granted an emergency protection order (for the duration of the order)
Note: *Parental responsibility, once acquired, remains even after parents divorce and step-parents do not automatically acquire parental responsibility.* *Adapted from Hope et al. 2008.*

treatment to children under the age of 16. The clinician must be satisfied that:

- the young person understands the medical advice
- the young person cannot be persuaded to inform their parents
- the young person is likely to begin, or to continue having, sexual intercourse even without contraception
- unless the young person receives contraception, their physical or mental health, or both, are likely to suffer
- the young person's best interests require them to receive contraceptive advice or treatment with or without parental consent.

The Gillick case arose in response to a Department of Health and Social Security circular that advocated the preservation of confidentiality when the patient was requesting contraception, even if the patient was less than 16 years old.

Mrs Gillick had 10 children, a number of whom were girls under the age of 16, and went to court to challenge the reasonableness of the Health Authority's ability to give contraceptive advice to her children without her knowledge or consent. The case went all the way to the House of Lords, which finally decided against Mrs Gillick. It was asserted that:

- the parental right to 'control a child' existed for the benefit of the child not the parent; it was thus only justified in the best interests of the child. In terms of the law in the UK at least, children are not the property of their parents
- the parental right should yield to the child's right when the child reaches a sufficient understanding and intelligence
- the sufficient understanding and intelligence may be present in a child under the age of 16 years; it is up to the doctor to assess whether the child is capable of understanding the medical, social and moral aspects of the proposed treatment. In effect, this applies an adult test of capacity to children (see above).

This judgement allows only mature children under the age of 16 to *consent* to medical treatment.

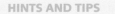

HINTS AND TIPS

Remember: Gillick competence may apply to any child under the age of 16 who demonstrates sufficient maturity in agreeing to any type of medical treatment. The Fraser guidelines refer to contraceptive treatment and advice and protect the clinician from being an accessory to a crime under the Sexual Offences Act 2003.

Children and the refusal of treatment

If a person has the capacity to consent to treatment, then it follows logically that they should also be able to refuse treatment (Fig. 3.4). This can be problematic when adolescents refuse necessary or life-saving treatment.

Legal action was withdrawn in Hannah Jones' case in 2008 and the case was not 'tested' in the courts. According to Johnston (2009), the courts have tended to conclude that a young person who makes an 'unwise' decision is thereby not competent to make it. Competence is assessed on a sliding scale in proportion to the importance or seriousness of the outcome and the ratio of risks-to-benefits of the treatment. Court decisions demonstrate that a high standard is required for a minor to be considered competent to refuse. In the case of *Re E* [1993], for example, a 16-year-old who refused blood transfusions on the basis of his religious

Fig. 3.4 The case of Hannah Jones.

In 2008, Hannah Jones, aged 13, came to public attention in the UK when she refused to consent to a heart transplant. The operation carried significant risks and a recurrence of her leukaemia could be prompted by the postoperative medication. Hannah convinced a child protection officer, called in by her local primary care trust, that she was able to make an informed decision having endured six operations in the previous 2 years. Legal action was withdrawn and her refusal was respected. Hannah was assessed to be competent to make the decision, even though she was only 13 years old. Her understanding of the treatment was enhanced by her experience of illness and this had more impact than her age alone. Although the heart transplant could perhaps be considered a 'one-off', recognition was given to the fact that ongoing postoperative medication was needed, which could have adverse side-effects. While the treatment was potentially life-saving, it also had risks and the long-term effectiveness was not certain. Most important was the issue of the practicality of enforcing treatment against the wishes of a competent young person, who was supported by her parents.

Adapted from Johnston 2009.

beliefs was not considered sufficiently competent to refuse blood transfusions.

Controversially, case law in the 1990s (*Re A* [1992] 3 Med LR 30 and *Re W* [1993]) has shown that in some circumstances, a refusal by a competent young person can be overridden and treatment can be authorized by a parent or the court. In the case of *Re W* [1993], this appeared to be on the basis that the state has a duty to see that children survive to the age of 18. Following the 1998 Human Rights Act however, a failure to respect refusal by a Gillick-competent minor could be in breach of Articles 2, 3, 5 and 8 (see Chapter 1).

Child abuse

As far as the law is concerned, the interests of the child are 'paramount' and this principle is enshrined in legislation. Because of their relative physical and emotional vulnerability, like other vulnerable groups (e.g. the very old and sick and people with diminished mental capacity), children are at risk of abuse. Child abuse includes:

- Physical abuse
- Emotional abuse
- Sexual abuse
- Neglect

Medical professionals may become involved with cases of child abuse as a result of:

- a member of the public reporting their suspicions about abuse
- treating a child and becoming suspicious of abuse
- being asked by the local authority to investigate a child for evidence of abuse.

If abuse is suspected, a *senior clinician should be consulted*, preferably one with expertise in child abuse. Making allegations or reporting the suspicions to other agencies can be a difficult decision. This is because an incorrect allegation of abuse can be devastating for families and inappropriate examinations can be devastating for the child. Collier et al (2006) list three 'dangerous' ethical questions:

1. Could proving of abuse be more destructive of abuse itself?
2. Is it better for a child to be loved and battered than neither?
3. Is help from extended family better than help from the law?

Collier et al (2006) remind us that even if the answer to the above questions is Yes, society places a (legal) duty to report abuse. The first aim is to avoid a child's death or significant harm.

The responsibility for investigating abuse lies primarily with the social services. The welfare of the child is of paramount importance.

If you are worried that a child is at significant risk of harm, what should you do?

- Clearly communicate your concerns with appropriate members of your healthcare team and document them clearly.
- Call the appropriate child protection worker. Social services and a member of the child protection team can be contacted 24 hours a day.
- Be familiar with your local guidelines and your duties as a healthcare worker (www.everychildmatters.gov.uk).
- Hospital admission may allow a full assessment and provide a protective environment.
- If necessary (e.g. if parents refuse to have the child assessed), social services may instigate an emergency protection order (see below) or the police can remove a child into police protection.

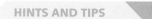

HINTS AND TIPS

Remember: As far as the law is concerned, the safety of a child is more important than other considerations such as confidentiality.

Child protection orders

There are two key sections of the Children Act 1989 (2004), which are relevant to child safeguarding:

- Section 47: Children at risk of significant harm (allows parents to be overruled, e.g. in cases of child abuse)
- Section 17: Children in need of assistance to flourish (parental consent is required for social services to become involved).

The Children Act 1989 gives power to the courts to issue a number of different orders that aim to safeguard children.

Specific issue order

This addresses a specific question that is in dispute. The courts will resolve the issue by saying what they think should be done. For example, if parents and doctors disagree about the treatment a child should receive, the courts will consider the question and decide one way or the other (usually in favour of the doctors).

Care and supervision order

The courts may make this order to place a child at risk of harm, or suffering actual harm, in the care of a local authority and to give parental authority to the local authority.

Emergency protection order

This is issued where there is an urgent need to move a child at risk to a safe place.

Child assessment order

This allows a court to have a child, believed to be at risk, assessed by a doctor for evidence of abuse. However, if the child is of sufficient understanding, the child can refuse to submit to any such medical or psychiatric assessment.

Other laws relevant to child welfare

The Sexual Offences Act 2003 clarifies what is a sexual offence against a child, especially what may be classed as a sexual offence. The Forced Marriages Act 2007 protects children, among others, from becoming coerced into marriage. The Education Act 1981 provides legal guidance on education standards and provision of assistance for children with special educational needs.

LEGAL AND ETHICAL ASPECTS OF MEDICAL CARE OF OLDER PEOPLE

In some older patients who may have mental or physical frailty, there may be numerous ethical and legal issues to consider. Coni et al (2004) summarize legal and ethical issues associated with age and aging:

- Driving in later life (legal issues, balancing public safety against the benefit to the patient)
- Mental capacity for treatment (see above) and research (see Ch. 2)
- Consent (see above)
- Restraints including the use of sedation (see above)
- Testamentary capacity and powers of attorney (see above)
- Advance decisions (see above and Ch. 4)
- Ethical issues relating to life-supporting interventions (see Ch. 4)
- Euthanasia (see Ch. 4)
- Age discrimination
- Elder abuse
- Breaking bad news
- Death Certification and when to refer to the Coroner (see Ch. 10).

Most of the above list is covered elsewhere in this book. We will briefly examine driving, testamentary capacity, age discrimination and elder abuse. Confidentiality is also a perennial issue, because whether a person is competent or incompetent, there may be concerns about how much personal information is shared with carers.

Driving in later life

UK law obliges everyone to surrender their driving licence at the age of 70. A new licence is then issued, which must be renewed every 3 years and requires a written declaration of good health. Insurance companies may insist on a physical examination and the Driver's Vehicle Licensing Authority (DVLA) must be advised *by the patient* of changes in health status. Certain conditions will render someone unfit to drive. These include:

- Any episodic impairment of consciousness (e.g. epilepsy or poorly controlled diabetes)
- Fluctuating or declining cognitive ability
- Cardiac arrhythmias and angina (even after a myocardial infarct or stroke with good recovery, a transient ischaemic attack or pacemaker insertion means that a person needs to avoid driving for at least 1 month).

Coni et al (2004) identify two common scenarios:

1. A patient refuses to accept advice to stop driving in spite of a condition which makes them unfit to drive.

2. A patient has some cognitive impairment, and while their condition is not clearly on the DVLA's list of conditions which proscribe driving, the doctor is convinced that they are unsafe on the road.

In the first instance, the doctor has a clear legal obligation to inform the DVLA, in the event that the patient really cannot be persuaded – and they should let the patient know that they plan to do this. In the second instance, Coni et al (2004) recommend involving relevant family members or seeking advice from the DVLA or a professional driving instructor. In both circumstances, doctors need to consider why an older person is keen to continue driving and whether there is a compromise or solution, e.g.:

- Geographical or social isolation (is there any other form of transport available?)
- Loss of independence and status (e.g. could the patient get their weekly shopping delivered?)

The GMC has produced supplementary guidance on confidentiality and disclosure of lack of fitness to drive to the DVLA. This may be accessed at: http://www.gmc-uk.org/Confidentiality_reporting_concerns_DVLA_20|09.pdf_27|49|42|14.pdf

Testamentary capacity

Testamentary capacity is the mental capacity required in order to draw up (or revoke) a will or lasting power of attorney. In order to do any of the above, a person needs to understand the nature of the act, have a reasonable understanding of their assets and be aware of who might have a claim on them, and be free from delusions which might distort their judgement. The Mental Capacity Act (see above) has clarified this area, especially with regard to healthcare decisions. The Mental Capacity Act has been discussed earlier.

Age discrimination

Age discrimination, according to Coni et al (2004), may be based on three rational and humane misconceptions:

1. Older people are denied access to high-tech medical interventions on the basis that they do much less well than younger people. Coni et al argue that there is clinical evidence of the benefits of many such interventions for older patients, and to use age to discriminate rather than an appropriate medical or mental-state assessment is unjust.
2. It is sometimes argued that the potential quantity and quality of life is too low to justify the procedure under consideration. The counter argument is that life-expectancies for a healthy older person may be surprisingly good, and that quality of life is best assessed by the person living it. Coni et al (2004)

add that doctors persistently underestimate the quality of life of older patients. Older people (like disabled people) may be discriminated against by measures like quality-adjusted life-years (see Chs 5 and 6).
3. Making high-tech interventions and healthcare resources available to older patients denies them to younger people. Coni et al (2004) argue that resource allocation on the population level should be the responsibility of elected politicians and not doctors (this idea is explored further in Chapter 5). Another argument is that today's younger person will be tomorrow's older person.

Elder abuse

This may take the following forms:
- Physical (e.g. pushing, hitting, deliberate overdosing or withholding medication)
- Psychological (e.g. verbal abuse, blaming, humiliation)
- Sexual
- Neglect (e.g. withholding basic needs such as food and drink)
- Financial (e.g. taking away an older person's assets in a way which does not benefit them)
- Cultural (e.g. forcing a vegetarian to eat meat).

Risk factors for elder abuse may relate to the victim, the carer or be shared by both:
- *The victim*: Dependency; communication difficulties; behavioural problems
- *The carer*: Drug or alcohol misuse; lifestyle adversely affected by caring role; divided loyalties (e.g. older relative and young child); physical or mental health problems; role reversal (e.g. ageing child and aged parent) and isolation (real or perceived)
- *Shared*: Poor housing; poor long-term relationship.

Warning signs may be difficult to substantiate and may include:
- Unexplained injuries or recurrent accidents
- Bruises or burns in unusual areas or shaped like an object
- Odd patient behaviour (e.g. anxious, frightened or withdrawn)
- Difficulty gaining access to the patient or refusal of necessary support services by the patient or carer.

Elder abuse can be an ethically difficult area for clinicians. On the one hand, a competent older person has the right to choose to remain in a vulnerable setting. On the other hand, social services and/or the police may need to be involved if a doctor suspects that a patient's autonomy is compromised by reduced capacity or coercion and elder abuse is suspected.

MENTAL HEALTH AND MENTAL ILLNESS

The question of what is mental illness is itself deeply problematic. As with other problematic areas in medical ethics, it is a question of what we believe to be true rather than one of which acts are right or wrong. For example, what we believe to be mental illness can determine whether or not someone has their liberty restricted or compulsory treatment given to them:

- The boundaries of mental illness have changed over time: In 1851, 'drapetomania' was described as an illness from which negro slaves suffered; it manifested as a tendency to run away from their masters. Homosexuality was listed as a mental disorder in the US Diagnostic and Statistical Manual of Mental Disorders, until 1973. Neither drapetomania or homosexuality are now considered to be psychiatric disorders in Western medicine.
- Those who maintain mental illness is a myth, argue that people with such 'problems' – while they should receive treatment if they so wish – should not be forced to have treatment as they do not recognize mental illness as a 'real' disease. The most prominent advocate of this argument, Thomas Szasz, considered mental disorders to be 'problems with living' – dependent on the environment or individual reaction to stressors – without a biological cause. However, it has become progressively more difficult to maintain the assertion that mental illness is a myth, given what is now known about the biological correlates of illnesses such as depression and schizophrenia and their responsiveness to psychotropic drugs.
- A particularly problematic aspect of mental illness, is that it is arguably more value-laden and contains more issues of morality than physical illness. Mental illness excuses behaviours that might be considered antisocial, immoral or criminal. Consequently, many societies have sought psychiatric opinion to inform decisions about who should be punished, who should be subjected to compulsory medical treatment, and who is so disabled by their beliefs, perceptions or behaviours that they require assistance in daily living. A danger associated with this deference to psychiatry is that, in the twentieth century, particular political regimes used psychiatry to suppress dissent and to imprison or kill those who did not fit with their vision of a perfect society.

The ethical justification for psychiatric treatment

Some conditions render people out of touch with reality and cause suffering to the extent that they are the concern of the medical specialty of psychiatry. Most Western countries have special legislation to allow patients to be detained and treated against their will. Such legislation, according to Hope (2004) addresses two issues:

1. When can treatment be imposed on patients with a mental illness for their own sake, in situations where they are refusing treatment?
2. How can society be protected from dangerous people with mental illnesses?

So, how can society be protected from dangerous people with mental illnesses? Hope argues that mental health legislation discriminates against those with mental illness. Mental illness does not generally make people dangerous to others. Mentally disordered people, if they are considered to be dangerous to others (or to themselves), may be kept in a secure place for an indefinite period. Those without a mental disorder, however dangerous they may be, cannot be kept in a secure place if they have either not yet committed a crime, or if they have committed a crime and have served their prison sentence (Hope 2004, Hope et al 2008). This criticism appears weaker in countries where similarly dangerous criminals receive less humane treatment or are executed (historically this was also the case in the UK).

Why should treatment be imposed on patients with a mental illness for their own sake, in situations where they are refusing treatment?

- If we say that someone is mentally ill, we imply that they are not in control of their thinking; thus patient autonomy appears less stable as a foundation from which to base ethical reasoning. However, strange behaviour is not conclusive evidence of incompetence or necessarily a sign or symptom of mental illness.
- Powerful psychopharmacological treatment and (much more rarely) surgical treatments such as deep brain stimulation can be used to change the personality, and perhaps the identity of patients. This can raise issues of whether this is a benefit. Furthermore, treatments such as deep brain stimulation may ease distress but render patients less autonomous – is this right?
- Others who accept mental illness as a real phenomenon argue that psychiatric treatment is only effective when the patient consents to treatment. This view holds that coercion is never justified in the treatment of the mentally ill.

But:

- this ignores the effectiveness of coercion in some situations. An analogy could be drawn with an ill child who refuses treatment because he fears needles. Mental illness can reduce some individuals to a similar child-like state, where long-term goals are not considered. In addition, experience shows that many patients who are coerced into treatment are grateful for such treatment after recovery, even if they refused treatment at the time (adapted from Peele & Chodoff 1999).

Historically, the mentally ill have been a vulnerable section of society. A core element of psychiatric ethics is about not abusing this vulnerability. Psychological therapy represents a relationship of unequal power between doctor and patient, by encouraging patients to reveal more highly personal and intimate details about their life. Even today, media portrayal of the mentally ill is predominantly negative, leading to stigma and increased isolation of people with mental illness. It seems unlikely that the stigma of mental illness can be entirely eradicated (although this does not mean we shouldn't try).

> **HINTS AND TIPS**
>
> *Remember*: People with mental illness may be vulnerable to harm or coercion. A key element of psychiatric ethics is the prevention of this vulnerability being exploited.

Psychiatrists have been portrayed as 'double agents'. On the one hand, they aim to help the distressed patient, and on the other, they are responsible for informing court decisions on who is punished and who is treated, who is told to work and who receives benefits. Even patient confidentiality may cause difficulties. Such a situation was addressed in *W v. Egdell* [1989]. In the case of Egdell (an English case and therefore binding on subsequent decisions) a psychiatrist voluntarily disclosed to the authorities, a report on a person with paranoid schizophrenia, who had been convicted of manslaughter but had requested the report in order to seek less severe detention. Public interest in disclosure that W was dangerous was held to outweigh W's private interests.

The Mental Health Act 1983 (2007)

In England and Wales, the major piece of mental health legislation is the Mental Health Act (MHA) 1983 (amended 2007) and in Scotland, it is the Mental Health (Care and Treatment) (Scotland) Act 2003. These Acts enable the state to enforce the assessment and treatment of patients with mental disorders with powers that go beyond those of the 'common law'. They also provide mechanisms to ensure that these powers are not abused.

The MHA primarily deals with compulsory assessments and, if necessary, treatment or detentions of patients with a mental health disorder.

There are two main justifications for the compulsory detention of people:

1. To protect patients from harming themselves
2. To protect patients from harming others.

Compulsory admission is governed by two sections of the MHA:

- **Section 2** allows for admission for the purpose of *assessment* – it cannot exceed 28 days. Patients can be admitted if:

> **HINTS AND TIPS**
>
> *Essential Update*: The 1983 Mental Health Act had four categories of mental disorder which might come under the Act: mental illness, severe mental impairment, mental impairment and psychopathic disorder. These categories were removed from the legislation when the 2007 Mental Health Act came into force. Only those who suffer from a mental disorder are covered by the act – treatment of people with learning disability and mental impairment (such as from dementia or a stroke) is now covered by the 2005 Mental Capacity Act.

- the patient is 'suffering from mental disorder of a nature or degree that warrants the detention of the patient'
and
- the patient ought to be so detained in the interests of his own health or safety or with a view to the protection of other persons
- admission is supported by two registered medical practitioners (often the psychiatrist and the patient's GP) and an approved social worker or relative.
- **Section 3** allows for admission for the purpose of *treatment* – which in the first instance should not be for longer than 6 months (this can be extended after a review tribunal first for another 6 months, then 3-yearly extensions are possible – someone may be detained under Section 3 for life). Patients can be detained if:
- the patient is suffering from a mental disorder of 'a nature or degree which makes it appropriate for him to receive medical treatment in a hospital'
- in the case of psychopathic disorder or mental impairment, 'appropriate treatment is available'; this has replaced the 'treatability requirement'; patients should not be detained simply to protect themselves or others, rather there must be some treatment available. This has generated some discussion as to whether it allows people with psychopathic disorders to be detained because treatments are available, regardless of whether they themselves respond to treatment – which would amount in effect to detaining someone purely for protection (Hope et al 2008)
- it is for the protection of the health and safety of the patient or for the protection of others

- treatment cannot be provided unless the patient is detained
- admission is supported by two registered medical practitioners (often the psychiatrist and the patient's GP) and an approved social worker or relative.

In addition, special note is made that patients cannot be detained on the grounds of the following:

- Dependence on drugs and/or alcohol
- Promiscuity
- Sexual deviancy.

So why do we need a Mental Health Act in addition to a Mental Capacity Act?

Surely if someone's capacity (see above) is affected by physical or mental illness, they should be treated in their best interests? Why are two laws needed in the UK?

When someone is not being detained for the assessment or treatment of a mental disorder, the preferred legislation is generally the Mental Capacity Act. Also, where there is a requirement for treatment of someone (who lacks capacity) for a physical disorder, the Mental Capacity Act should prevail. There will, however, be individuals who lack capacity and require treatment for mental disorder and therefore, may be subject to the provisions of either of the Acts.

Circumstances where the Mental Health Act may be required to detain and treat somebody who lacks capacity to consent to treatment, rather than use the Mental Capacity Act are as follows (adapted from Brindle & Branton 2010):

- The relevant person is under 18 (the Children Act 1989 may be appropriate)
- It is not possible to give the person the care or treatment they need without depriving them of their liberty
- Treatment cannot be given under the Mental Capacity Act because the person has made a valid and applicable advance decision to refuse an essential part of treatment
- The treatment would conflict with a decision of the relevant person who has lasting power of attorney, court-appointed deputy or a court ruling
- The person may need to be restrained in a way that is not allowed under the Mental Capacity Act
- It is not possible to assess or treat the person safely or effectively without treatment being compulsory, perhaps because the person is expected to regain capacity to consent and then to refuse to give it
- There is some other reason why the person might not get treatment and they or somebody else might suffer harm as a result.

Perhaps the key difference is that:

- the MCA 2005 aims primarily to ensure the best interests and maximize the liberty of people without capacity
- the MHA 1983 (2007) primarily is for the purpose of compulsory assessment and treatment of people who (because of their mental disorder) may be a danger to themselves or others.

Key questions

- What are the legal requirements for valid consent?
- What is the difference between invalid consent and obtaining consent in a negligent manner?
- What are the five main principles of the Mental Capacity Act?
- What key ethical issues arise in the treatment of children?
- What does the Children Act 1989 say about the welfare of the child?
- Define Gillick competence?
- When do the Fraser guidelines apply?
- What ethical and legal issues may be associated with the medical care of the older patient?
- Why is the treatment of mental disorders ethically problematic?
- What justifications are there for the compulsory detention of the mentally ill?
- What is the purpose of Section 2 of the Mental Health Act?
- What are the key differences between the Mental Capacity Act and the Mental Health Act?
- We have discussed issues linked to care of the elderly, children and people with mental disorder – can you think of any other vulnerable group in society and the ethical and issues associated with this group?

References

Appleton and Others v. Garrett, 1997 8 Med L R 75.

Brindle, N., Branton, T., 2010. Interface between the Mental Health Act and Mental Capacity Act: deprivation of liberty safeguards. Advances in Psychiatric Treatment 16, 430–437.

Chatterton v. Gerson, 1987 1 All ER 257.

Chester v. Afshar, 2004 UKHL 41.

Collier, J., Longmore, M., Brinsden, M., 2006. Non-accidental injury. In: Oxford Handbook of Clinical Specialties, seventh ed. Oxford University Press, Oxford.

Coni, N., Nicholl, C., Webster, S., et al., 2004. Legal and ethical aspects of medical care of elderly people. In: Lecture Notes on Geriatric Medicine, sixth ed. Blackwell, Oxford.

De Zulueta, P., 2010. Choosing for and with children: consent, assent, and working with children in the primary care setting. London: Journal of Primary Care 3, 12–18.

Garside, J.P., 2006. Consent. In: Law for doctors: principles and practicalities, third ed. Royal Society of Medicine Press, London, pp. 49–60.

Herring, J., 2010. Consent to treatment. In: Law Express: Medical Law, second ed. Pearson Education, Harlow.

Hope, T., 2004. Inconsistencies about madness. In: Medical Ethics: A Very Short Introduction, Oxford University Press, Oxford.

Hope, T., Savulescu, J., Hendrick, J., 2008. Children. In: Medical Ethics and Law: The Core Curriculum, second ed. Churchill Livingstone Elsevier, Edinburgh.

Johnston, C., 2009. Overriding competent medical treatment refusal by adolescents: when 'No', means 'No'. Arch. Dis. Child. 94, 487–491.

Johnston, C., Holt, G., 2006. The legal and ethical implications of therapeutic privilege – is it ever justified to withhold treatment information from a competent patient? Clinical Ethics 1, 146–151.

NHS Trust v. T, 2004 EWHC 1279 (Fam).

Pearce v. United Bristol Healthcare NHS Trust, 1999 ECC 167, CA.

Peele, R., Chodoff, P., 1999. The ethics of involuntary treatment and deinstitutionalization. In: Bloch, S., Chodoff, P., Green, S.A. (Eds.), Psychiatric Ethics, third ed. Oxford University Press, Oxford, pp. 430–431.

R v Tabassum, 2000 Lloyds Rep Med 404.

Re C (Refusal of treatment), 1994 1 All ER 819; noted in [1993] 4 Med LR 238.

Re E (A Minor) (Wardship: Medical Treatment), 1993 1 FLR 386.

Re T (Adult: refusal of treatment), 1992 3 Med L R 306.

Re W (A Minor) (Medical Treatment: Court's Jurisdiction), 1993 Fam. 64.

Re W v. Egdell, 1989 EWCA Civ 13.

Rogers, W., Braunack-Mayer, A., 2010. Why do children raise particular ethical issues? In: Practical Ethics for General Practice. Oxford University Press, Oxford, pp. 154–155.

Sidaway v. Board of Governors of the Bethlem Royal Hospital and the Maudsley Hospital, 1985 AC 871.

Further reading

Brazier, M., 1992. Medicine, Patients and the Law, second ed. Penguin, Harmondsworth.

Grubb, A., 1997. Consent. In: Boyd, K., Higgs, R., Pinching, A.J. (Eds.), The New Dictionary of Medical Ethics, BMJ Publishing, London, pp. 56–58.

Hoggett, B., 1996. Mental Health Law, fourth ed. Sweet and Maxwell, London.

Re R (A Minor) (Wardship: Consent to treatment), 1992 1 FLR 190.

Medical ethics is often identified with issues at the beginning and at the end of human life. This chapter explores issues around the 'beginning' of life, such as contraception, sterilization, abortion and reproductive technologies. The second part of the chapter deals with end-of-life decisions, euthanasia, the definition of death and organ transplantation.

CONTRACEPTION

As far as the law in the UK is concerned, this is any treatment which prevents fertilization of the human egg or implantation of the fertilized egg in the womb. However this definition causes ethical difficulty for people who believe that human life begins at conception (see below). The National Health Service Act 1977 requires the Secretary of State for Health to ensure that reasonable requirements for treatment and advice on contraceptive issues are met (see Chapter 1 for brief look at the statutory basis of Medicine in the UK).

Ethical objections to types of contraception tend to fall into two categories: a) One argument goes that contraception is wrong because it interferes with a natural process (fertility) and promotes promiscuity (also seen as wrong) by breaking the link between sex and reproduction. b) The other main (consequentialist) argument is that many forms of contraception fail to protect the user against sexually transmitted diseases and other consequences of sexual intercourse.

Contrasting arguments may be deontological, e.g. that at the ecological level humankind has a duty to contain its population so as not to exceed available resources. Utilitarian arguments may include the idea that at an individual level prospective parents may wish to limit their family to size which they can support. A utilitarian viewpoint might consider that undesired pregnancy is a 'harm' and that therefore it is a benefit that sex can be enjoyed without pregnancy as a consequence.

There is a third key issue regarding the provision of contraception and contraceptive advice: Is the person using contraception in a position to give informed consent to a) the contraception, b) sexual intercourse? This is an issue regarding capacity rather than contraception and is considered in Chapter 3.

A legal distinction between contraception and abortion?

In 2002 the Society for the Protection of Unborn Children (SPUC) challenged the legality of government regulations permitting the sale of the 'morning after pill' without a prescription. The 'morning after pill' can be given up to seventy-two hours after unprotected sexual intercourse and its contraceptive action is in preventing the successful implantation of an embryo in the womb lining. The SPUC claimed that the medication caused a miscarriage or abortion, and therefore could only be used lawfully if the criteria in the Abortion Act 1967 (see below) were met, such as the requirement for signature by two doctors. The government argued that the medication was a contraceptive. The judge ruled that a miscarriage could only occur once a fertilized embryo had implanted in the womb, and that there would be harmful social consequences if emergency contraception had to be subject to the same criteria as abortion in the UK. Therefore the 'morning after pill' can be provided without a medical prescription, and is often referred to as 'emergency contraception'. In effect the case also underlines the legal principle that pregnancy begins at implantation rather than conception (*R (Smeaton on behalf of SPUC) v The Secretary of State et al* [2002] 2 FCR 193).

> **HINTS AND TIPS**
>
> *Remember*: According to UK case law, pregnancy begins when the fertilized embryo is implanted in the womb. This means that the Abortion Act 1967 (amended 1990) does not apply to drugs which prevent implantation of the fertilized embryo.

STERILIZATION

Sterilization is a medical treatment intended to make a person permanently infertile. While a person may have capacity, and autonomously decide to be sterilized, the decision will also affect that person's partner – especially if they want to have children. Sterilization can be ethically problematic:

- Some religious groups consider sterilization to be a form of bodily mutilation that goes against the natural function of humans to reproduce (similar to the argument against contraception above).
- Some people who are sterilized may change their mind, and regret the decision. Fully informed consent is therefore crucial.
- Sterilizing particular people in society such as the mentally incompetent, people with a history of substance misuse, or ethnic minorities, can be criticized as a form of unacceptable eugenics. Coercing any type of person to be sterilized is generally seen as unacceptable. However, do incentives (e.g. giving substance misusers a one-off cash payment on the condition that they are sterilized) amount to a kind of coercion? If the incentive is something a person desperately needs, then this is arguably coercive.

Failed sterilization

Some of the issues surrounding sterilization are illustrated by cases of 'failed sterilization', which have gone to court. These are considered as 'negligence' cases (see Ch. 1) in the civil courts. The key issues here are:

- is consent fully informed?
- can conception (as a result of failed contraception) be considered to be a harm?

As with other medical negligence cases, information given must be in accordance with a *responsible body of professional practice*. In the case of sterilization, this means telling the patient both that 1) the operation is permanent and may be non-reversible and 2) there is a failure rate of the operation, i.e. while sterilization is effective, it is not an *absolute guarantee* of never conceiving.

Failure to give the above information would be considered a 'breach of duty' to warn about a foreseeable risk of the woman becoming pregnant. While courts are reluctant to award damages in the case of a failed sterilization (or failed abortion) resulting in the birth of a healthy child for the living costs of the child, they may more readily consider the discomfort and financial loss resulting from either a subsequent abortion or pregnancy and delivery. However, courts are much more prepared to award damages towards the upkeep and treatment of handicapped children born as a result of failed sterilization and abortion. They are sometimes referred to as 'wrongful conception' and 'wrongful birth' cases (Kennedy & Grubb 2000).

HINTS AND TIPS

Remember: A failed sterilization operation on a man (if negligence is alleged) may result in a case being brought to court by the woman who is his sexual partner.

Sterilization and the mentally incompetent

As discussed in Chapter 3, lawful treatment for a mentally incompetent adult can only be given if what is proposed is in their 'best interests'. Consequently, sterilization for 'best interests' appears more likely to be considered 'on behalf of' mentally incompetent women than men. This is because pregnancy and indeed menstruation have been seen as potential harms for women with severe mental incapacity. By contrast, it is harder to argue that a man with significant mental incapacity gets a similar benefit from being sterilized.

The sorts of things that law courts have considered, in deciding what is in the patient's best interests include:

- The likelihood of pregnancy – that is, is the individual engaging or likely to engage in sexual intercourse?
- How well is the patient able to understand the concept of pregnancy and its relation to sex?
- Would the patient be able to cope with parenthood?
- Would this patient be able to use any other form of contraception?
- How would a sterilization operation affect the other medical problems of the patient – e.g. will sterilization stop heavy periods from causing a female patient distress?
- What other support is available to the patient?

THE HUMAN EMBRYO

A common thread of argument may run through a number of the issues in reproductive ethics. A person's ethical stance on abortion, *in-vitro fertilization* (IVF), cloning and genetic screening may largely be determined by his/her view on the moral status of the embryo or fetus. Gillon (2001) goes so far as to say that this question is not so much ethical (to do with right and wrong) but epistemological (based on what you believe, in this case about the status of the fetus).

HINTS AND TIPS

Remember: Two people may agree that killing people is wrong, but disagree over what counts as a person.

According to the law in England and Wales (adapted from Herring 2010):

- a fetus is not a legal person
- a fetus is not simply part of the mother either
- it is not possible to bring legal proceedings in the name of the fetus

- a fetus has interests which are protected by the law
- a fetus is not directly protected by the European Convention on Human Rights.

The legal status of the fetus is clear: it has no legal rights. However, the human embryo (or fertilized egg) does not become a fetus until about the 6th week of pregnancy. How should we determine the *moral* status of the embryo as it develops into a fetus and progresses towards birth? A number of views, and objections, are presented below.

The embryo is morally valuable because it is a human organism

This view holds that the value of the embryo is situated in the fact that it is *human* and as such deserves moral recognition. Therefore, as it is morally wrong to kill an adult, it would have been equally wrong to kill that same person when he or she was a child, fetus or embryo. All of these entities are part of a continuous individual identity that can be traced back to conception.

But:

- is killing a zygote, or a primitive embryo, really as morally bad as killing a child? One way of thinking about this is to imagine a scenario where you are able to save either an embryo (in a test-tube) or a 5-year-old child from a fire in a laboratory. Would you be morally justified in preferring to save the embryo? If not, why not?
- why are human embryos more important than other embryos? What characteristics do early human embryos (e.g. at the 8- or 16-cell stage) have that distinguish them from other mammalian embryos, apart from potential to develop into humans?

The embryo is morally valuable because it is a potential human being

This view accepts that the embryo is not morally valuable in and of itself. However, because it can potentially develop into a human child, it deserves moral concern. Killing an embryo is wrong because it deprives the child that could have potentially lived its existence. This view also generally holds that moral concern starts at conception.

However:

- if it is potentiality that important, are gametes deserving of moral concern as well? For example, a couple that uses contraception is effectively preventing a number of potential children being realized.

The embryo/fetus is morally valuable if it is a 'person'

This view holds that there is some characteristic or characteristics that morally valuable entities have. Common characteristics of personhood include: consciousness (or perhaps *self-consciousness*), sentience, rationality, the ability to form future plans and the capacity to value one's own life. Various religious views may hold that embryos are not persons until the soul enters the body, which may be at conception or at a later stage.

In this context, 'being *a person* is not necessarily the same as 'being a *human being*'. Some humans may not qualify as persons, and some non-humans may qualify as persons!:

- Some of these characteristics will confer the status of personhood on embryos beyond a certain stage of development; e.g. after 24 weeks, a fetus can probably feel pain, so would qualify as a person if sentience was the criterion being used. However, others, like self-consciousness or the capacity to value one's own life, require a far greater degree of development, and indeed may exclude newborns and infants from 'personhood'.
- Some characteristics may also exclude individuals with severe learning difficulties, leaving some questions as to how these individuals are to be treated and their interests protected.
- Some characteristics may include other animals; we have no reason to doubt that all other mammals are able to feel pain in a similar way to humans, and some higher primates may be self-conscious.

The embryo is morally valuable because it is valued by others

This view holds that embryos are morally valuable because they are the objects of moral concern to others. This means that the value of the embryo is not *intrinsic*, but is conferred by others. Thus, the wrong in killing an embryo, fetus or even an infant is not the wrong done to that entity, but is wrong because there exist individuals (e.g. the parents) who care for it, and do not wish it to be harmed. There also exists a broader concern that the killing of such entities would diminish the concern for older children and human life in general.

But:

- does this mean it would be acceptable to kill newborns if no-one around them cared? This idea appears to clash with the idea of a right-to-life for all humans from birth. Western society in general is protective towards all children (see Ch. 3).

The moral value of the embryo increases as it continues to develop

This viewpoint accepts that the moral value of the zygote is less than that of the embryo, which in turn is less than that of the newborn. This view does not specify a particular stage of development that is of overriding importance. This, however, does not provide practical guidance on whether abortion at 12 weeks, 24 weeks or at term, is morally acceptable.

ABORTION

Abortion is the intentional termination of pregnancy with the resulting death of the embryo or fetus (Hope et al 2008). While the Hippocratic Oath appears to forbid abortion in ancient Greek and Roman times both abortion and infanticide were practised. The fetus and infant were seen to be products of the mother and as such 'owned' by the husband, who was free to dispose of the infant in any way he saw fit. In general, Christianity forbade abortion, although arguments were put forward between the fifteenth and eighteenth centuries that claimed abortions prior to the mother feeling the fetus move (a time known as the 'quickening') were permissible on the grounds that 'ensoulment' was yet to happen. In the eighteenth and nineteenth centuries, 'medical opinion' accepted 'preformism' – the idea that spermatozoa contained a fully formed, miniature, human being (known as a *homunculus*) and that the uterus simply provided a fertile environment for a diminutive person to grow. Such a view was used to bolster anti-abortion arguments and persisted into the first-quarter of the twentieth century. However, abortion remained illegal in most Western countries until the 1960s.

Abortion legislation

The Abortion Act 1967 (amended 1990) sets out circumstances in which clinicians have a defence to what would be considered in law to be a crime.

Important statutes to consider in the law on abortion:

1. Offences Against the Person Act 1861, *ss*.58–59: these sections make illegal:
   a. The self-induction of miscarriage
   b. A second person helping a woman to procure an abortion
   c. The supply or procurement of an abortifacient.
2. Infant Life Preservation Act 1929:
   a. Makes it illegal to destroy the life of a child capable of being born alive
   b. The destruction of a 'child capable of being born alive' is not a criminal offence if this is done with the intention of saving the life of the mother.
3. Abortion Act 1967, amended by the Human Fertilisation and Embryology Act 1990.

The Abortion Act 1967 was designed to tackle two key problems. The first was that illegal abortions carried out in secret by often untrained and poorly qualified 'abortionists', were leading to significant injury in women. The second was the result of a common-law decision that suggested that abortions were acceptable if the doctor believed a continuation of the pregnancy would cause severe harm to the physical or mental health of the mother. This decision led to the problem of doctors thinking they were carrying out abortions in good faith, but at the same time, running the risk of facing criminal charges.

Figure 4.1 shows an important section of the Abortion Act 1967 (as amended 1990). The following points are important:

1. In general, the opinion of two doctors is needed – only one doctor in an emergency.
2. *ss*.1,(1a) allows an abortion to be carried out before the 24th week of pregnancy for a wide variety of reasons, including preventing harm to a woman's existing children. This clause is sometimes referred to as the 'statistical clause', as statistically *any* normal pregnancy carries more risk than a standard early termination – according to some, it effectively allows any abortion to fulfil the criteria of the Act. Most abortions take place under this section.
3. The Abortion Act does not give women the *right* to demand an abortion. The power to decide whether a woman qualifies for an abortion lies with the medical practitioner. The woman's *consent* is necessary and she can of course *refuse* to have an abortion, even if it is thought necessary to save her own life.
4. If the woman is unable to give consent, then an abortion can still be carried out if it is in the woman's *best interests* and in accordance with good medical practice.
5. After the 24th week of pregnancy, risk to the life of the woman, the prevention of serious disability or fetal disability (most common) is required for an abortion to be carried out.
6. The fetus does *not* have any legal rights.
7. The father of the fetus has no legal right to prevent the woman from having an abortion.
8. The Abortion Act gives doctors the right to make a 'conscientious objection' to participating 'in any treatment authorized by [the] Act' except in an emergency. However, the doctor must not prevent the woman from obtaining access to abortion services. For example, if a patient sees her GP and requests an abortion, the GP must either refer her (if she meets the criteria of the Abortion Act), or be sure she has access to information about abortion services and the ability to use the

---

Fig. 4.1 The Abortion Act 1967 ss.1,(1–2).

1. Subject to the provisions of this section, a person shall not be guilty of an offence under the law relating to abortion when a pregnancy is terminated by a registered medical practitioner if two registered medical practitioners are of the opinion, formed in good faith:

   a. that the pregnancy has not exceeded its 24th week and that the continuance of the pregnancy would involve risk, greater than if the pregnancy were terminated, of injury to the physical or mental health of the pregnant woman or any existing children of her family

   or

   b. that the termination is necessary to prevent grave permanent injury to the physical or mental health of the pregnant woman

   or

   c. that the continuance of the pregnancy would involve risk to the life of the pregnant woman, greater than if the pregnancy were terminated

   or

   d. that there is substantial risk that if the child were born, it would suffer from such physical or mental abnormalities as to be seriously handicapped.

2. In determining whether the continuance of a pregnancy would involve such risk of injury to health as is mentioned in paragraph (a) or (b) of sub-section (1) of this section, account may be taken of the pregnant woman's actual or reasonably foreseeable environment.

---

information if she wishes, even if the GP personally thinks abortion is morally wrong.

9. If in a late abortion the fetus is born alive, then doctors have a legal obligation to try and save it, if it is the newborn's best interests. This is because a child gains independent human rights upon birth.

The ethical arguments for and against abortion

The ethical argument tends to be framed by opposing positions:

- The *'pro-life'* position: the extreme version of this view holds that all human life is sacred and an embryo counts as a human life from the point of fertilization. Therefore, abortion is the moral equivalent of murder. Arguments are in general made either from the position that all human life is valuable and that the fetus is human, or that the fetus is a potential human being and should be protected for that reason (see above for the different views about the human embryo).
- The *'pro-choice'* position: this view holds that ending a pregnancy is a choice that ought to be made by the individual woman involved. The value of the life of the fetus is not always seen as zero, but as being subordinate to the rights of the mother to determine what happens to her own body. There are consequentialist and rights-based reasons for this argument:

Consequentialists argue that harms that may occur if there was no legal option of a safe termination including the following:

- Increasing the poverty of women and their existing children

- Pregnancy may be a risk to the health of some mothers
- Women may seek unsafe terminations – putting themselves at even greater risk.

Rights-based arguments include the idea that: restricting access to abortion is an infringement of a woman's autonomy to exercise control over her own body and that to refuse an abortion also infringes a woman's right to health and the pursuit of a satisfactory life. The validity of these arguments in part depends on the acceptance of the 'pro-choice' perspective that fetuses are not human *persons* with rights of their own, or at least not rights that are equivalent in force to those of the pregnant woman.

The mother–fetus conflict

Clinical dilemma: Part I

Miss F has a history of mental disturbance and drug abuse. She is pregnant for a second time – her first child is currently in care. She wishes to continue smoking, drinking and taking drugs throughout this pregnancy. She has not been found to be incompetent. Can (and should) the unborn child be made a ward of court in an attempt to curb the mother's harmful behaviour towards it?

This scenario is based on a real case, *Re F (in utero)* [1988]. It is an example of where the autonomy of the mother (to live the lifestyle she wishes) conflicts with the interests of the fetus to be born healthy. Smoking and excessive alcohol consumption have the potential to cause a number of problems in the baby that will continue outside of the uterus. Drug use may lead to withdrawal symptoms in the newborn and may also be associated with problems of child development.

As we have discussed above, the fetus does not have personhood or rights as far as the law in the UK is concerned. The *Congenital Disabilities (Civil Liability) Act 1976* (as amended by the Human Fertilization and Embryology Act [HFEA] 1990) holds that a mother cannot be held liable for any harm that occurs to the fetus *in utero* (apart from harm due to negligent driving). UK courts have expressed the view that if the behaviour of pregnant women was to be controlled in order to safeguard the health of their unborn children, this would have to be expressed by an Act of Parliament.

It has been said that if we agree that termination is ethically acceptable how can we object to harmful behaviour to the fetus that doesn't kill it? However, this objection ignores the difference between a pregnant woman going to term, and a pregnant woman who is going to abort. The former is responsible for harmful consequences to both the fetus *and* the future child. The latter is only responsible for the harmful consequences to the fetus. There is arguably a much greater moral duty upon the woman who intends to give birth.

Clearly from a virtue or consequentialist perspective, it would be 'better' if Miss F did stop smoking, drinking and taking drugs, not only for the health of her unborn child, but also for her own health. However, this does not necessarily mean that such a moral duty should also be a legal one. Imagine a further development in the scenario.

Clinical dilemma: Part II

Miss F is now 2 weeks past her due date; the baby is in a breech position and is showing signs of fetal distress. It is thought that a caesarean section is the only way of saving the life of the baby. Miss F refuses to have the operation, saying she wants a 'natural' birth. She is still found to be competent. What should her doctor do?

A number of cases have gone to court in order to force women to have caesarean sections – either to preserve the mother's life or the life of the unborn child. Legally, if the woman is competent, then her refusal (whatever her reasons) is sufficient to prevent the operation. However, the moral acceptability of refusal may depend on the nature of her reasons. Is it morally acceptable for the woman to refuse a caesarean because she does not want a scar? What about religious reasons? What about no reason at all?

There is a growing consensus among Western clinicians and bioethicists that overriding a competent woman's refusal is almost never justified. The following are a few reasons why:

- A caesarean might involve some risk to the mother (though in a complicated labour, the procedure may reduce the overall risk to the mother).
- Courts would not order a mother to donate a kidney to an ill child in need of a transplant. So it seems unfair to force a woman to undergo a caesarean section (consider whether a caesarean section and operation to donate a kidney are fair comparisons).
- If a woman continued to object would doctors be expected to forcibly restrain and anaesthetize a pregnant woman?

ASSISTED REPRODUCTION

To begin with, there are problems relating to whether 'infertility' or 'sub-fertility' are 'illnesses', and whether treatment should be provided for anyone who needs it, irrespective of the ability to pay (Chapter 5 considers: What is need?). The answers to this sort of question may turn on whether or not we consider that people have a *right* to have children, and whether such a right applies equally to everyone (including same-sex couples, single women, poor women, post-menopausal women or even single men).

> **HINTS AND TIPS**
>
> *Remember*: Whether or not we believe people should have a right to assisted conception depends on whether we believe that there is a right to have a child or whether infertility is an illness – AS WELL AS whether the particular method of assisted reproduction is ethically acceptable.

What then are the different ways in which infertility can be treated?

Gamete donation

This can take the form of egg donation or artificial insemination (AI), either from the husband/partner (AIH) or from a donor (AID). Some of the ethico–legal problems of gamete donation are concerned with:

- the number of children a man can father by AI
- whether or not payment can be made for donor sperm or eggs
- who the father of the child is if donor sperm is used
- who the mother of the child is when one woman provides the genetic material, and another gives birth to the child.

In-vitro fertilization

This requires the fertilization of an egg outside of the human body. In-vitro fertilization (IVF) requires the stimulation of ovulation in the woman and the harvesting of eggs. The eggs are incubated with the sperm in a petri dish, and in some cases a single spermatozoon may be injected under the covering of the egg. Finally, the fertilized egg (usually more than one) is transferred to the woman's uterus. The ethical problems particular to IVF include:

- The production of excess embryos that must subsequently either be stored (by cryopreservation) or destroyed
- The increased likelihood of multiple pregnancies and the subsequent increased demand for obstetric and neonatal services
- The potential for embryo selection to avoid genetic disease, but also potentially to choose the sex, or other characteristics of the embryos
- Discrimination in the provision of the service against poor, single or older women.

Surrogacy

This can be either of the following:

- *Partial* – in which the surrogate (or carrying) woman's ovum is fertilized by the husband/partner from the commissioning couple, either via IVF, AID or sexual intercourse, so she not only carries the baby, but has a genetic link with it
- *Full* – in which the commissioning couple provide both the ovum and the sperm, so that while the surrogate carries the child, it is not genetically related to her.

The ethical problems of surrogacy include:

- It represents a separation of genetic, gestational and social parenting
- It raises the issue of the commodification of human life and the threat of 'baby selling'
- There are fears of the exploitation and/or coercion of women into being surrogates.

General arguments against in-vitro fertilization and other reproductive technologies are given below.

Assisted reproduction separates sex from reproduction

This argument generally relies on an underlying belief either in natural law theory or a religious principle. A version of natural law theory might claim that the function of sex is reproduction and, therefore, the separation of the two represents an unnatural use of medical technology. But:

- the problem with this and all '*it's unnatural*' arguments is that nature is not always a good guide in showing what is ethically right and wrong. Much of modern medicine is in a sense unnatural, but this does not mean it is *wrong*. Similarly, argument-based principles from any one religious viewpoint may be

considered unsuitable for basing social policy in a pluralistic society.

Assisted reproduction alters the nature of traditional relationships

IVF and the other reproductive technologies enable single women or lesbian couples to have children. The claim has been made that such individuals are less suitable parents than a heterosexual couple. An additional argument is sometimes made that each partner in homosexual relationship is not necessarily infertile and therefore could have simple donor insemination.

However, it is yet to be conclusively shown that heterosexual couples are 'better' parents or raise 'better' children, however that may be measured. It is accepted that children thrive in a loving environment, but it has not been shown that either single parents or same-sex couples are unable to provide such an environment. In the face of such a lack of evidence, we should be cautious in denying the ability to raise children to these sections of society.

Assisted reproduction perpetuates negative social attitudes towards infertile women

This is the argument that there are positive social attitudes towards women who have children, and negative attitudes towards those who either do not have children or do not want children. Such attitudes place pressure on women to become mothers. The presence of IVF and other reproductive technologies increases this pressure. Rather than perpetuate such attitudes, the state should encourage acceptance of childlessness within society.

However, while there is the possibility of social attitudes factoring in the reasons why a woman might wish for IVF, it is not clear that this would be an overriding reason. Furthermore, it seems to disregard the autonomy of individual women to make their own reproductive choices.

Assisted reproduction leads to the exploitation of women

IVF is an expensive technology and occasionally, patients have been asked to donate eggs in return for treatment. Furthermore, surrogates might ask for large sums of money to cover the costs of 'being pregnant'. This argument focuses on the danger of less-well-off women being exploited.

However, the plausibility of this argument relies on how one thinks about luxury goods and capitalism in general. Most luxury goods are provided by the less well-off for consumption by the well-off; whether or not this is exploitation is debatable.

Assisted reproduction is not sufficiently important to be provided on the NHS

This argument focuses on the resource issue surrounding the provision of IVF and related services on the NHS. Does providing infertility treatment deny resources to other more urgent and worthy NHS services? Indeed, what obligation, if any, does the NHS have to provide treatment for infertility?

Being infertile however, is a profoundly distressing condition for many individuals. Being able to become pregnant, give birth and raise a child can be substantial 'goods' in leading a fulfilled life. The provision of IVF *may* lower the associated psychological morbidity of being childless.

Also, IVF is provided by medically qualified personnel in a clinical setting. This suggests that it is a medical treatment. Infertility is characterized as a health problem. Therefore, it is arguable that IVF should be considered with other treatments for provision in an NHS setting.

Assisted reproduction will lead to social and eugenic selection

IVF enables embryos to be screened. At present in the UK, this is allowed in order to prevent embryos that will manifest a genetic disease from being implanted. In the case of X-linked diseases, IVF can be used to select only female embryos. However, the potential exists for sex selection for social reasons. In the future, there may be the potential to select embryos on the basis of height, intelligence, sexuality, hair or eye colour. The creation of such 'designer babies' is considered wrong because it plays into the idea that children are a commodity.

The social selection of embryos argument uses the threat of a *slippery slope* – it implies that by allowing one type of selection now, we will end-up with an unacceptable eugenic programme. However, the fact that we allow some kinds of selection does not mean that we will *inevitably* allow all kinds of selection – sex selection is currently legal in the UK on medical grounds (to avoid sex chromosome-linked serious disease), but not on social grounds.

To an extent, eugenics is already practiced when genetic disease is screened for. If better (normal) embryos can be selected, then why shouldn't embryos with genes for attributes like intelligence, long life and disease resistance be selected?

General ethical approaches to assisted reproduction

A useful way of thinking about the ethics of assisted reproduction is to consider the interests of:

- *the (potential) child*: for example, what are the consequences to the child of being born to a particular couple? The HFEA 1990 endorses this approach (see below), requiring that account be taken of the *'welfare of any child who may be born'*. This approach may be criticized in that it assumes that it is better for a child *never to have existed* rather than to be born in a particular set of circumstances.
- *the parents*: is having children who are genetically related a *human right*?
- *the state*: assisted reproduction is an expensive treatment. Are the state's limited resources best spent on this sort of health care? Is infertility a *disease*? Should the state only allow those individuals who are financially capable of supporting a child to have IVF? Is IVF more expensive than supporting children with disabilities into adulthood?

HINTS AND TIPS

Hint: A useful way of thinking about the ethics of assisted reproduction is to consider the interests of the potential child, the parents and the state (or society in general).

Assisted reproduction and legislation

The most important piece of legislation in the area of reproductive medicine is the Human Fertilization and Embryology Act (HFE Act) 1990.

The HFE Act governs:

1. The creation of embryos *in vitro*, i.e. outside the human body
2. The storage and use of embryos and gametes.

This means it forms the basis for legislation on artificial insemination (in a clinic), egg donation and IVF.

The HFE Act 1990 (*s*.5) stipulates the creation of the Human Fertilization and Embryology Authority (HFEA): a body charged with the responsibility of:

1. reviewing information about activities governed by the Act
2. granting licences to carry out activities specified in the Act
3. publicizing the services provided to the public
4. providing appropriate advice to licensed clinics.

Artificial insemination

Artificial insemination from the husband/the male partner (AIH)

- No licence required unless gametes need to be stored or frozen. This usually occurs only if the husband is to undergo treatment that may render him infertile (e.g. chemotherapy).
- The HFE Act 1990 requires that adequate *written* consent is obtained. It is good practice for clinics to ensure couples consider and agree on what should happen to gametes in relation to:
  A. the couple splitting up prior to implantation
  B. one of the couple dying
  C. neither one of the couple losing the capacity to revoke consent
  D. how long they would like them stored (the amended HFE act stipulates a maximum time limit of 10 years for gametes and 10 years for embryos).

The case of *R v. HF&E Authority, ex parte Blood* [1997] involved a married man who had developed meningitis and lapsed into a coma. His widow, Diane Blood convinced the doctors treating her husband to remove sperm from her unconscious husband prior to his death: *this act was considered to be unlawful* as there was no *evidence* of consent. The sperm were stored at a licensed clinic and thus came within the remit of the HFE Act. The HFEA refused her permission to use the sperm in order to conceive a child – even though Diane Blood claimed she and her husband had been trying for a child. The Court of Appeal held that insemination in Britain would be illegal, but agreed that under European Law, Diane Blood was entitled to seek medical treatment in another member state. A Belgian clinic agreed to carry out artificial insemination, and the HFEA agreed to allow the transport of the sperm to that clinic. However, the Court of Appeal stated that this case should not set a precedent, as the taking and storing of the sperm without consent was illegal.

Artificial insemination with sperm from a donor (AID)

- Does require a licence when it is done in a clinic under *s*.4 of the HFE Act 1990
- Does not always require a licence: all it requires is a suitable male to 'donate' sperm and the woman to self-inseminate; this is often referred to as the 'turkey baster' method or 'do-it-yourself insemination'. If no clinic is involved, it is unregulated. The UK court case, *MacLennan v. MacLennan* [1958] asked the question of whether such donor insemination constitutes adultery. The courts found that without a sexual relationship, it does not

- Sperm donors should be over 18 years and under 55, and egg donors over 18 years and under 35.
- Must be screened appropriately if used in a clinic setting; *s*.44 of the HFE Act amends the *Congenital Disabilities Act* making it possible to bring an action against a clinic should negligent screening of gametes take place. Potentially, donors can also be liable if they lie about their family/medical history when they donate.
- Is dealt with in *ss*.27–29 of the HFE Act regarding the parental status of the parties involved:
  - If a married couple have AID, the husband/civil partner is the legal parent
  - If a cohabiting couple both seek AID, the partner is the legal parent
  - If a woman receives treatment without the consent of her partner, even if she is in a relationship, there is *no* legal father
  - If treatment occurs outside the remit of the HFE Act, for example do-it-yourself inseminations or AID in another country, then the donor becomes the legal father
  - Treatment carried out within the remit of the HFE Act accords no rights and no responsibilities to the gamete donor.
- The child's right to access information is dealt with under *ss*.31–35 of the HFE Act:
  - At 18, an individual who suspects they may have been fathered by donor insemination can find out if their suspicions are true.
  - At 16, an individual who wishes to get married and suspects they may have been fathered by donor insemination can find out if they are related to their intended spouse.

Activities which are unlawful under the HFE Act 1990 (Amended 2008)

The Amended HFE Act prohibits certain activities:

- The creation or use of any embryos outside the human body (however they are created) except by licensed clinics
- The creation of 'human admixed embryos' except for research in licensed facilities
- Use or storage of embryos beyond the 14 days after the gametes have been mixed
- Placing a human embryo in an animal
- Placing a non-human embryo or gamete in a woman
- Modification of the genetic structure of any cell which is part of an embryo
- Sex-selection of offspring for non-medical reasons (sex selection to avoid having a child with a serious sex-linked disease is allowed).

Section 13(5) requires clinics to take account of: the welfare of any child who may be born as a result of the treatment, including the need of that child for 'supportive parenting' (replaces 'a father').

Section 38 of the 1990 HFE Act states that: no person who has a conscientious objection to participating in any activity governed by the Act is under any duty, however arising, to do so.

GENETIC COUNSELLING AND SCREENING

Clinical dilemma

Huntington's chorea is a hereditary disease caused by a single gene inherited as a dominant characteristic. The children of patients with this condition have a 50% chance of having the disease, which does not appear until later in life. A GP has cared for a woman during the early stages of Huntington's chorea. Her son, also a patient and aged 48 years, has repeatedly refused any test to establish whether or not he is affected. He remains asymptomatic.

The man is on the point of re-marrying. His fiancée is a 34-year-old woman who also happens to be a patient of the GP, and the GP knows that she desperately wants to have children. The man angrily rejects an invitation from the GP to discuss matters.

The man's daughter from his first marriage is 20 years of age. She too is a patient of the GP. She approaches the GP and asks to be tested for Huntington's chorea before starting a family herself. She does not want her father to know. She does not want the results put in her clinical records, as it may affect her application for a life insurance policy.

We can try to approach this scenario by looking at the duties of care and confidentiality the GP has to each of his patients involved.

The father

The father in the scenario does not wish to be tested. At face value, it seems that in order to treat this patient as an autonomous agent, his wishes should be respected. To remain ignorant of his genetic status with regards to Huntington's chorea is a valid stance.

But:

- respect for autonomy can be challenged by competing moral obligations, as when respecting someone's autonomy would cause significant harm to another, or where one person's autonomy inhibits or diminishes that of another. We are told the man is about to re-marry and his fiancée is desperate to have children. So, does the father have any responsibility to tell his fiancée of the increased risk of Huntington's that any of their children may have? If the father is a carrier of the Huntington's chorea allele, then any of his children have a 50% chance of inheriting it. He

himself has a 50% chance of being a carrier; as his status is unknown, the probability of any of his children being carriers is 1 in 4 or 25%.

However:

- we do not know whether the man wishes to have further children at all. If he does not and discusses this with his fiancée and takes the necessary precautions to avoid the situation, there is no reason why the father should be tested or even why he should tell his fiancée of his family history of Huntington's chorea. (Although, many would argue he has a duty to his fiancée to be truthful – in order to establish a relationship based on trust.)
- if the man does decide he wishes to have more children with his new wife, and does not inform her of his family history of Huntington's, then the GP is faced with a conflict of moral duties.

The fiancée and future children

The fiancée is one of the GP's patients, so the obligation of veracity asks of the GP to be truthful with her. We can assume that the fiancée is keen to be informed of all the possible risks to her children. The GP possesses some information that is relevant to the woman and child, but perhaps ought not to disclose it. Were the woman informed of all the facts she might feel it prudent to have a pre-natal screening done for Huntington's should she fall pregnant. Perhaps by choosing to have further children, in the knowledge that there is a 1 in 4 chance of them being affected by Huntington's, the father's autonomy and thus his right to confidentiality, are diminished in favour of the children, as the health and autonomy of third parties are introduced.

The daughter

The daughter is a fully autonomous individual and, therefore, does not require consent from her father to be tested – even though a positive test result will indicate that the father also is positive for Huntington's. Although he does not wish to know his status, he cannot prevent his daughter from finding out hers. If the daughter is determined to know whether or not she is a carrier of Huntington's, there is no reason why the GP cannot encourage her to discuss the implications of the testing with her father, although if she does not wish to do so, she cannot be coerced into this or have her test made conditional on this.

If her test result is positive for Huntington's, the daughter introduces a greater degree of certainty into the scenario. It will be known to both the daughter and the GP that the man is also a carrier and thus any future child of the man will have a 50% chance of developing Huntington's. The daughter now possesses knowledge about her own condition that implies information about her father's genetic status. Her father has no rights over this knowledge – it is information that is 'owned' by his daughter. The father's right to privacy has been curtailed because of the third parties involved and the fact that his carrier status is deduced via a test on relatives rather than actually on him. For the daughter to discuss this with her father's fiancée could be seen as a breach of his privacy, although perhaps the fiancée's right to be informed overrides this. This right to be informed, however, may not override the GP's duty of confidentiality, so it may be that there is less of a moral dilemma if the daughter informs the fiancée of her family history of Huntington's, rather than the GP doing it. With regards to situations like this, John Harris (1994) says that: 'While it will always be open to individuals to refuse tests for themselves, they may not be able to so effectively shield themselves from the increased knowledge of their own chances, which will come from relatives who do opt for the test. They will also have to consider whether they are justified in having children who will certainly, or probably, have the disease'. This shows that the greatest responsibility lies with the father – it is he who must decide if he is justified in having children that may have Huntington's.

The end of the scenario mentions the daughter's wish for the test not to be recorded on her clinical records, as it might adversely affect her life insurance. If the test is done, it seems important that it is recorded. There is no reason for the GP to break any confidences and inform any insurer – it is up to the patient what information they give to the insurer. On a broader scale, we can ask whether genetic screening should cause people to be liable for higher insurance premiums. If we are happy for this to occur with other diseases such as familial heart disease and diabetes, should genetic tests not be just as acceptable? This debate would of course depend on the reliability of such tests.

CLONING

On 23 February, 1997, aged just 6 months, Dolly the sheep was revealed to the world's media by the Roslin Institute, Edinburgh. Dolly had been cloned directly from a single cell from the breast tissue of an adult sheep. In December 2001, the UK Parliament passed the *Human Reproductive Cloning Act* to make human cloning illegal. Given this apparent consensus against cloning, how as medics, should we approach the ethical debate?

One starting point is a variation of Mill's Liberty Principle. We can reasonably argue that individuals should be free to act as they please as long as their actions do not harm anyone. Along these lines, John Harris talks of a 'procreative autonomy', which extends to reproductive cloning. This is the idea that individuals should be allowed to control how they reproduce. Such a freedom

is especially important when the choices made cause little harm to either the children produced or society as a whole, and in addition, extends a principle such as respect for autonomy. In essence, this argument, when applied to the question of cloning, requires that in order to restrict choice and freedom, we present a strong case as to why cloning is unacceptable for human reproduction.

The following are a few commonly given suggestions:

Cloning is wrong because:

- the technology is unsafe at present, and could give rise to a large number of fetal abnormalities, and children with a shortened lifespan or who suffer
- it prevents genetic variation
- it is unnatural
- it deprives clones of the right to be unique
- it would be a psychological harm to those born as a result of it
- it treats children as commodities.

The loss of genetic variation argument

The loss of genetic variation argument runs that sexual reproduction is essential in producing variation within the human species; cloning removes this variation and, thus, reduces genetic diversity – this may in the long-term threaten the survival of the species.

But:

- if only used in situations where infertile parents wished for genetically related offspring, it is likely that only a minority of people would use cloning technology, and this surely would not be sufficient to threaten species survival
- even if everyone in the world were to be cloned, genetic diversity would not change from what it is now – in fact it would stay exactly the same. (This assumes that only one clone of each person is made.) However, problems involving reduced diversity could arise if some individuals produce vast numbers of clones, e.g. if a 'crazy dictator' decides to create clone armies.

But:

- this objection is really to do with a misuse of a technology rather than an objection to the technology itself. Baseball bats can be used when mugging someone, but this doesn't mean we should ban baseball.

If reproductive cloning were to be used, then it would have to be regulated, as IVF and abortion are currently regulated. At the root of this sort of concern may be the fear that once we allow certain procedures that involve tampering with the human genome, there is a slippery slope to unacceptable eugenic policies being introduced. This type of concern affects a number of genetic techniques, including sex selection, pre-natal genetic diagnosis and selective terminations.

The 'it is unnatural' argument

A more common accusation is that cloning is 'unnatural' – it arouses a feeling of uneasiness that cannot easily be clarified. This is sometimes called the 'yuck factor'. However, 'unnatural' does not always mean 'morally wrong'. An objection to cloning must involve something over and above a sense of being unnatural, or simply prompting a sense of disgust. The crux of the 'it is unnatural' argument may be to defend the notion that technological developments should be used in such a way as to improve humanity without destroying or detracting from what it is to be human.

Clones are not 'unique'

Can clones be unique if they are 'copies' of other people? We know that identical twins have identical copies of DNA, and at the same time they exist as unique individuals with differing personalities. If we think of clones as 'vertical twins', rather than 'horizontal' ones, there is no reason to suppose that they will be any less unique from their vertical twins than identical twins are from their horizontal twins. In fact, given the different environments in which they are raised, we could suppose that clones would be rather more different than horizontal twins are.

Psychological harm to the clone

Next, there are those who object to human cloning on the grounds of the harm that might be inflicted on the child. Indeed, the HFEA, which governs IVF treatment and the use of embryos, indicates that the *good of the child is paramount*. The sentiment of the Act is clear, but what exactly is the nature of the harm that may be visited upon a clone? The harm is often described as psychological and may have at least two aspects.

First, there is said to be the burden a child would have of seeing exactly how they would appear at various ages, by seeing photographs (or home videos) of their 'parent' at those ages. However, many sons and daughters already look at their parents and resign themselves to the same fate, without suffering too greatly for it. Granted, the similarity will be greater between clones, but the idea that that fact will lead to *intolerable* suffering, such that we consider it is better that child doesn't exist, is unsubstantiated.

Second, there is the objection that the 'parents' may expect too much of their clones. For example, a concert pianist may clone himself and expect (to an unreasonable degree) his clone to possess a similar talent for music. Many parents may place unreasonable demands on their children in this way. The children of doctors often feel pressurized into medical careers, but no-one suggests that doctors don't have children; what they suggest is that children be accorded the freedom to flourish in areas of their own choosing. Parents of clones may be more likely to expect too much of them (because of certain preconceptions), but this is not an *inevitable* consequence of cloning. Any harm that is isolated, if it exists, is located in the parenting, not the act of cloning. Indeed, it may be that *a planned* child who is cloned may be more cherished than one conceived accidentally.

The commodification of children

Finally, there is the objection that cloning represents a commodification of children and this in itself is wrong. Implicit in this claim, is that there is no morally admirable reason for producing a clone. The standard reason given for wanting to clone oneself is that cloning represents the only chance that a particular individual can have a genetically related child. The strength of this reason depends on whether people have a *right* to have genetically related children. Thus, is the desire to have a genetically related child simply a selfish one – a desire that treats children simply as a consumer product? Is there in any sense a healthcare *need* for cloning that cannot be satisfied by the reproductive technologies already available? Tied in with this question is that of what kind of person would desire to have a clone? And, are they the kind of people who should be able to have clones? It may be that while cloning *in principle* is morally acceptable (i.e. for *good* purposes), *in practice* the only people who would want clones would want them for morally unacceptable reasons (e.g. *unreasonably* wanting to replace a dead child).

THE END OF LIFE

The treatment of those people of advanced age or with terminal illnesses is perhaps one of the more distressing aspects of medicine. Ethical questions in this area not only include when it is appropriate to stop treatment, but whether hastening death is something which should take place in a clinical setting. The definition of death is another 'epistemological' question, which has major implications, such as when efforts to maintain a body's vital functions can be withdrawn and whether organs may be taken from a body for use in transplants.

The sanctity of life or the value of life?

Is life 'sacred' or intrinsically valuable? Is it always wrong to deliberately end someone's life?

The most extreme version of the principle of sanctity of life is sometimes referred to as vitalism. According to vitalism, human life is of absolute value and should be maintained whenever possible and by whatever means, irrespective of the quality of a person's life. A less extreme version of the principle holds life to be a basic but not an absolute good. This still means that there is value to a person simply being alive, no matter what state that person is in.

Other thinkers, such as Doyal, think that the value of life is self-determined in accordance with respect for autonomy. In addition to this, Doyal and others think that life is only instrumentally valuable. We can say that something is instrumentally important if its value depends on its usefulness for something else, e.g. pleasure, money or medicine, and some lives are therefore not worth living.

'Quality of life' arguments are also used in a similar manner to 'value of life' arguments. Some people argue that their quality of life is so poor, either because of pain and suffering or because their ability to flourish as individuals is so diminished (e.g. because of a severe disability), that continued existence is not in their best interests. Consequently, they may argue that life-saving treatment should not be provided, or ask for assistance in dying.

Acts and omissions

The act/omission debate centres on the question of whether actions are more culpable than omissions. In the euthanasia debate, the question is whether there is a moral difference between killing someone (actively) and allowing them to die (passively), where their death is avoidable. The distinction between killing someone and allowing someone to die is maintained in English Law.

The reasons for maintaining the act/omission distinction are:

- intuitively, there seems to be a difference between killing and allowing to die
- we make omissions all the time, e.g. by *not* giving £50 per month to charity, I may consequently allow the deaths of five people overseas, yet this does not seem as bad as actively killing five people
- in practice, the courts are easily able to distinguish acts from omissions, and find it useful to do so.

The reasons for ignoring the act/omission distinction are:

- to the consequentialist, it does not matter whether the death was brought about by an act or an omission; both are choices we make and are ultimately responsible for
- some omissions can be relabelled quite easily as acts and vice versa. For example, is switching off a ventilator an act or an omission? If this is done by a

patient's relative, it would be an act (and the relative could be charged with murder). If done by a doctor, it is seen as an omission (see below).

Withholding and withdrawing life-sustaining treatment

The deliberate omission of care in order that (i.e. it is 'intended') someone dies (in that person's best interests) is referred to as 'passive euthanasia'. However, the ethical and legal justifications for withholding or withdrawing a treatment are more likely to be on the basis of futility, refusal of consent (such as an advance decision) or an argument that the burdens of the treatment are disproportionate either the benefits or the likelihood of success.

Remember that if a competent adult refuses treatment, even if this is life-saving, the law in the UK states that the refusal must be respected. Consequently, many of the decisions discussed below are for people who do not have capacity (see Ch. 3).

The BMA, in-line with the decisions of the courts, has produced guidance on withholding and withdrawing life-sustaining treatment (including artificial nutrition and hydration). According to the guidance, use of nasogastric tubes, percutaneous gastrostomy and IV fluids are considered to be medical treatment. There is no obligation to provide treatment which will not benefit the patient and it is also permissible to withdraw treatment which is not benefiting the patient. Where there is any disagreement regarding what is beneficial or the patient's wishes, it may be advisable to seek court approval before doing so.

> **HINTS AND TIPS**
>
> *Remember*: No method of feeding is risk-free: oral feeding may result in choking or aspiration. NG tubes may be associated with risk of reflux and aspiration and gastrostomies with skin infection and tube blockage.

Two recent legal cases illustrate the idea that a patient may refuse life-sustaining treatment even if it will result in death, but cannot demand any treatment which the medical team deem not to be beneficial:

- In *Re B* [2002]: a 41-year-old woman was paralysed from the neck down and dependent on a ventilator. She asked for the ventilator to be switched off. The medical team felt unable to comply on the basis that they felt she had a worthwhile life. The court held that Miss B was competent and well informed and therefore her refusal of ventilation had to be respected, even if this meant her death.

- In *R (Burke) v. GMC* [2005]: Mr Burke, a man with cerebellar ataxia predicted that at some point in the future, he would need artificial nutrition and hydration (ANH). He was concerned that if he lost capacity a doctor would decide that ANH was no longer in his best interests and he would die of thirst and starvation. He wanted to be able to demand these in advance. The court held that a patient has no right, whether he is competent or incompetent, to demand a treatment which is not in his best interests.

Treatment and basic care

Since the decision of the House of Lords in the case of Airedale NHS Trust v. Bland [1993], artificial nutrition and hydration (ANH) are considered in law to be a form of treatment, which can be withdrawn (see above). Basic care includes oral feeding (where appropriate) as well as washing and maintaining the basic dignity of patients who are unable to do this for themselves. Whether ANH is treatment or basic care has been hotly debated in medical ethics circles for decades. However, classifying ANH as treatment means that it can be given as part of treatment for conditions such as severe anorexia nervosa.

Do not attempt resuscitation orders

The 'do not attempt resuscitation' order (DNAR) involves making an advance decision to withhold cardiorespiratory resuscitation from a patient in the event that they have a cardiac or respiratory arrest. DNAR should be considered only when:

- resuscitation is *not* in the best interests of the patient; that is, it is likely to cause a quality of life that is considered to be worse than death
- resuscitation is likely to be *futile*
- resuscitation is contrary to the informed wishes of a competent patient; that is, resuscitation is not *consented to*
- resuscitation is contrary to an *advance directive*.

HINTS AND TIPS

Remember: a DNAR order is not the same thing as withdrawing all treatment. It only relates to cardiorespiratory resuscitation. In fact there have been suggestions (Sokol 2009a) that DNAR should be replaced by 'Allow natural death' (AND).

Futility

The usual reason for considering a request for a bed in the intensive care unit is to provide artificial ventilation for life-threatening respiratory failure, e.g. due to pneumonia or drug overdose. The dilemma is to avoid deaths when the condition is reversible (such as asthma or Guillain–Barré syndrome) but also to avoid the prolongation of life when the outlook is hopeless (such as end-stage motor neurone disease). The other considerations are similar to those governing CPR – the enduring wishes of the patient and an assessment of the quality of life (advice from friends and family as to what an unresponsive patient would have wanted is also relevant, see Chapter 3). Many illnesses which end in respiratory failure, such as chronic obstructive pulmonary disease, have a long course, so an advanced care plan may be put in place and the patient's wishes ascertained.

Jonsen et al (2010, adapted from Sokol 2009b) distinguish three types of futility:

1. *Physiological* futility is when the intervention cannot physiologically achieve the desired effect. This is the most objective, and least controversial, type of futility. If a patient is in cardiac arrest, for example, it would be physiologically futile to administer shocks from a defibrillator for a 'non-shockable' rhythm such as asystole, or pulseless electrical activity.
2. *Quantitative* futility is when the intervention has very little chance of achieving the desired effect. If a patient goes into cardiac arrest and CPR is initiated, it may be quantitatively futile to continue if the patient remains in asystole after several minutes. The probability of achieving the goal, namely restoring breathing and circulation, is minimal.
3. *Qualitative* futility is when the intervention, even if successful, will produce such an undesirable outcome that it is best not to attempt it. In the above example, doctors may decide that, even if the patient's breathing and circulation are restored after 30 min of CPR, the extent of the neurological damage will be such that the patient's quality of life will be unacceptable.

Neonates

There have been a number of cases where disabled newborns have had treatment withdrawn or withheld. The courts have tended to take the approach that aggressive treatment for gravely handicapped children need not be pursued, especially if there is only a short gain in life expectancy anticipated from treatment.

Adults

In the case of *Airedale NHS Trust v. Bland* [1993] Tony Bland was injured at the Hillsborough football ground in April 1989 after being crushed in the crowd. He was diagnosed as being in a persistent vegetative state (PVS) with no signs of recovery. He was not ventilated, but was fed via a nasogastric tube. The hospital treating him sought court approval to discontinue nasogastric feeding, on the basis that this was a form of treatment and not in his best interests. His family were in agreement. The case was finally decided at the House of Lords.

Key points of the Bland case were as follows:

- This case confirmed the *act/omission distinction in law* (see below for an ethical discussion).
- Withdrawal of treatment is not a legally culpable omission *if in the patient's best interests*.
- The case was decided on 'futility' of care, although some would argue feeding is not futile.

Euthanasia

Euthanasia is often defined as a gentle and easy death or the act of bringing about this, especially in the case of incurable or painful disease. It comes from the ancient Greek for 'good' (*eu*) and 'death' (*thanatos*). The term has changed its meaning over time. Huxtable (2007) provides a modern working definition: The intentional ending of life (whether the recipient wants this or not) of someone which is motivated by the belief that this will be in some way beneficial for them.

The act of euthanasia is conventionally classified in the following ways:

1. The person whose life is at stake: may want help in dying, not want help in dying or be unable to form or communicate any decision on the matter; these positions are, respectively, called voluntary, involuntary and non-voluntary euthanasia.
2. Positive acts (active) euthanasia vs. negative omissions (passive) euthanasia; e.g. intentionally failing to provide hydration to a patient so that they die might be considered passive and giving someone a lethal injection with the intention that they die is clearly active. However, what about pulling out a nasogastric feeding tube with the intention that a patient dies? Is the action of pulling out the tube active or does ceasing to feed the patient make this passive euthanasia?

In Huxtable's definition there are six versions of euthanasia: active voluntary, active involuntary and active non-voluntary, passive voluntary, passive involuntary and passive non-voluntary. To be called euthanasia, rather than murder, this must always be considered to be in the best interests of the person who dies (in technical legal terms, euthanasia remains indistinguishable from murder, as it is the intentional killing of another person). In addition, there is assisted suicide: one may passively or actively facilitate the suicide of another. To commit suicide is defined as to kill oneself intentionally. To commit suicide oneself is not illegal, but to encourage or assist the suicide of another is a

crime according to the 1961 Suicide Act, as amended by the Coroners and Justice Act 2009. Assisted suicide may include a variety of acts including giving advice on ways to commit suicide; prescribing a medication with the intention that the patient will choose to take it in lethal dosage; as well as setting up devices to deliver a lethal drug which are activated by the patient, rather than the clinician.

> **HINTS AND TIPS**
>
> *Remember*: Arguments about the rightness or wrongness of different types of euthanasia may depend on: what we consider to be alive or dead; who we consider to be a person; what we consider to be a medical treatment and even what we consider to be an intention.

Ethical arguments for and against assisted suicide and euthanasia

Arguments for euthanasia (adapted from Hope et al. 2008)

Consistency

- *Suicide is accepted*: it is commonly held that it is possible to rationally decide to kill oneself. Why then, should those who are unable to physically kill themselves be denied the right to choose how and when they should die, if in their opinion their life is no longer worth living? Perversely, it is the most disabled and ill who are least able to end their own lives. Do these people not deserve assistance if they wish to die?
- *From passive to active euthanasia*: the law currently allows the withdrawal and withholding of life-saving medical treatment. In the case of withholding nutrition (as in the Tony Bland case) death comes about due to dehydration and may take days or weeks to occur. If this kind of death is morally permissible, why should we not also permit active euthanasia, which by common intuition would seem to cause less suffering?
- *From painkillers to lethal injections*: if we allow the giving of painkillers that shorten life as well as relieving pain, and are unconvinced by the doctrine of double-effect (see above), then why should we not give drugs that simply shorten life?

Appeal to principles

- *Autonomy*: respect for autonomy should mean assisting patients in bringing about their death when they so request.
- *Beneficence*: euthanasia is often described as 'mercy' killing. Death is seen as preferable to continued life with a high degree of suffering.

Arguments against euthanasia (adapted from Hope et al 2008)

Improvements in palliative care mean euthanasia is unnecessary

- It is argued that palliative care is adequate to prevent suffering, and if the major argument for euthanasia is the reduction of suffering, the need for it is obviated.

Availability of euthanasia means advances in medicine are less likely

- It is argued that, if people with terminal or distressing illnesses are helped to die, there will be less of a drive to find cures and treatments for those diseases, especially if those new treatments are initially expensive or burdensome.

Exploitation by others

- It is thought that some elderly or disabled people would consider themselves to be a burden on their family and carers, and while they may personally prefer to continue living, would request euthanasia in order to relieve their carers. It is also suggested that some people would be encouraged to request euthanasia by their families.

Slippery-slope objections

- A slippery-slope argument starts with something that some argue is acceptable, e.g. assisted suicide for capacitous, able-bodied people and ends with something we currently consider unacceptable such as involuntary euthanasia (murder) of people with mental illness and old people. So if we permit assisted-suicide then people who cannot take their own life will ask that we permit voluntary euthanasia (for people who have capacity) – after all, to do otherwise discriminates against the disabled. If we permit voluntary euthanasia, then people will ask that they have this service at a time when they are have lost capacity. Society will ask if people who are capable can have this as a good thing, then why should this not be provided to people who have poor quality of life but cannot ask for it, such as people with dementia or severe learning needs. If we permit non-voluntary euthanasia on the basis that it is a good thing, perhaps we should also provide this benefit to all people who have a poor quality of life and are a financial burden on society, such as people with mental health problems and the elderly or even unwanted children? If we accept that people who are a burden to society should be helped to die, perhaps we should also arrange a painless death for people who are using resources that could be much better used by healthier people, even if those who are a burden to society object.

Contrary to the aims of medicine

- Some healthcare professionals are opposed to assisted-suicide and euthanasia on the grounds that it is not what they consider to be part of the aims of medicine. In their view, health care is about prolonging life and reducing suffering, not causing death. Furthermore, patients may not trust their doctors, if part of their role is carrying out euthanasia. Participating in assisted suicide and euthanasia may consequently result in demoralized clinicians who try less hard to heal and cure patients.

The law and euthanasia

The key legal issue with euthanasia is that it represents the intentional killing of another human being. If a clinician, whether through an act or an omission, caused the death of a person, they could face a number of criminal charges, most notably: murder or attempted murder, manslaughter or aiding and abetting suicide.

Someone is guilty of murder if they caused the death of the victim, and intended to kill or to cause the victim grievous bodily harm, and cannot raise a defence (a reason which is acceptable in the eyes of the law for doing so, such as self-defence). Because murder, manslaughter and aiding and abetting suicide are all criminal charges, a jury must be convinced beyond all reasonable doubt before a conviction occurs. There are two key issues in a murder charge against a clinician:

- Did the clinician cause the deceased to die? This includes hastening the death of a patient by a few hours. However, it can often be uncertain whether the patient has died because of a doctor's actions or despite them (i.e. from natural causes). If cause of death cannot be proved, e.g. in the case of *R v. Cox* [1992], the patient had been cremated before the charges were brought, then a conviction for attempted murder can still be sought.
- Did the clinician intend the death of the patient? This is mainly direct intention, where it was the clinician's purpose or aim to kill the patient. The courts may also recognize indirect intention, where the clinician realizes that death or grievous bodily harm will arise as a result of his actions. In theory, indirect intention may be relevant to treatments, where death or the hastening of death is virtually a certain side-effect of the treatment.

Important cases in the development of case law on euthanasia

- In the case of *R v. Carr* (1986), Dr Carr was charged with murder of a terminally ill adult after he administered a massive dose of phenobarbitone. Though the prosecution drew attention to Dr Carr's interest in voluntary euthanasia, he was acquitted on the basis that the overdose had occurred 'by mistake'; the judgement held that 'every patient was entitled to every hour that God had given him, however seriously ill he might be'. In this case, the courts did not find intention (see above).

- In the case of *R v. Cox* [1992], Dr Cox gave a 70-year-old woman with rheumatoid arthritis and multiple other pathologies an injection of potassium chloride (at her repeated request to die). He was convicted with attempted murder and given a 1-year suspended prison sentence. The GMC cautioned him, but allowed him to continue practice conditional on additional training in palliative care, as it believed him to have acted in good faith. The court found intention (in part because the drug used in order to end the patient's life was not one with well-known and accepted painkilling properties. Had Dr Cox used an opiate or sedative, he might have tried to argue that his intention was to relieve pain and hastened death was a side-effect or 'double-effect').

In 1994, a House of Lords committee considered the ethical legal and clinical implications of end-of-life decision-making. Their recommendations were as follows:

- The law should not be changed to permit active euthanasia
- The right of competent patients to refuse medical treatment was strongly endorsed
- The law on suicide (and assisting suicide) should not be changed
- There should be no new offence of 'mercy killing' (as opposed to murder)
- The mandatory life sentence for murder should be dropped.

The government at the time accepted all but the last recommendation. An example of a lesser offence would be that 'Assisting suicide' (maximum penalty of 14 years imprisonment, whereas murder carries a mandatory life sentence).

The law on encouraging or assisting suicide

The 1961 Suicide Act was recently simplified and modernized in line with recent case law by the Coroners and Justice Act 2009. Sub-section (2) of the Coroners and Justice Act 2009 replaces Section 2(1) of the Suicide Act 1961. It provides that a person commits an offence if he or she does an act which is *capable* of encouraging or assisting another person to commit or attempt to commit suicide, and if he or she *intends* the act to encourage or assist another person to commit or attempt to commit suicide. The person committing the offence need not know, or even be able to identify, the other person. So, for example, the author of a website promoting suicide who intends that one or more of his or her readers will commit or attempt to commit suicide is guilty of an offence, even though he or she may never know

the identity of those who access the website. The offence applies to whether or not a person commits or attempts suicide.

Further changes and clarifications are summarized as follows:

- Arranging for someone else to encourage or assist suicide is also an offence.
- Even if the encouragement or assistance does not result in suicide, it is an offence to attempt to assist or encourage suicide.
- The act does not *actually* need to be capable of encouraging or assisting a suicide attempt if the person committing the offence *believes* it to be so (i.e. the wrong advice is given or a harmless medication is prescribed).
- Encouragement or assistance of suicide may include threatening of another person or otherwise putting pressure on another person to commit or attempt suicide. This may include a course of conduct.
- Providers of information society services (such as 'right to die' websites), established in England, Wales or Northern Ireland, are covered by the offence of encouraging or assisting suicide even when they are operating in other European Economic Area states. *There are exemptions* for internet service providers from the offence in limited circumstances, such as where they are acting as mere conduits for information that is capable, and provided with the intention, of encouraging or assisting suicide or are storing it as caches or hosts.

The Director of Public Prosecutions is responsible for instigating public criminal charges. In 2010, he published guidance (see paragraph below) on the prosecution policy relating to charges brought under the Suicide Act 1961 in England and Wales (as amended by the Coroners and Justice Act 2009). There is a potentially heightened risk of prosecution that doctors now face.

Public interest factors (summary) affecting the decision over prosecution with potential relevance for doctors (Director of public prosecutions guidance)

Factors tending in favour of prosecution
- The victim was under 18 years of age.
- The victim did not have the capacity (as defined in the Mental Capacity Act 2005) to reach an informed decision to commit suicide.
- The suspect gave encouragement or assistance to more than one victim, and these victims were not known to each other.
- The suspect was acting in his or her capacity as a medical doctor, nurse, other healthcare professional, a professional carer or as a person in authority, such as a prison officer, and the victim was in his or her care.

Factors tending against prosecution

- The victim had reached a voluntary, clear, settled and informed decision to commit suicide.
- The actions of the suspect, although sufficient to come within the definition of the offence, were of only minor encouragement or assistance.
- The suspect had sought to dissuade the victim from taking the course of action that resulted in his or her suicide.
- The actions of the suspect may be characterized as reluctant encouragement or assistance in the face of a determined wish on the part of the victim to commit suicide.

Assisted suicide and human rights: The case of Dianne Pretty

Probably the most important recent case in the law courts was that of Dianne Pretty. This case went beyond the House of Lords and was heard in the European Court of Human Rights (ECHR). Dianne Pretty was suffering from motor neurone disease and wanted a declaration from the DPP (see above) that her husband would not be prosecuted if he assisted her to die. The court considered her argument in terms of the European Convention on Human Rights (see Ch. 1).

Herring (2010) summarizes the findings of the House of Lords and ECtHR:

- Article 2 (The Right to Life) could not be interpreted to include the right to control the manner of your death.
- Article 3 (The Right Not to Suffer Torture or Inhuman or Degrading Treatment): The ECtHR held that even if a medical condition amounted to torture or inhuman and degrading treatment, it could not be argued that the state was inflicting it. For the state to authorize killing would also bring it into conflict with Article 2.
- Article 8 (The Right to Respect for Private and Family Life): The ECtHR held that even if prohibiting assisted suicide did interfere with this, it was a justifiable interference. The state had a right to protect vulnerable people from being manipulated into committing suicide.
- Article 14 (The Right to Protection from Discrimination): Mrs Pretty argued that if she was able-bodied, she would be able to kill herself and that the law would not be able to prevent that, but now that she needed assistance, the law prohibited it. She claimed that this amounted to discrimination on the grounds of disability. The ECtHR held that if there was discrimination, then this was justified by the need to protect vulnerable people.

Doctrine of double-effect

Much ethical and legal debate around end-of-life decision-making, and whether it is a criminal act to cause or hasten a person's death, revolves around the concept of intention (see above). By doing something, does the doctor intend that the patient will die, or is this merely a foreseeable consequence?

This doctrine of double-effect (DDE) is first notably mentioned in English Law in *R v. Bodkin Adams*. The DDE, in essence, claims that it is sometimes morally permissible to carry out an action that has bad consequences which are foreseen but not intended. In the case of end-of-life treatment, this means that doctors may give strong painkillers to alleviate pain (intended consequence), even though such medication may shorten life (foreseen, but unintended consequence).

The DDE holds if, and only if, four conditions are met (Hope et al 2008):

1. The action (e.g. relieving pain) is good in itself
2. The intention is solely to produce the good effect (i.e. the intent is to relieve pain, not to kill the patient)
3. The good effect is not achieved by the bad effect (i.e. killing the patient isn't the method by which the pain is relieved – it is a side-effect of giving the pain medication)
4. There is sufficient reason to permit the bad effect (i.e. the relief of pain – that is the increase in quality of life – justifies the reduction in quantity of life).

There are a number of criticisms of this doctrine put forward by Glover (1977). The DDE has a *distinction without a difference*. This is a criticism often levied by utilitarians who claim that the DDE creates a distinction between foreseen and unintended consequences in scenarios where the outcomes are without difference. For example, if a pregnant woman with carcinoma of the uterus required the surgical removal of the uterus to save her life, with the foreseen but not intended death of the fetus, the doctrine would find this morally permissible. However, if treatment involved the direct killing of the fetus, this would not be acceptable, even though the consequences (death of the fetus and life-saving treatment of the mother) would be the same.

The DDE also suffers *the problem of clarity*. Acts can be described in different ways according to one's viewpoint. For example, a suicide bombing on a bus may be described as making a political protest or as killing a busload of innocent people. Furthermore, it is unclear as to whether the deaths of the people on the bus are *intended* or merely *foreseen* consequences.

Painkillers and the DDE

In the case of *R v. Bodkin Adams* [1957], Dr Adams was tried for murder after the death of a patient who had made him a beneficiary of her will. He had prescribed heroin and morphine to an 80-year-old woman following a stroke. It was not the first patient who had left him items in their wills. The judge in this case held that:

The defence in the present case was that the treatment given by Dr Adams was designed to promote comfort, and if it was the right and proper treatment, the fact that it shortened life did not convict him of murder.

Huxtable (2007) argues that the legal doctrine is unhelpful in four ways:

1. It is uninformed, in that the incidence of double-effect is overstated and the dangers of appropriate medication are overplayed.
2. 'Double-effect' has unclear legal status: Does it mean there is no intention to kill, there is no killing or there is a justified killing?
3. It is unfair in that it appears to be applied selectively by courts.
4. It is dangerous in that it may overlook killing patients (where painkillers or sedatives are used) or deprive patients of relief from pain or distress through inadequate analgesia or sedation (because staff are afraid of being accused of murder).

DEATH: WHEN DOES 'DEATH' OCCUR

Doctors traditionally diagnose people as dead on the basis that they are pulseless, apnoeic, with fixed pupils and no heart sounds. However, in order to be able to diagnose someone on a ventilator as dead, the concept of brain-death or brainstem death was developed. From a legal point of view in the UK, death is equated with irreversible loss of brainstem function. The UK Medical Royal Colleges put forward criteria for brainstem death in 1976 (Anonymous 1976, 1979). Hypothermia and drug intoxication must be ruled out as differential diagnoses, and the tests must be repeated (criteria include the absence of spontaneous respiration or brainstem reflexes). The doctor making the diagnosis must be a consultant and a second opinion must be sought from another doctor (both must be 5 years post-full GMC registration). The official time of death is the time of completion of the second set of tests. The concept of brain death was accepted as the legal definition of death in the UK in the legal case *Re A* [1992].

In the USA, the term 'brain-death' infers that the neocortex has also been destroyed (the concept of 'whole brain death'). 'The Harvard Criteria', a protocol for defining brain-death, includes four major criteria for 'brain-death':

1. Absence of cerebral responsiveness
2. Absence of induced or spontaneous movement
3. Absence of spontaneous respiration
4. Absence of brainstem and deep tendon reflexes.

No patient meeting The Harvard Criteria has ever recovered.

Brainstem death (the UK version of brain-death) is a compromise between two views:

1. That a person (or 'self') ceases to exist when they irreversibly lose the capacity for consciousness
2. The human *organism* dies *only* when it ceases to function in an integrated way (biological death).

HINTS AND TIPS

Remember: Brainstem death criteria are generally applied to patients who cannot be pronounced dead without switching off a ventilator, NOT to everyone who dies. Confirmation of death is usually done by junior doctors or specially trained nurses in UK hospitals. But think – what makes you decide to pronounce one person dead, and call the cardiac arrest team for someone else?

Is brain-death a sufficient condition for defining death?

McCullagh (1993) summarized the reasons for thinking of the brain as the organ critical to identifying the death of the individual. They are:

- after irreversible cessation of brain function, all other organ systems will inevitably cease to function
- unlike other organ systems, brain function, once lost, is irreplaceable
- irreversible loss of brain function is synonymous with permanent loss of consciousness
- loss of sentience is a feature of loss of brain function
- the integrative function of the brain is lost if the brain ceases to function
- death on the basis of loss of brain function is doing no more than recognizing overtly the reason underlying the traditional diagnosis of death following cessation of the blood circulation. In other words, someone whose heart or lungs fail, dies when the brain dies – in theory, the heart and lungs can be replaced
- if a patient is brain-dead, but their body is maintained on an artificial ventilator, the cardiovascular, gastrointestinal and urinary systems continue to function. The body is warm, consumes oxygen and has a pulse. This is not a 'dead body', even if the patient is categorized as dead. The patient as *a person* is dead, but the body in some very important senses, is alive. A brain-dead, ventilated body is still recognized as a living organism.

ORGAN TRANSPLANTATION

Organ transplantation is considered here in terms of end-of-life issues, consent and other issues concerning the process of transplantation in and of itself. It is also considered as a resource-issue in the Chapter 5.

Notably, the 1998 Department of Health code of practice for diagnosing brain-stem death also deals extensively with the issue of seeking organs for transplantation. The most suitable cadaveric donors are brainstem dead individuals who have died in intensive therapy units (ITU), who are younger than 35 years (40 for women), and who have no history of organic heart disease. In the UK during 1989 and 1990, an audit (Gore et al 1992) found that of 24 000 people dying in intensive care, 3200 had a possible diagnosis of brain-death by conventional definition. However, only 37% of these went on to become organ donors. Some of the reasons given for the loss of potential donors included:

- Brainstem death tests were not carried out in 39% of the cases
- Relatives refused in 27% of the cases
- Relatives were not asked in 6% of the cases.

Willingness to receive

A majority of patients in the UK would accept a transplant if they really needed it; only a small minority would refuse one on cultural, moral or other grounds.

Willingness to give

A number of surveys asked respondents about their willingness to donate *their own* organs and their findings were very consistent, with 7 in 10 people (70%) willing to donate, and only 14% against donating their own organs. This indicates a widespread willingness among the UK population to donate their organs after they die. However:

- only one in five people regularly carried a donor card in the early 1990s (shown consistently throughout the three surveys), and approximately 70% did not have a donor card. The OPCS survey showed that only 27% of people without a card at that present time would think about getting one in the future. This leaves a large section of people who claim to be in favour of organ donation, but are unwilling to act
- The NHS central organ donor register was launched in October 1994, yet 5 years later, less than 14% of the population had registered.

The law and organ transplantation

The legislation governing organs and tissues has been incorporated into the Human Tissue Act 2004:

- The Human Tissue Act 2004 is a framework for regulating the storage and use of human organs and tissue from the living, and the removal, storage and use of tissue and organs from the deceased, for specified health-related purposes and public display. It extends to England, Wales and Northern Ireland.
- The Human Tissue Act 2004 repeals and replaces the Human Tissue Act 1961, the Anatomy Act 1984 and the Human Organ Transplants Act 1989 as they relate to England and Wales, as well as legislation in Northern Ireland.

The Human Tissue Act 2004 – summary

- The Act was produced in the wake of the Alder Hey Inquiry, and as a result, places emphasis on the importance of consent when storing or utilizing tissue samples.
- Cell-lines are excluded from the Act, as are hair and nail from living people. Live gametes and embryos are excluded as they are already regulated under the Human Fertilisation and Embryology Act 1990.)
- The Act provides for the institution of the 'Human Tissue Authority', a regulatory body charged with the responsibility of inspecting and licensing those organizations involved in the storage and use of human tissue.
- The Act specifies criminal punishments for those acting outside the legislation.
- The Act prohibits the sale of any human material, thereby making a transplant organ market illegal.
- The Act permits cold perfusion of cadaveric organs to improve the success of subsequent transplants
- The Act does not affect the rights of coroners to demand a post-mortem and retain tissue without consent if they deem it necessary.
- A new offence of DNA 'theft' applies throughout the UK, as the act makes it illegal to take samples (including gametes and embryos, hair and nail) without consent for the purpose of analysing someone's DNA.

The Human Tissue Act and organ transplants

It is legal to remove organs for transplantation if:

- the deceased gave express consent during their lifetime, provided that: there is no suspicion they may have changed their mind, and the deceased did not have religious views forbidding the removal of organs from the body after death. There is no legal requirement to respect the wishes of the next of kin if they object and the deceased is on the organ donors' register, but this is respected in relevant codes of practice

- the person 'lawfully in possession of the body' may authorize transplantation if there is no recorded declaration by the deceased. This can occur only when 'having made such reasonable enquiry as may be practicable' he/she can be sure neither the deceased nor the 'surviving spouse, or any surviving relative' has any objection.

It should be noted that:

- the person 'lawfully in possession of the body' is usually the Hospital Authority – it is *not* the relatives, until the deceased's legal representative (e.g. relative) has claimed the body
- what 'reasonable enquiry' entails is vague and, technically, '*any*' surviving relative – however remote – can object to transplantation. As can a 'surviving' spouse, even if the couple has been separated for many years. In practice, hospitals usually seek the opinion only of those they consider to be 'close relatives'
- there is no specific penalty for breach of this statute. However, healthcare professionals are most likely to be sanctioned by the GMC for professional misconduct, should they act in a manner inconsistent with professional guidance.

HINTS AND TIPS

Remember: A person has no legal right in common law to determine what happens to their body after death. A body, or part of it, cannot be the subject matter of ownership.

The ethics of organ transplantation

The field of organ transplantation raises a huge number of ethical questions. One way of thinking about the ethical dilemmas raised is by considering the problems caused by:

- cadaveric organ donation
- organ donation from living people
- xenotransplantation
- methods of increasing organ supply
- resource allocation (see Ch. 5).

Cadaveric organ donation

There are ethical questions about the *definition of death*. Should the point of death be brainstem death or death of the entire brain cortex? Should we be allowed to keep brain-dead patients indefinitely ventilated, if there is no need for their organs at the time of their death or to use them as self-replenishing blood banks? Should we choose to intubate dying patients in order to ventilate them when they die – even if it is of no benefit to them? There are also questions about *supply*. Cadaveric donation has often in the past relied on young healthy people who have died as a result of accidents – now fewer accidents as a result of better safety measures (e.g. laws on seatbelts and motorcycle helmets) mean fewer available organs for transplantation.

Organ donation from living people

Organ transplants legislation is strict with regard to unrelated donations – perhaps because it assumes that altruistic donation is less likely between unrelated individuals. However, it seems plausible that family members may be under significant pressure to volunteer to donate an organ to an ailing relative. Children in particular may be pressured into donating to an ailing sibling. This is chiefly problematic, in that it may undermine autonomy and consent, and tissue donation. This and other ethical issues must be considered when thinking about how to increase organ supply.

Methods of increasing organ supply

There are a number of different propositions for increasing organ supply. These include:

Mandated choice
One of the problems with the current system (an 'opt-in' system) is that often no-one knows how the donor would have felt in life about donating organs, so relatives are consulted at a time when they are newly bereaved. The mandated choice would force citizens to answer whether or not they wish to donate their organs after death; this choice would be held on a central register and then held to be binding in the event of their organs being suitable for donation. People could be asked when registering with a GP or via electoral registration.

Presumed consent (an 'opt-out' system)
This system would not require everyone to be asked, rather it would assume that organs will be available for donation after death, unless individuals had registered the choice *not* to donate organs after death. At present, the wishes that the deceased had expressed in life are usually subordinate to those of the relatives. There has traditionally been more concern for the grieving process of the newly bereaved rather than for the need of those on the organ waiting list. Yet, if we weigh the

interest of the relatives (in not having organs removed from their loved one) against that of patients who need organ transplants *in order to remain alive*, we are hard-pressed to justify being in favour of the relatives.

Organ markets

There are a number of ways this might work. Money could be paid to living donors – to donate kidneys for example. Or certain rewards could be given to the families who agree to the donation of organs from their relatives, e.g. help with funeral expenses. Utilitarian arguments would support an organ market if it led to more lives being saved at a reduced cost; such a system might well benefit donors (or their families) and those in need of treatment. However, arguments against this method include:

- It is contrary to human dignity to commodify the human body by allowing the sale of organs
- It would lead to exploitation of the poor by coercing the least well-off to sell their body parts. This is currently illegal in the UK.

Xenotransplantation

This is the transplantation of organs from animals to humans. Disadvantages of xenotransplantation may include:

- The cost of producing sterile transgenic animals (probably pigs) – which will have to be researched, tested and pass stringent safety requirements.

Research questions will include:

- Whether it is appropriate to spend limited resources researching this technology when there are other methods to increase organ supply – such as an 'opt-out' system
- Whether the risk of introducing animal pathogens into the human population is justified
- The ethics of treating animals as disposable commodities in this manner – raising animals simply as a source of spare organs. However, the widespread acceptance of factory farming and other livestock practices demonstrates a readiness to treat animals as commodities (although this is not necessarily an ethically justifiable position).

Key questions

- Outline five views on the moral worth of the human embryo.
- What are the ethical and legal issues in contraception and sterilization?
- Outline the pro-life vs pro-choice abortion debate.
- Outline the legislation which regulates reproductive technologies

---

- What are the flaws in the '*it is unnatural*' argument in cloning and other reproductive technologies?
- What is the difference between voluntary, non-voluntary and involuntary euthanasia?
- Explain the *doctrine of double-effect*?
- What is the key legal guidance for doctors on the issue of assisting suicide?
- What is the difference between an act and an omission in health care?
- When is the DNAR acceptable?
- What is the relevance in ethics and law of having a definition of death?
- What are the key ethical issues in human organ transplantation?

References

Airedale NHS Trust v. Bland, 1993 AC 789.

Anonymous, 1976. Diagnosis of brain death. Statement issued by the honorary secretary of the conference of Medical Royal Colleges and their Faculties in the United Kingdom on 11 October 1976. Br. Med. Bull 2 (6045), 1187–1188.

Anonymous, 1979. Diagnosis of brain death. Memorandum issued by the honorary secretary of the conference of Medical Royal Colleges and their Faculties in the United Kingdom on 15 January 1979. Br. Med. Bull. 1 (6159), 332.

Coroners and Justice Act, 2009. Explanatory Notes: Section 59. Online. Available at: http://www.legislation.gov.uk/ukpga/2009/25/notes/division/5/1/2/1/8 (accessed 15.04.12.).

Department of Health, 1998. A Code of Practice for the Diagnosis of Brain Stem Death. HMSO, London.

Gillon, R., 2001. Is there a 'new ethics of abortion'? J. Med. Ethics 27, 5–9.

Glover, J., 1977. Causing Death and Saving Lives. Pelican Books, Harmondsworth (Chapter 6).

Gore, S.M., Cable, D.J., Holland, A.J., 1992. Organ donation from intensive care units in England and Wales: two year confidential audit of deaths in intensive care. Br. Med. J. 304 (6823), 349–355.

Harris, J., 1994. The Value of Life. Routledge, London.

Herring, J., 2010. Death and dying. In: Law Express: Medical Law, second ed. Pearson Education, Harlow, pp. 96–107.

Hope, T., Savulescu, J., Kendrick, J., 2008. Medical Ethics and Law: The Core Curriculum, second ed. Elsevier, London.

Human Tissue Act, 2004. Explanatory notes. The National Archives. Online. Available at: http://www.legislation.gov.uk/ukpga/2004/30/notes/contents (accessed 02.01.12.).

Huxtable, R., 2007. Euthanasia, Ethics and the Law: From Conflict to Compromise. Routledge-Cavendish, London.

Jonsen, A., Siegler, M., Winslade, W., 2010. Clinical Ethics, seventh ed. McGraw-Hill, New York.

Kennedy, I., Grubb, A., 2000. Actions for damages by children and parents arising from occurrences before birth. Medical Law, third ed. Butterworths, London.

MacLennan v. MacLennan 1958 SC 10.

McCullagh, P., 1993. Brain Dead, Brain Absent. Brain Donors. John Wiley & Sons Ltd, Chichester.

Re A, 1992 3 Med LR 303.

Re B (Adult: Refusal of Medical Treatment), 2002 2 FCR 1.

R (Burke) v GMC and Others, 2005. EWCA Civ 1003.

R v. Bodkin Adams, 1957 Crim LR 365.

R v. Carr (1986), Sunday Times, 30th November

R v. Cox, 1992 12 BMLR 38.

Re F (in utero), 1988 2 All ER 193; 2 WLR 1288.

R v. Human Fertilisation & Embryology Authority, ex parte Blood, 1997 2 All ER 687.

R (Smeaton on behalf of SPUC) v. The Secretary of State et al., 2002 2 FCR 193.

Sokol, D.K., 2009a. The death of DNR: can a change of terminology improve end of life care? BMJ 338, 1043.

Sokol, D.K., 2009b. The slipperiness of futility. BMJ 338, 1418.

Further reading

Harris, J. (Ed.), 2001. Bioethics. Oxford University Press, Oxford.

Harris, J., Holm, S. (Eds.), 1998. The Future of Human Reproduction. Oxford University Press, Oxford.

McHale, J., Fox, M., Murphy, J., 1997. Health Care Law: Texts and Materials. Sweet & Maxwell, London.

Healthcare commissioning and resource allocation ⑤

This chapter takes a broader look at the rights and wrongs of the provision of health care in society. To a certain degree, all healthcare professionals will have to make healthcare allocation decisions in the context of finite available resources. The first decade of the twenty-first century has seen a global financial recession, with cuts to many public services, including health care. While this book cannot predict what will happen over the next 10 years, it is worth considering the ethics of commissioning and resource allocation in health care.

This chapter examines the difference between commissioning and rationing, and examines relevant ethical concerns with the commissioning process. The chapter then looks at the ethics of resource allocation and concludes with a suggestion of how these kinds of decisions might be challenged (and defended) in court.

COMMISSIONING AND RESOURCE ALLOCATION

Commissioning is more than just a resource allocation process: it involves four stages:

1. Identify the need (referred to as needs assessment)
2. Identify capacity to meet the need (referred to as tendering)
3. Delivery of service from that capacity (referred to as procurement)
4. Evaluation of the service (referred to as contract management). Evaluation should be linked to ways of improving or replacing a service which is inadequate.

By contrast, resource allocation is concerned with catering to established need as much as possible, using existing resources. 'Rationing' is a word which implies that there are not enough resources to meet everybody's wants or needs, and, therefore, however well resources are allocated, someone will be dissatisfied. Consider for example the idea that resources are best allocated according to local priorities. If local priorities mean that, e.g. people in Oxford do not get a service that is provided in London, a dissatisfied person in Oxford might use a phrase like 'postcode lottery' to describe the unfairness of being denied something because of where he lives.

What is need?

A need is what is necessary for a person to exist (e.g. air, food, shelter) or to flourish (health). As well as biological needs, there are culturally specific needs such as education. Needs are often contrasted with desires. Many religions and world views endorse the idea that people with excess have a duty to help the needy. The concept of need is linked to the concept of justice and rights (see below). For example access to health care has been argued to be a human right. Consider how we decide what is a need and what is a desire. If there is a need, then who should address that need? For example the need for health care in the UK is addressed by the State and funded by means of taxation. This can then raise the question of what is a healthcare need? Is, for example, the ability to found a family a healthcare need on the grounds that infertility treatments are delivered by healthcare professionals? Who should address this need and to what degree? These are questions debated when deciding the proportion of NHS resources allocated to infertility treatments.

What should count as health care?

There are a number of things which contribute to public health which are not in the remit of healthcare providers, and therefore are not paid for out of money allocated for health care. These might include:

- Enforcement of legislation to reduce air pollution in cities
- Traffic calming measures such as speed bumps to reduce road traffic accidents
- Long-term care to assist the elderly and chronically infirm with activities of daily living
- Health education in schools, advocating healthier lifestyles and the avoidance of risky behaviour.

However, there are a few areas that are open to dispute, either because they are provided in the healthcare setting but not necessarily seen as part of health care (e.g. chaplaincy services in hospitals) or where the theoretical basis for the treatment or evidence of effectiveness is questioned (e.g. homeopathy or crystal healing).

The two levels of resource allocation

1. *Micro-allocation*: decisions about treatment between patients. Doctors tend to be concerned with decisions of micro-allocation, i.e. deciding which patients get which treatments.
2. *Macro-allocation*: decisions over the share of a society's total resources that are devoted to health, and the division of the healthcare budget between possible uses. Health authorities and the government make decisions regarding macro-allocation.

Decisions about commissioning and rationing must be ethically 'sound'. According to Gillon (1994) we should:

- exclude decisions with no justification – would our reasoning stand up to public scrutiny?
- resources must not be wasted – e.g. do not give treatments we know do not work
- respect patients' rights (e.g. to receive what they are entitled to) and respect their choices as far as possible
- obey morally acceptable laws. Gillon suggests that the best way to change morally unacceptable laws is via the democratic process, e.g. lobby the government to change the law or vote for a government that will change the law.

Consider the overlap between ethics and law: if a decision followed the above points well, it might be harder to challenge that decision in court.

Are there any particular ethical concerns regarding commissioning?

Conflicts of interest

Providers of services should not direct the commissioning process. This is because they may prioritize their own service or their own patients over those of others without valid justification. Sheehan (2011) and others argue that doctors should act as patient-advocates rather than prioritize resources at a financial level, as this might compromise the doctors' desire to obtain the best care for each and every patient.

Transparency

If resource allocation in the UK previously depended on implicit choices between which patients and which diseases to prioritize, choices made by committees behind closed doors, then it was surely associated with a high degree of trust in the people who made the decisions (often but not always doctors). While trust in UK GPs remains high, at a personal level, dilemmas of funding are increasing as individual patients are denied healthcare interventions on the basis of cost-effectiveness or finite resources. Spicer (2010) suggests that trust may not survive an environment of financial constraint if GPs motives are unclear. Patient involvement in decision-making may assist in this spirit of openness. Part of the problem is that the patient depends on the provider for information about which service or treatment is needed. The provider (who is trained in medicine) has a potential influence over the choices made by the patient (who usually is not).

Patient involvement in decision-making

The closer commissioning and resource allocation is to the end-user, the better, surely? But should people be allowed to make selfish decisions, whether the commissioning agenda is dominated by one powerful lobby group, or more local decisions determined by the loudest and most articulate people rather than the neediest? Sheehan (2011) argues that choice and empowerment are irrelevant in decisions about scarce resources. He uses the following scenario:

> A baker has one loaf and three customers. Each customer has autonomously chosen to purchase a loaf of bread before they enter the bakery. In selling the loaf to any one of his customers, the baker would respect that customer's autonomy. His problem is precisely that he cannot respect all of their autonomous choices. He must decide which customer gets the loaf and so which person's autonomy he should respect. He might sell the loaf to the first person into the shop, adopting a first come, first served principle of justice. He might divide the loaf into three so that everyone gets an equal but unsatisfying share. One might argue that he should sell the loaf to the hungriest customer!

There are many more ways of approaching distributive justice here, each of which decides between autonomous choosers rather than respecting their choices. Resource allocation decisions in the NHS are necessarily decisions between patients and so do not involve considerations of respect for patient choice. Instead, justice is a relevant consideration in deciding how to distribute resources fairly (Fig. 5.1).

The role of the private sector

The key concern with the involvement of commercial companies in a health service provided by the state for patients, is a conflict of duties and interests. The primary legal duty of company directors in the UK is to act, 'for the benefit of the members [of the company] as a whole' (Companies Act 2006 *s.172*) and non-financial considerations are made subsidiary to this within (*s.172*). The only benefit from a company for shareholders is financial; profits paid out as dividends.

Fig. 5.1 An example of public participation.

In 1989, the State of Oregon (USA) passed the Basic Medical Service Act. The Act required all those in employment to be covered for health insurance by their employers, and extended state health insurance provision cover for the poor unemployed from 42% to 100% of healthcare costs.

The price of this universal coverage was an explicit, democratically led, system of healthcare rationing. Around 700 medical conditions were paired with treatments, and a state Health Services Commission decided on priority setting between them. In doing so, they used a measure of cost utility analysis, but also input from community meetings and 'Citizen's juries' to aid their deliberations.

The State of Oregon embraced at least two ethical approaches to distributive justice: *cost-utility* and *public participation*, in a way that had not been done before. This was done in an open and transparent manner, in that the way decisions were made was open to scrutiny.

Safeguarding local NHS services

The BMA's 'Look after our NHS' (2011) campaign argues (adapted from www.lookafterournhs.org.uk) that:

- private providers favour more routine treatments, like hip replacements and cataract operations, leaving the NHS to deal with more complex, costly treatments, and have often been guaranteed payments, even if they have not treated enough patients
- private companies pay dividends to their shareholders, taking money away from patient care or investment in training or research
- as NHS hospitals lose routine procedures to commercially run clinics, students and junior doctors get fewer opportunities for practical training.
- having more providers of care than is actually needed is wasteful and an expense the country cannot afford. Some NHS Trusts may have to advertise to attract patients, money which should and could be spent on patient care
- patients are now able to choose where to have any elective treatment. Included in this choice will be commercially run clinics or private hospitals which are contracted to provide NHS work. If a patient chooses to have that treatment in one of these private hospitals or clinics, the funding for that treatment is taken out of the NHS. A possible consequence may be that some NHS services do not have enough funding to continue

- the private sector is also involved in the building and running of NHS hospitals in England under a scheme called Private Finance Initiative. They build the hospitals which the NHS then pays for over a period of 25–30 years. But these costly contracts have left many hospitals with crippling debts.

WHY IS RESOURCE ALLOCATION NECESSARY?

The usual answer to this question is that resources (money, doctors' and other health professionals' time, equipment and so on) are not infinite. When demand exceeds the available resources, there comes a need to decide who receives treatment and who does not.

While resources are not infinite, a budget can be traded off other budgets – priorities can be reassessed – so if this year, the budget for the NHS is £130 billion, it could be increased next year if people are happy to pay higher rates of tax. Demand for a service is not inevitably infinite – rather, 'the amount demanded of a free service is determined at the point where customers see no additional benefits to be gained from additional recourse to the service in question'. This could be at quite modest levels (Harris 2001).

Having said this, it is generally accepted that some decisions have to be made with regard to the allocation of resources. If this is the case, what are the grounds (Fig. 5.2) upon which rationing decisions could be made?

Fig. 5.2 Some theories of Justice.

Hippocratic duty – prioritizing the common good over the individual is morally wrong! The hippocratic doctor makes the care of his patient his first concern
Aristotle: treat equals equally and unequals unequally according to morally relevant inequality
Utilitarianism: act to maximize welfare for the greatest number (at the least cost)
Libertarianism: (the right not to be killed and to possess property) – in simplistic versions, each for him/herself
Marxism: (not communism) – take from each according to ability and give to each according to need
Rawls theory of justice: A rational person who makes a decision behind a veil of ignorance (without knowing who will benefit) will look after the least well-off

The following are some suggestions regarding the grounds upon which we could choose between claimants upon resources (these grounds are more specific to health care rather than the bakery example used above):

- Increase in *quantity* of life as a result of treatment
- Increase in *quality* of life as a result of treatment
- *Prognosis* – treat those with the best *chance* of a successful outcome
- Past *contribution* or future (expected) *contribution* to society – who has paid the most taxes? Or will do in the future? Should criminals receive poorer health care?
- *Personal responsibility* – should smokers and alcoholics have equal access to health care to people without such harmful habits? What about skiers and people injured while, e.g. quad biking? What about risky professions, such as firemen?
- *Moral character* and fault – de-prioritize treatment for those seen to be at fault or make them pay more, e.g. would you charge a person for attendance at an emergency department for a minor complaint (e.g. nausea or cuts and bruises) related to alcohol overuse?
- *Triage* – will immediate treatment help? Can wait but needs treatment? No point treating?

A number of alternative theoretical foundations for deciding how to allocate scarce resources will be explored below.

Utilitarianism and quality-adjusted life years

The quality-adjusted life years (QALY) theory is an approach to cost-effectiveness and is a *utilitarian* theory (see also Ch. 1), in that it attempts to assign numerical values to types of health care so that the interventions producing the *cost-effectiveness and therefore the greatest good to the greatest number* may be identified. It attempts to bring two considerations into a single framework when assessing the cost-effectiveness of healthcare interventions:

1. Quality of life

and

2. Quantity of life.

These two criteria are used because both are thought to be central to the purpose of health care. Medicine is not seen simply as a method of saving lives (increasing *life years*); part of its role is to alleviate suffering, that is improve *quality*. QALYs combine both criteria in a single measurement.

This theory was developed by Williams, who wrote:

The essence of a QALY is that it takes a year of healthy life expectancy to be worth 1, but regards a year of unhealthy life expectancy as worth less than 1. Its precise value is lower the worse the quality of life of the unhealthy person (which is what the 'quality-adjusted' bit is all about).

(Williams 1985)

This theory allows healthcare interventions to be scored according to how many QALYs they result in. When this is considered along with the cost of an intervention, health interventions can be considered in terms of *cost per QALY*. This allows cost-effective analysis to take place. Without such a system, it can be hard to compare widely divergent medical treatments.

QALYs allow two sorts of decisions to be made when choosing health care. These are:

1. to determine which therapy is given to an individual patient: this is effectively a decision made according to the rules of evidence-based medicine
2. to determine which patients receive treatment at all: a cost-effective analysis.

Like utilitarianism, QALYs are popular because they tap into two main moral intuitions. First, that we *ought* to promote *well-being* as measured – the 'quality' part, and, second, that we *ought* to *maximize* the amount of well-being – the 'quantity' part. They are also useful to health economists, who can assign a financial cost per QALY.

Objections to quality-adjusted life years

Two of the major problems with QALYs are:

1. QALYs are arguably *unjust*. They favour younger, healthier people.
2. QALYs are arguably *difficult to calculate practically*. The quality part can be derived from conducting surveys of a large number of people to determine what is beneficial, and this can vary depending on who you speak to.

The argument from justice claims that QALYs are systematically biased against certain sections of the population and that this means they are an unfair basis upon which to allocate resources. Those groups which are not favoured by the QALY system include the disabled, the chronically ill and the elderly. This bias is illustrated by considering the following scenario.

Imagine Tom, Dick and Harry are in a car crash. Tom is 20 years old, with no previous disabilities. Dick is also 20 years old and is blind. Harry is 40 and was previously well. The car crash results in all three sustaining similar injuries. They all arrive at the Accident and Emergency (A&E) department at the same time, but the hospital has enough resources for only one patient to be treated.

Assuming that all three patients could be returned to the same level of health they had before the accident, the

QALY system would oblige the hospital to treat Tom over the other two. The reasons for this are that Tom will live longer than Harry (assuming both have an average life-span), therefore, even though both can be returned to perfect health, treating Tom will lead to a greater number of QALYs being accrued. (Assuming the average life expectancy to be 75, treating Tom will lead to 55 QALYs vs 35 QALYs for Harry.) While many people think that we should treat children in preference to the very old, it becomes less clear whether we should treat 20-year-olds instead of 40-year-olds, or indeed 30-year-olds instead of 35-year-olds.

Tom will also be treated in preference to Dick, although both have the same life expectancy. Because Dick already has a disability, treating him will not restore him to *perfect* health. Each year of life after treatment will be worth less than 1 on the QALY scale – so his total expected QALY score will be less than 55. John Harris (1995) has called this problem 'double jeopardy'; not only does Dick have the misfortune to be blind, but this disability can also, under the QALY system, adversely affect the priority assigned to him in receiving treatment for an unrelated injury.

The problem *of calculating* QALYs is a more practical difficulty. For example, how can we compare the quality of life of being blind as against that of being paralysed? The answer tends to depend both on how the question is asked and which groups of individuals answer the question. Disabled groups tend to rate the quality of life of disabled people much higher than do non-disabled groups.

Rawls' theory of justice

John Rawls (1972) utilizes a hypothetical device he calls the *'veil of ignorance'* – this is part of an explanatory model to explain an ideal social contract – for Rawls this is the type of contract it would be rational to choose if we had been given the chance. Unlike the QALY theory, the supreme goal in Rawls' theory of justice is not maximization of welfare as such, but treating those who have the greatest need for treatment. This theory emphasizes fairness rather than absolute welfare.

Rawls supposes:

- humans are rational
- humans are self-interested.

Thus, in order to further fairness (justice), steps must be taken to avoid selfish interest in the original position (from which the social contract is made) as follows:

1. If people are self-interested, they will seek advantages at the expense of others whenever they can

but

2. If people did not know how to advantage themselves, they would not 'rationally' try to advantage themselves

hence

3. The veil of ignorance disguises salient information that they could use to advantage themselves

therefore

4. If we can suppose what the social contract would have been, had it been designed from behind a veil of ignorance, it would be fair

and

5. If we could be sure of this, it would also be fair to hold people to this in the real world.

Working under this model, Rawls produced two important principles:

- People would choose to have an equal right to the most extensive basic liberties compatible with everyone having those liberties: that is, there would be MAXIMUM FREEDOM.
- As people don't know where they will be in society, they will accept the prudence of making the situation of those on the lowest rung as good as possible (MAXImum welfare for the MINimally well off). Because people are rationally self-interested, they will adopt a MAXIMIN POLICY (i.e. a worst-case scenario).

A theory of resource allocation in the healthcare setting

Len Doyal (adapted from Berney et al 2005) argues that the following principles should apply to healthcare resource allocation:

- Healthcare needs should be met in proportion to prevalence of the needs
- Within treatment areas, resources should be prioritized according to extremity of need
- Those in similar need should have an equal chance to access health care
- Scarce resources should not be provided for ineffective health care
- Lifestyle should not determine access to health care
- The public should advise but not determine policy
- Healthcare rationing should be explicit.

Exceptions

If rules have to be set up to guard NHS resources by not providing or restricting particular services to particular cases, patients or their advocates (and that may be you) need to argue why the rule is unreasonable or the case is exceptional. In the UK, funding panels (sometimes called 'low priorities panels') often decide whether a case should receive NHS funding.

While it is unlikely that medical students could be tested on this in a multiple-matching question, this can be discussed in class, or tested in a short answer or essay in the following way:

Exercise

You are on a funding panel and have been asked to consider the following cases:

- A 34-year-old woman has developed an apron of skin after successful weight reduction treatment. She says that she is depressed by the effect of this on her body image and she has undergone counselling. She states that it is also affecting her marriage.
- A 14-year-old girl wants leg-lengthening surgery. She would like the chance to be an air-hostess when she is older and her short stature is likely to prevent this being a possibility.
- A 48-year-old married father of three children wants to be given a new chemotherapy drug for lung cancer. Local oncologists think this may improve his 5-year survival chances by 10%.
- The mother of a 2-year-old boy with eczema which is affecting his development and is unresponsive to standard treatments, would like to take him to a homeopathic hospital.

You have the funds for one of the above treatments. Why would you fund any of the above cases' treatment and what would be your reasons for not funding the others? Remember that your decisions should be consistent and fair. This is helped by having a process (such as using the four principles of bioethics to look at each case), and having consistent policies (such as only funding treatment for which there is an evidence base unless you have a good reason to make an exception). Remember that you need to have rules in order to make exceptions!

Organ transplantation and resource allocation

The ethics of transplantation has been discussed in Chapter 4 from the point of brain-death, end-of-life decision-making, consent and the law. Here, organ transplantation is discussed in terms of resource allocation. Transplants are often seen as expensive, heroic experiments, rather than life-saving or life-improving procedures; it is perceived that they drain resources from routine and more cost-effective treatments. One argument against allocation of resources to transplant surgery would be that many of the diseases which lead to the need for transplants are modifiable by lifestyle and early intervention.

However:

- kidney transplants were quoted as costing £4710, whereas hospital/home haemodialysis costs an *extra* £21 970/£17 260 (respectively).
- a heart transplant costing £7840 may be the only recourse to save a patient's life, whereas to remove a malignant tumour from the brain (which is a regularly performed life-saving intervention) would cost £107 780.

Although these figures (prior to 2004) are relatively crude, they show that transplantation compared well with other interventions that NHS resources already covered. If you consider the earlier argument about fairness and consistency, this makes it harder to argue that kidney transplants should not be provided based on cost-efficiency alone. If you argue against organ transplantation based purely on economic cost efficiency, then, by the same argument, heart transplants and brain tumour surgery should be abandoned as well.

Transplant organs are a good example of a resource which has to be rationed, as there are many more people who claim a need to them than can have them. At the end of March 2011, 7800 patients were on the waiting lists in the UK (with a further 2783 temporarily suspended because they were unfit or otherwise unavailable for a transplant). Several thousand more who could benefit were not on the waiting list. This is because only those who are considered to have a 'reasonable chance' of receiving a transplant are put on the list. The figure of about 1000 people dying per year (or three deaths per day) due to the shortage of donor organs is usually quoted (BMA Medical Ethics Committee 2012).

HINTS AND TIPS

Organs for transplantation are a good example of a resource which has to be rationed, as there are many more people who can claim a need for them than can have them. While it is worth thinking about ways to decrease the demand on organs, and/or to increase the supply of organs, it is essential to have a fair and consistent way to decide who receives an organ for transplantation (i.e. to ration them) while the need exceeds the supply.

Given that there is a shortage of organs, who should get priority in receiving a transplant? Currently, children receive organs in preference to adults, on the basis that they will derive greater benefit. So a 16-year-old will receive a new kidney in preference to a 19-year-old. However, a 19-year-old will not be treated in preference to a 59-year-old. Both are adults and therefore have an equal right on the basis of age to an organ transplant, as the age of 60 has been the arbitrary age at which someone is deemed too old to receive a transplant on the NHS. This seems inconsistent, as the 59-year-old has less life to gain and greater chances of surgical complications. However, the 59-year-old might argue that he has an equal right to life, and should not be discriminated against solely on the basis of age, and the 60-year-old may argue that he is healthier than many 59-year-olds, with just as much life expectancy.

Challenging resource-allocation decisions in the courts

If a decision about resource allocation in healthcare were to be challenged in court, two key questions would be asked about that decision:

- Was the procedure for making the decision reasonable? (This might suggest the decision-making *process* is consistent and fair)
- Were the *grounds* for making the decision reasonable and relevant?

According to Hope et al (2008) there are some key ways that the courts might be involved.

Judicial review

For example a patient might claim that in not funding a particular service, the NHS failed in its statutory duty. If the claim succeeds, the court would strike down the decision not to fund and ask the decision-maker to re-think the decision using relevant criteria and with due process. Judicial review may also be used to question legislation as well as policy (see Ch. 1).

Negligence

This would involve a private claim to the effect that the decision-making process had been negligent in some way, in that it fell below the standard of a reasonable and responsible body. While there would not necessarily be an obligation to reverse the decision, a successful claim would necessitate compensation for the claimant's loss.

The Human Rights Act 1998 brings the articles of the European Convention on Human Rights into British law and could also conceivably be invoked in challenging resource allocation decisions:

- Article 2 (right to life) could be used to challenge refusal of life-saving treatments
- Article 3 (protections from inhuman or degrading treatment) could be used to challenge refusal of treatment to alleviate conditions which cause pain and suffering
- Article 8 (right to respect private and family life) could be used to challenge refusal of treatments like assisted conception, or resources which allow privacy (such as those which protect patient confidentiality or unreasonably restrict a patient's ability to follow their religious beliefs, see below)
- Article 9 (right to freedom of thought, conscience and religion) might be used to challenge refusal of treatments that unreasonably restrict a patient's ability to follow their religious beliefs (e.g. funding for chaplains, prayer spaces in hospital)

- Article 14 (protection from discrimination) could be used to challenge any decisions which appear based on discrimination such as on the basis of age, gender, lifestyle or sexuality.

Increasingly, doctors need to be able to justify any controversial decision, often to patients and their representatives, and possibly even to a court (see Ch. 1). As with clinical decisions, resource allocation needs to be consistent and fair (process). They also need to be reasonable (grounds) – you must be able to justify your decision, whether it is to give someone a cheaper medication or to make regional resource decisions.

Key questions

- What is need and how is this linked to rights and justice?
- What does commissioning involve how does this differ from rationing?
- What ethical issues can arise when commissioning healthcare services?
- What are the advantages and disadvantages to patient involvement in healthcare commissioning?
- Outline some theories of justice.
- What are the advantages and disadvantages of QALYs?
- What interventions can you think of which the state provides in order to improve health but which are not provided by the health service?
- Would you choose to fund more services for the medical management of diabetes or put more money into the national transplant service? Outline reasons for and against.
- What are the ways in which commissioning and rationing decisions might be challenged in the courts?

References

Berney, L., Kelly, M., Doyal, L., et al., 2005. Ethical principles and the rationing of health care: a qualitative study in general practice. Br. J. Gen. Pract. 55 (517), 620–625.

BMA, 2011. Look after our NHS. Online. Available at: www.lookafterournhs.org.uk (accessed 25.07.11.).

BMA, Medical Ethics Committee, 2012. Building on Progress: Where Next for Organ Donation Policy in the UK? British Medical Association, London.

Gillon, R., 1994. Four principles plus attention to scope. BMJ 309 (6948), 184–188.

Harris, J., 1995. Double jeopardy and the veil of ignorance – a reply. J. Med. Ethics 21, 151–157.

Harris, J., 2001. Micro-allocation: deciding between patients. In: Singer, P.A. (Ed.), Companion to Bioethics. Blackwell, Oxford.

Hope, T., Savulescu, J., Hendrick, J., 2008. Resource allocation. In: Medical Ethics and Law: The Core Curriculum. Churchill Livingstone Elsevier, Edinburgh pp. 202–216.

Rawls, J., 1972. A Theory of Justice. Oxford University Press, Oxford.

Sheehan, M., 2011. Personal view: it's unethical for general practitioners to be commissioners. BMJ 342, d1430.

Spicer, J., 2010. Oregon and the UK: experiments in resource allocation. London Journal of Primary Care 2, 105–108.

Williams, A., 1985. The value of QALYs. Health Soc. Serv. J. (Centre 8 Supplement), 3–5.

Introduction to sociology and disease

The second half of this book deals with another area which students are sometimes tempted to give less priority to but is nonetheless an important part of the undergraduate curriculum. Chapters 6–8 deal with some key areas in *sociology*, as applied to medicine. Chapters 10 and 11 introduce two areas which overlap with sociology in undergraduate teaching: *public health and clinical governance*.

WHY IS SOCIOLOGY IMPORTANT TO MEDICAL STUDENTS?

We are born into a society. Society provides: language and values; influences our knowledge; and influences our thoughts and behaviour. Sociology is accordingly the scientific study of society. Its wide scope contributes to the study of medicine as, arguably, the role of healthcare professionals is to provide holistic care – that is caring for the *whole person*; therefore, medical students ought to be learning how to accomplish this. Armstrong (2003a) outlines three key aspects of sociology:

1. Sociology *in* medicine: Sociology takes a look at the ways in which social factors impinge on individuals and groups to influence their health and behaviours. For example: How do people decide that they are ill or whether to consult a doctor?
2. Sociology *of* medicine: Sociology can explore how the concepts of health, disease and medicine are themselves socially established. For example different societies have different concepts of health and illness.
3. Sociology can look at the ways in which health care is provided and evaluated. This may overlap with epidemiology, social policy and economics, among other disciplines.

Sociology research can involve both *quantitative* (e.g. surveys) and *qualitative* (e.g. interviews and focus groups) data. Qualitative data tend to involve closer analysis of smaller sample sizes, and thus rely on different measures of validity to quantitative studies.

HINTS AND TIPS

Being an effective doctor means being able understand the different social processes that lead patients to

present in a particular place and time and in a particular way. Knowing that particular social groups' lifestyles predispose them to particular illnesses is one of many ways in which an understanding of society can assist medical practice. At a more strategic level, an understanding of how social groups might behave can assist in the planning and delivery of effective healthcare services.

SOCIAL CAUSES OF DISEASE

Western medicine has been based upon what is known as the *biomedical model*. This makes the following assumptions:

1. The mind and body can be treated separately – *mind–body dualism*
2. The body can be treated as a machine – *the mechanical metaphor*
3. Technological interventions are generally successful in the treatment of disease – *the technological imperative*
4. Explanations of disease focus on biological changes rather than social and psychological factors – that is, they are *reductionist* in nature
5. In the nineteenth and early twentieth centuries, educationist explanations led to the *doctrine of specific aetiology* – where it was assumed that every disease is caused by a specific identifiable agent or 'disease entity' (the biomedical view has since become considerably more nuanced).

The success of the biomedical model has been, in part, attributed to its claim that it is an *objective* science – with a gradual increase in the truth of explanations provided. Medicine has, thus, claimed to be the only valid response to the understanding of disease and illness. *Sociology* has sought causes of disease beyond the reductionistic – or simply biological – level (Fig. 6.1).

What is a 'cause' of disease?

A cause is generally understood to be the one thing that brings about a change in another. For example we can

Fig. 6.1 Challenges to the biomedical model.

The efficacy of the biomedical model has been exaggerated
The reduction in disease in the Western world has more to do with improved social conditions, i.e. sanitation, housing, availability of fresh food, etc., than with medical advances such as vaccinations and antibiotics
The causes of disease are multifactorial
Focussing on the biological changes has underestimated the links between material circumstances and illness. An under-appreciation of the social factors may have led to a failure to account for the inequalities of health
Biomedicine has failed to account for sociocultural interpretations of disease that influence an individual's perception and experience of health and illness
Sociologists have suggested that some disease is socially constructed, and, therefore, by attempting to examine only the biological dysfunction, biomedical models miss much of the cause and, therefore, potential cure. Even apparently biologically based disease may be directly brought about by social factors

Source: *adapted from Nettleton 2003.*

say atheroma causes ischaemic heart disease. This is a *monocausal* model. It can be written as:

A → B : where A is the cause and B is the effect.

Of course, the causality of ischaemic heart disease is more complicated than atheroma – because this simple model begs the questions: 'What causes atheroma?' and 'How does atheroma cause ischaemic heart disease?' Atheroma can be increased or decreased by promoting or inhibiting factors. A *multicausal* model is more appropriate. Factors such as genetic predisposition, poverty, poor diet, smoking, diabetes and oral contraceptives may be promoting factors, whereas physical activity, access to medical health care and polyunsaturated fats may be inhibitors. The possible multicausal model is illustrated in Figure 6.2.

In order to establish a cause, there are three conditions that need to be fulfilled:

1. Temporal sequence: the cause must precede the effect – if it does not, the relationship cannot be causal
2. Association between cause and effect: the effect should vary with the cause – so increased atheroma should lead to increased incidence of ischaemic heart disease
3. There should be no confounding variable: e.g. cases of gout might increase with the number of cars

owned per family. The third variable here might be increased affluence, which may lead to a richer diet which may be a factor in symptomatic gout (Fig. 6.3).

Theories of disease causation

The following is adapted from Locker (2008, p. 20).

Germ theory

- Germ theory was established during the late 1800s, when scientists such as Ehrlich, Koch and Pasteur isolated various disease-causing organisms.
- Koch (who isolated the bacillus that causes TB) established the idea that a disease agent must always be found with the disease in question, rather than be found with other diseases.

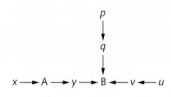

Fig. 6.2 A multicausal model for disease.

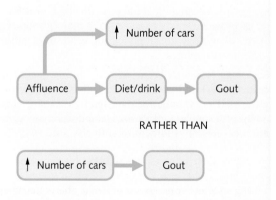

Fig. 6.3 Confounding variables.

- The purpose of medical practice was to identify these agents, then neutralize them.
- This is a 'monocausal' model.

Epidemiological triangle

- This refined the 'germ theory'.
- Disease is seen as an interaction between three entities:
  - The host
  - The disease agent
  - The environment.
- Exposure to the disease agent is necessary for the disease to manifest – but not sufficient.
- The disease can be prevented by modifying factors that influence exposure and susceptibility. This is a 'multicausal' model.
- More useful in understanding causation of infectious diseases than chronic, degenerative ones.

Web of causation

- Disease results from the complex interaction of many risk factors.
- Any risk factor can be implicated in more than one disease.
- Disease can be prevented by modifying these risk factors.

General susceptibility

- This theory has grown out of the observation that certain groups (e.g. the lower social classes or people who have been divorced) are more susceptible to a number of diseases (see Ch. 7).
- It is not concerned with the individual risk factors – rather the general susceptibility to disease and death.
- General susceptibility is probably a result of the complex interaction of environment, lifestyle, behaviour and genetic predisposition.

Socioenvironmental approach

- This refinement of the 'general susceptibility' theory recognizes social and physical environments have a heavy effect on health and disease.
- Identifies socioenvironmental risks, physiological risks, behavioural risk and psychosocial risks
- The interaction between the above types of risks affects health status.
- Suggests the importance of protective/vulnerability factors that help to explain why some people are less/more at risk than others.

SOCIAL STRUCTURES AND HEALTH

Social integration, support and life events

The sociologist *Emile Durkheim* argued that industrialization had led to a loss of social integration, due to an emphasis on individualism, division of labour and specialization of tasks. He supposed that suicide could be explained in terms of how individuals were integrated into their social group and that suicide would be associated with very excessive or very deficient social integration. In industrialized societies where under-integration is a primary hazard, the greatest risk of suicide would be in those who were most isolated. He hypothesized that:

- single people, widows and widowers would show a higher rate of suicide than similar, married individuals
- suicides would decrease in wartime when community spirit was more prevalent
- protestants, who were less well integrated into their religious community, would have a higher rate of suicide than Jews or Catholics.

Other studies have also shown the wider benefits to health of social support. Gove (1973) showed that the single, widowed and divorced people had higher rates of mortality, and a number of diseases (Fig. 6.4).

There are a number of reasons why marital status might make an indirect difference to health:

- Married couples may be happier, or experience less stress and are less likely to be socially isolated.
- Marriage might confer meaning upon the lives of individuals imbuing them with a sense of purpose.
- The trauma of separation or not being married may lead to risky behaviours such as smoking or drinking.
- The presence of a partner may encourage medical advice to be sought early on in disease.

Fig. 6.4 Marital status and mortality.				
	Married	**Single**	**Widowed**	**Divorced**
Mortality	1.00	1.95	2.64	3.39
Lung cancer	1.00	1.45	2.24	3.07
Diabetes	1.00	2.69	2.46	4.32
Liver cirrhosis	1.00	3.29	4.61	8.84
Leukaemia	1.00	1.07	0.91	1.28
Source: *Gove 1973.*				

- Single, never married people may have started off as less healthy – thereby failing to get married.

Other studies have looked into social support and its effect on health:

- Social support was defined in terms of marital status, *number* of contacts with friends/relatives and membership of religious/social groups – to give a social network score.
- Low social network scores were associated with increased risk of early mortality (two to three times above those with high network scores).
- Church attendance was related to low mortality scores Berkman and Syme (1979). (Armstrong 2003b, cites other work which suggests the effect may not be as simple as perceived social support.)
- Increased heart disease was associated with low social support.
- Increased complications in pregnancy were associated with low social support.
- Increased emotional illness was associated with low social support.
- A lack of social support, social isolation and being unmarried reduced men's life expectancy following an initial myocardial infarction.
- A higher risk of suicide was found in divorced men and was twice that of married men.

However, in a study of women and depression, the following was found:

- Social support was protective in the context of a severe life event but was not so beneficial in other circumstances.

The lack of consistency and clarity of the findings may be due to the difficulties associated with accurate measurement of 'social support'. The relationship between social support and health may be due to the following factors:

- Increased provision of information about health
- Increased psychological support
- Support acts as a buffer against the negative effects of adverse life events (this suggests that social support is not beneficial in itself – rather it is protective against life problems).

Adverse life events

The association between severe life events, such as bereavement, and illness, such as depression, led to the idea that life events may be important in the aetiology of a variety of diseases.

Holmes and Rahe (1967) developed the Social Readjustment Rating Scale (SRRS). This consisted of a number of life events that were given a score depending on how life changing each event was, e.g.:

- Death of wife/husband: 100
- Divorce: 73

- Marriage: 50
- Retirement: 45
- Moving house: 20.

A number of studies have shown a correlation between the score of a life event and adverse health consequences. Problems with this scale include:

- Life events can be of variable meaning to individuals – moving house may be a positive or a negative experience, as could retirement.
- The scale neglects minor, but perhaps more frequent or chronic problems.

SOCIAL AND CULTURAL CHANGE

Some of the earliest social factors studied dealt with industrialization and the rural to urban migration of large populations. In Britain, this happened during the eighteenth century. (A similar process is now happening in much of the developing world.) Prior to that time, few families were entirely wage-dependent – rather, they worked the land tied to the home and exchanged produce for necessities. The industrial revolution transformed the workforce into large groupings of employees who were solely dependent on the wages they received. Subsistence became increasingly difficult – purchasing power became dependent on employment. Aside from the changes in employment, migration has further effects on health and disease.

Geographical mobility encourages the spread of infectious diseases, but its effect on non-communicable diseases is less clear-cut. This may be because people migrate for different reasons, and this may affect the impact of mobility on morbidity. Migrants are thought to suffer from higher levels of depression, insomnia and anxiety. This may be explained by factors such as language difficulties, hostility in the host country, new cultural practices and so on. However, this level of illness associated with migration may be dependent on the reasons for migration (more illness in refugees than economic migrants) and the ability of the migrants to adopt local lifestyles – a process known as 'acculturation'.

In a study looking at the health of Japanese migrants in California was compared with the health of Japanese people in Japan:

- Coronary heart disease was increased in the migrants.
- There was large variation within the migrants – with those continuing to follow traditional Japanese customs having lower heart disease.
- Coronary heart disease was increased in those who had adopted Western lifestyles.

Another study showed that the proportion of South Asians undergoing coronary artery revascularization was much lower than that of the Caucasian population, even though they suffer from more severe angina. In a UK study, it was shown that Asian, West Indian and African immigrants as a whole had about twice the rate of British-born subjects of having a first admission to the hospital for mental illness (Carpenter & Brockington 1980). From observations of women from ethnic minorities or from non-English-speaking backgrounds, another study concluded that these women should be regarded as a high-risk group for postnatal depression (Onozawa et al. 2003).

IATROGENESIS: DOES HEALTH CARE CREATE DISEASE?

Illich (1978) argued, in his famous book, 'Limits to Medicine', that there are three levels of iatrogenesis (doctor-induced disease). Medical treatment may obviously have adverse side-effects (Illich calls this 'clinical iatrogenesis'), sometimes as a result of negligence and malpractice (see Chs 1–5); sometimes as a result of error (see Ch. 11) and sometimes because it is currently impossible to a predict the effect that a medical intervention will have on every single person. However, knowledge is accumulating on the side-effects of treatments and investigations. Some iatrogenic disease may paradoxically represent therapeutic advances, which allow people to live longer, fuller lives. These people may have side-effects of the treatment (such as steroid therapy for Addison's disease) or experience greater problems when older.

Illich also argued that the greater availability of health care created an increasing dependence on doctors (social, cultural and structural iatrogenesis). In the past, people dealt with minor conditions themselves, whereas today patients attend healthcare settings for reassurance and advice, medications and a variety of services. According to Armstrong (2003c), GPs in the UK have found that when they attempt to reduce the pressure for appointments by taking on another doctor or extending the length of their clinics, the consultation rate tends to rise and the consultations tend to take longer. Illich argued that this gradual increase in dependence on health services is a form of sickness.

COMMUNICATION

Remember: Many of the treatments that doctors prescribe can cause direct harm to the patient, whether though a medical error or because of a recognized side-effect. However, a worse kind of harm might be caused by encouraging excessive dependence on medical services. Think about ways in which doctors educate patients to manage their own health.

There are two ways in which health care may make people feel less healthy:

- Unrealistic health goals, such as the World Health Organization's definition of health as a state of complete social mental and physical well-being, are used to convince people that they could be healthier or are 'by definition' unhealthy.
- Persuading people that good health equates to consumption of healthcare services. Screening (see Ch. 10) is one way in which 'healthy people' can become 'people at risk'. According to Illich, the main outcome has been increasing dependence on health care and iatrogenic disease.

While Illich's vision of a society where everyone is his or her own healer is probably not practical at present, Illich sounds a cautionary note and reminds us that health care can have negative as well as positive effects (Armstrong 2003c).

Key questions

- Describe the relevance of sociology to the understanding of health and illness.
- List the theories of disease causation and their key points.
- Outline the challenges to the biomedical model of illness.
- Discuss the changing patterns of disease from the pre-agricultural era to modern-day living.
- Briefly discuss the multifactorial models of disease.
- Compare and contrast the prevalence of diseases in the developing world with those in the developed world.
- Discuss the effects of family, marriage and life events on an individual's health.
- Describe how social and cultural change has led to a change in the patterns of disease.
- Define clinical iatrogenesis.
- Describe social, cultural and structural iatrogenesis.

References

Armstrong, D., 2003a. Introduction. In: An Outline of Sociology as Applied to Medicine, fifth ed. Hodder Arnold, London, pp. 1–2.

Armstrong, D., 2003b. Social support. In: An Outline of Sociology as Applied to Medicine, fifth ed. Hodder Arnold, London, pp. 34–36.

Armstrong, D., 2003c. Evaluating healthcare. In: An Outline of Sociology as Applied to Medicine, fifth ed. Hodder Arnold, London, pp. 125–137.

Berkman, L.F., Syme, S.L., 1979. Social networks, host resistance, and mortality a nine year follow-up study of Alameda County residents. Am. J. Epidemiol. 109, 186–204.

Carpenter, L., Brockington, I.F., 1980. A study of mental illness in Asians. West Indians and Africans living in Manchester. Br. J. Psychiatry 137, 201–225.

Gove, W.R., 1973. Sex, marital status and mortality. Am. J. Sociol. 79, 45–67.

Holmes, T.H., Rahe, R.H., 1967. The social readjustment rating scale. J. Psychosom. Res. 213–218.

Illich, I., 1978. Limits to Medicine. Caldar Boyars (subsequently published and reprinted by Penguin Books), London.

Locker, D., 2008. Social determinants of health and disease. In: Scambler, G. (Ed.), Sociology as Applied to Medicine. sixth ed. Saunders Elsevier, Edinburgh, pp. 18–37.

Nettleton, S., 2003. The Sociology of Health and Illness, second ed. Polity Press, Cambridge, pp. 5–6.

Onozawa, K., Kumar, R.C., Adams, D., et al., 2003. High EPDS scores in women from ethnic minorities living in London. Arch. Womens Ment. Health Aug(Suppl. 2), S51–S55.

Further reading

Donaldson, L.J., Donaldson, R.J., 2000. Essential Public Health, second ed. Petroc Press, Berkshire.

Fitzpatrick, R., 2008. Society and changing patterns of disease. In: Scambler, G. (Ed.), Sociology as Applied to Medicine, sixth ed. Saunders Elsevier, Edinburgh, pp. 3–17.

Gray, A., 2001. World Health and Disease, third ed. Open University Press, Buckingham.

Iphofen, R., Poland, F., Campling, J., 1998. Sociology in Practice for Health Care Professionals. Palgrave, Basingstoke.

Experience of health and illness

ILLNESS BEHAVIOUR AND THE SICK ROLE

In Chapter 6, we looked at how disease patterns have changed over time, and how social and environmental factors have played a causative role in the experience of disease. In this chapter, we look at the processes that motivate individuals to utilize health services and how people experience health and illness.

Hannay (1988) identifies five stages of illness:

1. The experience of symptoms (and illness behaviour)
2. Advice or consultation with friends/relatives – known as 'lay referral'
3. Consultation with a doctor – to confirm subjective *illness* and gain objective diagnosis of *disease*. This stage *legitimizes a sick role*
4. Being in the sick role as a dependent patient
5. Recovery.

Each of these stages can be affected by differing cultural and social factors, which are discussed below. However, it is first worthwhile noting how the biomedical model defines differences between illness, disease, sickness and problems of living or 'predicaments' (Fig. 7.1).

The traditional medical model held that when people experienced symptoms – that is they felt ill – they sought medical help to identify a disease process. However, work done in the 1950s illustrated that many individuals with symptoms – even potentially serious ones – did not seek medical help (Fig. 7.2). This was referred to as the 'clinical iceberg' to indicate that the majority of community illness was not seen by medical professionals. In addition, and somewhat conversely, it was noted that many people who do consult their GP do so with trivial or minor complaints.

COMMUNICATION

Remember: Patients may have 'consulted' friends and relatives, or sought advice from the local pharmacist before seeking medical advice.

Illness behaviour

The notion of 'illness behaviour' was introduced in 1960 by Mechanic and Volkart to describe the ways in which symptoms were evaluated and acted upon, or not acted upon, by different kinds of individual. Mechanic (1978) outlined a number of variables that influence illness behaviour. Each variable may be considered in relation to its impact on others, and in its impact on the 'patient':

1. *Visibility, recognizability, or perceptual salience of signs and symptoms*, i.e. how obvious the symptoms are. Individuals with a sudden headache or acute abdominal pain may consult their GP more frequently than those with a slow-growing lump. In the same way, if illness causes a change in behaviour, which is obvious to those close to the patient (e.g. expressed hallucinations), medical help may be sought more quickly than with an insidious change (e.g. increasing depression).
2. *The extent to which the symptoms are perceived as serious:* if a symptom is familiar, an individual may be more reluctant to visit a GP. Smokers may not attend a GP for a cough if they think 'it's just a smoker's cough', whereas a non-smoker might. Another example is if someone has a backache, and knows it was caused by heavy lifting, they may be less likely to attend the GP than if it had arisen 'out of the blue'.
3. *The extent to which symptoms disrupt family, work and other social activities:* the heavy drinker with a family is more likely to present to health services due to pressure from those around him, than a solitary drinker. Similarly, if an individual is unable to play his weekly round of golf because of breathlessness, he may consult a GP before a less active individual in a similar stage of disease.
4. *The frequency of signs or symptoms, their persistence or their frequency of recurrence:* frequent or persisting symptoms are more likely to lead to a consultation than rarely occurring ones.
5. *The tolerance threshold to the deviant signs and symptoms:* an individual's tolerance of pain and attitude towards it may determine when he consults a GP. This may be dependent on his cultural background. Zborowski (1952) showed that individuals of Irish or old-American descent were more stoical in their illness behaviour, compared with Italian and Jewish individuals, who more readily courted sympathy. However, more recent studies do not support this work.

Fig. 7.1 The definition of illness, disease, sickness and predicaments.

	Definition	Criterion
Illness	'the subjective component of disease as characterized by symptoms'	Subjective, medically and socially defined by doctor and patient
Disease	'an objective component confirmed by signs and investigations'	Objective and medically defined
Sickness	'the behavioural part of illness, e.g. obtaining sick notes from the doctor, or adhering to the sick role'	Objective or subjective – defined both medically and socially
Predicaments	'problems of living or situations which are socially defined, but are not accepted by the medical community as being part of disease'	Objective or subjective, socially defined

Adapted from Hannay (1988).

Fig. 7.2 Ratio of symptom episodes to consultations.

Headache	184:1
Backache	52:1
Emotional problem	46:1
Abdominal pain	28:1
Sore throat	18:1
Chest pain	14:1

Source: *adapted from Banks et al. 1975 (as reproduced in Armstrong 2003)*

6. *Available information, knowledge and cultural assumptions and understandings of the individual:* lay individuals have a wide range of knowledge about medical conditions. Those who are unaware of how changes in their body may relate to disease processes may take longer to present to their GP. Those who are more fearful of diseases such as cancer, arthritis and birth defects tend to know more about them and may present earlier. For example, people who present to hospital within 4 hours of chest pain are more likely to see themselves as at risk from a heart attack, know more symptoms of a heart attack and are less likely to use drugs to treat their symptoms than those who delayed presentation. Psychosis in the lower social classes shows a greater tendency to present to healthcare professionals via the courts or the police. Psychosis in the higher social classes tends to present via family, friends and self-referral.

7. *Basic needs that lead to denial:* anxiety, guilt and fear may lead individuals and their families to deny the existence of signs and symptoms of disease. However, this can be quite complex. Mechanic notes that, while anxiety about cancer can lead to shorter delay in presentation, high levels of fear may lead to the opposite.

8. *Needs competing with illness responses:* individuals may feel that their symptoms do not warrant over-riding other needs that may be more pressing.

9. *Competing possible interpretations that can be assigned to the symptoms once they are recognized:* friends and relatives may 'normalize' the symptoms of disease. Individuals who work long hours may not see tiredness as a symptom of illness – rather they expect it.

10. *Availability of treatment resources, physical proximity, and psychological and monetary costs of taking action:* the resumption of good health is not always a *supreme* priority – rather its attainment must be weighed against the other costs of going to see a doctor. The costs include (adapted from Mechanic 1978, pp. 268–87):
    a. Physical distance, time, money and effort
    b. Stigma, social distance and feelings of humiliation
    c. Self-blame and fear of being chastised for risky behaviour, e.g. smoking
    d. Concern that the doctor will form a negative judgement about them if they present with something 'trivial'.

The benefits of going to see the doctor are twofold. There is therapeutic benefit, and there is an endorsement of the 'sick role'.

> **HINTS AND TIPS**
>
> Illness behaviour is the process by which individuals with symptoms seek (or don't seek) medical advice.

Zola (1973) identified five 'triggers' that precipitate an individual with symptoms to consult a medical practitioner:

1. The occurrence of an interpersonal crisis (e.g. a bereavement)

2. Perceived interference with social or personal relations
3. 'Sanctioning' or pressure from others
4. Perceived interference with vocational or physical activity
5. 'Temporalizing of symptomatology' – the setting of deadlines before visiting the doctor, like 'if this headache comes back …' or 'if I still feel ill on Monday …'.

Lay referral and self-help

When an individual becomes aware of symptoms, they are presented with a number of options. They can:

1. ignore them
2. self-medicate without consulting anyone else
3. consult non-medical individuals
4. consult a medical professional.

This section deals with options (2) and (3). Given the quantity of symptoms in the community that do not lead to a consultation, it seems apparent that individuals undertake a great deal of self-care. Most people have ways of dealing with bruises, muscular aches and pains, headaches, cuts and colds without needing to consult a doctor. Hannay has shown that the proportion of people with significant medical symptoms who do not consult a doctor is higher than the proportion of people with medical symptoms who do consult a doctor. It has been reported that twice as many people take non-prescription medicine as prescription medicine, and this self-medication was associated with a lower consultation rate. Encouraging self-care for self-limiting illnesses has clear benefits for healthcare costs. However, Armstrong (1989) identified two problems that could arise if this policy were to be pursued too vigorously:

1. If people are encouraged to take responsibility for their health, they may also be seen as responsible for their illness. This 'victim-blaming' may be a particular problem for the lower socioeconomic groups, as they are least likely to be able to 'look after' their health.
2. Health is not just an individual problem – rather it is contingent on social and economic factors as well. The placing of responsibility upon the individual may deflect attention from the responsibility of wider society to prevent social deprivation and inequality.

Up to three-quarters of patients consulting a medical practitioner will have already discussed their symptoms with some other person. This 'lay referral' system can either increase or decrease the likelihood of an individual seeking professional help. One Scottish study showed high interlocking kinship and friendship networks 'inhibited' women from social class V seeking antenatal care. Lay members may also take it upon themselves to initiate medical consultation. This is more likely if the symptoms are serious, or if the sufferer is incapable of self-help (e.g. a parent acting on behalf of a child, or a wife acting on behalf of a husband with epilepsy).

Beyond the 'lay referral' system exists a vast number of *self-help groups*. Self-help groups 'gather together people with a similar problem in order to help them by a personal approach, preferably to solve the problem, and where that is impossible, to teach them how to live with their constraints' (Damen et al. 2000).

The first such group, Alcoholics Anonymous, started in 1935. Today, groups exist for a vast range of illnesses including multiple sclerosis, hypertension, all manner of cancers and depression. By the end of the 1970s, there were thought to be over half a million self-help groups in the USA alone. Previously, many self-help groups were both characterized as and perceived themselves to be anti-medical – an alternative to professional medicine. This perception has broadly changed, and self-help groups are widely seen to be supplementary to professional assistance – able to act as expert bodies in the *experience* of diseases that is unrivalled by healthcare professionals.

Self-help groups fulfil two main functions (Damen et al. 2000):

1. An informative aspect – they provide information about the condition, be this in leaflets, lectures, or through discussions with other individuals with the same condition.
2. An emotional aspect – they provide mechanisms to help the members to put their condition into perspective. Part of the role of such groups is to alleviate perceived stigma and aid narrative reconstruction (p. 98).

In general, self-help groups are seen as beneficial – reducing stress, increasing patient control and improving self-esteem. In particular:

- self-help groups are, next to family, the most important pillars for the chronically ill
- the long-term impact of group membership, e.g. in cancer patients, can lead to a significant reduction in anxiety and depression.

However, there have been some studies that have found the supportive or emotional side to self-help groups to be lacking. One study, reporting on newly diagnosed cancer patients, found that, although 66% used other patients as a source of support, only 39% found this to be a positive source. A number of factors could lead to negative experiences in such groups, e.g.:

- The presence of disruptive individual members at meetings
- The experience of loss when members left
- The potential for member dependency
- Individuals feeling threatened by the open communication.

Self-help groups for breast cancer have been found to be beneficial in relation to the informative aspect; however, in practical aspects of how to cope with breast cancer, many people found the emotional support aspect was less useful, for the following reasons (Damen et al. 2000):

- They perceived that such support from strangers was for people who had few other social ties (such as no partner or family)
- They felt no need for such support
- They wished to 'leave their cancer behind them'
- They felt there existed too great a gap of severity between themselves and the other group members
- They felt there existed too great a gap of age between themselves and the other group members.

Aside from self-help, individuals may choose to visit practitioners of alternative medicine or use complementary medicine.

Alternative and complementary medicine

As the names suggest, alternative is used as a replacement for conventional medicine and complementary is used alongside conventional medicine, often through referral (see http://nccam.nci.nih.gov/health/whatiscam for a full definition). Alternative medicine can be seen as part of a wider societal shift of attitude towards natural and 'organic' choices: this includes the green movements and the increased interest in organic foods vs pesticide-treated foods; holistic vs mechanistic approaches, and so on. Such popular support for alternative and complementary medicine has led to political support – with the appointment of junior ministers with responsibility for alternative medicine and the unveiling of plans to set up the Complementary Medical Council along the same lines as the General Medical Council.

There has also been a shift in perception by the medical community itself – with complementary medicine increasingly being practised in conventional medical settings – particularly with regards to acupuncture for pain, and massage, music therapy and relaxation therapy for mild anxiety and depression. This has largely been ascribed to the increasing amount of evidence in favour of certain complementary therapies.

Proponents of alternative and complementary medicine argue that the following benefits are offered:

- Care is health and not disease-oriented
- It respects the autonomy of the patient
- It allows freedom of choice
- It promotes self-treatment
- It encourages the patient to take on some individual responsibility for the outcome of the procedure and healing.

For patients, the common reasons given for attending a practitioner of alternative or complementary medicine include:

- *A greater amount of time and continuity in the consultation*: this allows the development of a deeper therapeutic relationship than the kind that can be forged in the average GP or hospital consultation
- *The attention to personality and personal experience*: treatment is 'individualized' in the sense of making it dependent on the patient's emotions, psychology and response to illness – rather than focussed on the disease itself
- *Greater patient involvement*: the patient is able to choose the type of therapist that they think would suit them, e.g. a homeopathist, reflexologist, acupuncture practitioner and so on. There is also the greater sense of being active in one's own treatment as compared with conventional medicine, which can make patients adopt a rather passive role to treatment
- *Hope*: patients may come to alternative or complementary medicine after having tried all that conventional medicine has to offer
- *Touch*: many of the alternative or complementary therapies involve a degree of physical contact with the patient that would perhaps be out of place in conventional medicine. This aspect can be important in facilitating a more open and trusting relationship between patient and practitioner
- *Dealing with ill-defined symptoms*: alternative or complementary medicine may be better placed to deal with nonspecific syndromes and symptoms, e.g. chronic fatigue and irritable bowel syndrome
- *Making sense of illness*: alternative or complementary medicine may provide explanations for patients' conditions that they find easy to understand. The treatment may fit with a patient's own personal beliefs or seem less threatening than 'orthodox' medicine by presenting a 'natural' alternative. The objectivity of such explanations may on occasion be questionable; however, if they accord with the prior beliefs of the patients, they may be beneficial
- *Spiritual and existential concerns*: such concerns are often not addressed by conventional practitioners. However, one study has shown that 66% of Americans would like their doctors to be aware of their religious or spiritual beliefs. Practitioners of alternative or complementary medicine may be more comfortable addressing these sorts of issues.

The above reasons represent a number of 'pull' factors towards alternative and complementary medicine; however, patients may experience a number of 'push' or negative factors that lead to a loss of faith in conventional medicine. These include being less confident about the conventional medicine, and less satisfied by it, as well as being more sceptical of its efficacy.

The negative aspects of alternative and complementary medicine include:

- Safety and competence: a lack of regulation may lead to unqualified practitioners. In addition, herbal medications are not subject to the same level of testing as conventional drugs – even though they may contain pharmacologically active components with significant side-effects
- Guilt and blame: when patients are encouraged to feel more responsible for their own health, they may be made to feel guilty for their past activities that have led to ill health, or to feel blame for not getting better
- Financial risk: there is a danger of exploiting the vulnerable who are willing to try multiple alternative or complementary therapies to find a successful outcome. Alternative medicine is a form of private practice
- Missed diagnosis or delayed presentation: conventional practitioners worry that alternative practitioners may miss serious diagnoses. This is only a risk in alternative medicine where it replaces the conventional medicine; however, most patients are most likely to consult conventional prior to alternative or complementary therapy
- Conflicting advice may lead to the abandonment of conventional therapy with potentially serious consequences
- The remedies provided by the alternative practitioner may react adversely with conventional medicines.

Normality in disease

When individuals talk about health, there are perhaps three commonly understood components of what health is. These are (Blaxter 1990):

1. A positive element: fitness and well-being
2. A functional element: an ability to cope with day to day life
3. A negative element: an absence of illness.

All these elements are overtly dependent on *social* values and criteria. However, when individuals talk about disease, it is in terms of *biological* criteria. Why does such a difference exist? A definition of 'disease' as a group noun, is more difficult than defining the criteria of individual diseases. This may be because: a) there is no agreed definition of disease; b) some diseases do not appear to have an apparent biological basis, e.g. some psychiatric diseases; c) if disease is simply some pathological state – that is some biological set of conditions – how can it be distinguished from a non-diseased biological state? That is, what differentiates a 'normal' biological state from an abnormal one?

Normality in medicine may be decided on a number of bases, as outlined below.

Statistical basis

One example of this is the 'normal' range of blood biochemistry, which is based on samples of the 'healthy' population and will fall in a 'normal' or Gaussian distribution. Levels that are outside a certain number of standard deviations from the mean are considered to be abnormal – even if they are not associated with symptoms. There are a number of problems with this approach:

1. The cut-off point may be somewhat arbitrary, e.g. diagnosis of diabetes or hypertension relies on what is effectively an arbitrary point in a spectrum of disease.
2. Certain biological states might be considered to be disease states, yet are statistically 'normal', e.g. the presence of atheroma is 'normal' in Western populations, but is still considered to be a disease process.
3. Certain biological states might *not* be considered to be a disease state, yet be statistically 'abnormal', e.g. being 7 ft tall, or having a 'genius' I.Q.

Bio-statistical basis

This is a variation of the statistical basis that aims to find a way around the problems mentioned above. This theory still holds that disease is an objective status, that not only can it be defined regardless of whether the patient 'feels' ill, but regardless of whether or not society negatively or positively values that particular biological state. This theory has been advocated by Boorse (1975). He asserts that disease is not an evaluative concept; rather, disease is an abnormality that hinders the attainment of 'natural goals'. An analysis of a large enough sample will lead to a bio-statistical analysis of what constitutes a natural and thus factual goal. This goal becomes the basis for judgements on what is and what is not a disease.

He claims that: an organism is healthy at any moment in proportion as it is not diseased; and a disease is a type of internal state of the organism which:

1. interferes with the performance of some natural function, i.e. some species-typical contribution to survival and reproduction, characteristic of the organism's age

and

2. is not simply in the nature of the species, i.e. is either atypical of the species or, if typical, mainly due to environmental causes.

(Boorse 1976)

However, a fundamental problem still exists. Namely, Boorse wishes to use terms like 'natural function' and 'biological disadvantage' as objective, descriptive terms, which are then used to elicit what doctors *ought* to treat without a need for moral analysis. However, it seems that inherent within the terms there is a moral judgement. 'Natural function' is that which is 'good' and 'biological disadvantage' is 'bad'. This assumption is not obviously true. As Toon (1981) writes: 'This tendency to find moral values creeping in under the cloak of a scientific definition is a central problem in the definition of disease, and it merely leads to confusion'. It is thus more prudent to accept that 'disease' in both its professional and its colloquial usage incorporates a degree of moral evaluation.

Normative basis

This view holds that normality is defined in the way in which society finds acceptable or desirable. It is often equivalent with those that are statistically normal, but not always. Some of the advantages of this approach are:

- it better accords with many of our intuitions about disease
- by defining normality in relation to socially accepted or desired criteria, disease becomes those states with socially deleterious consequences
- psychiatric disease, such as 'mania', is more readily understandable as a state that by (our) collective values is considered undesirable – even if the patient doesn't consider himself to be ill. Another example is homosexuality which, until the 1980s, was generally considered a mental illness.

Conditions such as 'dyslexia' only exist as 'diseases' in literate societies – the same biological state may exist in pre-literate cultures, but it is not a disease because it does not confer any social disadvantage.

The sick role

Social deviancy

With this conception of disease as a socially definable phenomenon, the sick role and illness can be understood as forms of social deviancy (deviancy in the sense of being different from what is the social 'norm', rather than in a pejorative sense or in the sense that the 'deviant' is morally responsible for 'not being normal'), as can certain diseases that carry with them considerable stigma – which essentially is social disapproval (see below).

Prior to the 1950s, deviance was simply used to describe those who were responsible for behaving in a way that did not accord with social and cultural norms, e.g. youth crime. Parsons (1951) defined deviance on the grounds that 'it disrupts the social system by inhibiting people's performance of their customary or normal social roles'. The sick role, according to Parsons, has the function of minimizing such social disruption, controlling the deviant illness behaviour. The sick role consists of two rights and two responsibilities (or duties).

The rights:

1. The sick are not obliged to perform their normal social roles.

2. The sick are not considered responsible for their own state.

The responsibilities:

1. The sick are obliged to want to get well as soon as possible.
2. The sick are obliged to consult and cooperate with medical experts.

Remember: According to Parsons' 'Sick role', someone who is ill gains rights, e.g. to medical help, sympathy and time off work, but also has duties, to comply with medical treatment and get better as quickly as possible.

Failure to successfully carry out the responsibilities of the sick role means that the sick may forfeit the rights associated with their role. Someone who appears not to want to get well may be considered a malingerer or a hypochondriac. Someone who does not cooperate with medical experts is seen as non-compliant. The non-compliant patient may be seen as responsible for his illness in a way that other patients are not, e.g. the patient who continues to smoke after bypass surgery.

The sick role is in general a temporary role into which all people can be admitted. The gatekeepers to the sick role are doctors who decide whether or not individuals have a disease. In doing so, they must draw upon general and objective criteria. However, it is possible to have a medical diagnosis, but not be admitted into the 'sick role'. For example, many people in Africa may suffer from constant diagnosable medical conditions such as malaria or malnutrition, however, because their economies cannot support non-productive individuals for any length of time, they are not considered sick and must carry out their social roles.

The main functions of the 'sick role' are to control illness and to reduce the disruptive effects on the social systems by returning the ill to good health as quickly as possible.

Labelling

Labelling refers to the process whereby individual characteristics are identified by others and given a negative label.

The act of making a diagnosis is the process by which people become 'patients' and are labelled as ill or deviant. In this sense, labelling *creates* disease. This should not be confused with *causing* disease, which it does not. Rather it enables the normal to be reaffirmed and the deviant to be identified. Labelling serves to delineate the boundaries of what are considered to be normal social values and behaviour.

Secondary deviance refers to the changes in behaviour as a result of labelling an illness (primary deviance). Strong social attitudes or stereotypes about how a blind, epileptic or alcoholic person should act may lead to self-fulfilling prophecies. The pressure upon patients derives from the expectations associated with the label (or diagnosis) a patient has been given. The blind may be seen as quiet and docile; the alcoholic as unkempt and incorrigible. People they encounter, and even medical professionals who deal with them, may present such stereotypic attitudes to the individual patients. This reactive attitude towards them may lead the patients to conform to the stereotype imposed upon them (either by others or self-imposed because they believe such stereotypical behaviour is appropriate for their illness).

The idea of secondary deviance has been most controversial in the field of psychiatry. Three main views exist as to the impact of labelling primary deviance, and secondary deviance:

1. *Psychiatric disease is a consequence of the labelling of primary deviance.* This view claimed that psychiatric illness only existed because certain behaviours were labelled as 'illness'; 'real' psychiatric illness did not exist.
2. *Psychiatric illness is a consequence of the labelling of primary deviance and the resulting secondary deviance.* This view holds that psychiatrists identify a slightly unusual behaviour in individuals (which is still within the normal range) and label it as psychiatric disease (that is primary deviance). The result of the labelling (that is secondary deviance) is the induction of the mental illness that was first diagnosed.
3. *Psychiatric illness can be exacerbated by labelling and secondary deviance.* This view holds that labelling and secondary deviance lead to some behaviours that are 'abnormal'. This is most evident in patients who have lived in institutions for many years. Such patients may develop certain behaviours that, while they are normal behaviours within the institute, may be seen as incongruous in the 'normal' world.

Stigma in disease

The concept of *stigma* requires us to accept that the labels given in a medical diagnosis have significance beyond the medical consultation and into wider society. 'Stigmatizing conditions [are] those that set their possessors apart from "normal" people [and] mark them as socially unacceptable or inferior beings' (Scambler 2008). Some of the most stigmatizing conditions are those that are generally visible, e.g. being deaf or blind or being seen to have an epileptic fit or being an amputee. However, many other non-visible conditions also have considerable stigma attached to them by virtue of strong social emotions related to the condition; for example, cancer (and the associated fear of dying), colostomies (and the social taboo about handling faeces) and HIV/AIDS (and the 'moral' condemnation of homosexuality and/or intravenous drug use) (Fig. 7.3).

Fig. 7.3	The four phases of the HIV stigma trajectory.	
At risk	Pre-stigma and the 'worried well'	This does not correspond to a stage of the disease trajectory. It denotes a time of uncertainty when an individual thinks behaviours might have put him at risk of HIV. He may cope through denial or disassociation. Much depends on the support available. The phase may end with testing for HIV.
Diagnosis	Confronting an altered identity	An individual may be diagnosed early or late in the disease trajectory. A typical stress response involves disbelief, numbness and denial, followed by anger, acute turmoil, disruptive anxiety and depressive symptoms. Identity and self-esteem may be threatened, stigma becomes salient and decisions on disclosure have to be negotiated.
Latent	Living between health and illness	This is when the disease is asymptomatic and perhaps at its least disruptive. Individuals may normalize, conceal and even deny their positivity. They may choose to pass as normal, thereby avoiding 'enacted stigma', but 'felt stigma' can exact a heavy price.
Manifest	Passage to social and physical death	There may be no fixed disease course because of widespread individual variation. However, there are fewer symptom-free periods and opportunistic infections accumulate. Stigma tends to be less salient as matters surrounding social and biological death become paramount. Intense felt stigma may, nevertheless, be associated with isolation and withdrawal as means of concealing 'abominations of the body'. Courtesy stigma may extend to carers who hesitate to reveal cause of death.

Adapted from Alonzo & Reynolds 1995.

Goffman (1963) described several strategies that a person with a stigmatizing condition could pursue. He described stigmatizing conditions as either:

- *discrediting* – if they were obviously visible (e.g. being in a wheelchair)

or

- *discreditable* – if they were relatively hidden (e.g. HIV).

Having a stigmatizing condition that was discrediting, limited one's options; however, the patient with the discreditable condition had the option of trying to keep the condition hidden. Coping with stigmatizing conditions could be achieved in one of the following ways:

1. Passing: by trying to 'pass as normal'. This would depend on the degree and nature of the stigmatizing condition. Problems that might occur revolve around the need for various forms of deception and the risk of being exposed.
2. Covering: a person with a discrediting condition could still try to hide the condition from view, or avoid situations where it is particularly obvious.
3. Withdrawal: at extremes, individuals may withdraw from social circumstances where attention may be drawn to their stigmatizing condition.

Scambler and Hopkins (1986) identified a distinction between two components of stigma:

1. *Felt stigma:* the shame associated with the condition, and the fear of being discriminated against because of the imputed cultural unacceptability or inferiority
2. *Enacted stigma:* actual discrimination of this nature.

The same authors noted that often the 'felt stigma' is greater than the actual or 'enacted stigma', and led to greater disruption of people's lives (in attempting to hide their medical condition) than probably would have been the case of enduring the enacted stigma.

THE DOCTOR–PATIENT RELATIONSHIP

Morgan (2008) refers to the meeting of patients with their doctors as the 'essential unit of medical practice'. There are estimated to be over half a million consultations between patients and GPs in the UK every day.

The utility and success of these consultations depends on the competence and expertise of the doctor, and the social relationship between doctor and patient:

- The doctor–patient relationship reflects and reinforces wider social relations and structural inequalities – especially those of gender, 'race' and socioeconomic class.
- The relationship and values maintained within them form a key dimension to social control.
- Historically, the view of the patient has been neglected.
- The quality of the doctor–patient relationship impacts on the health outcomes.

How the doctor–patient relationship is changing

In the eighteenth century, physicians treated upper class patients. The status difference and the need for physicians to compete meant that the doctor–patient relationship was characterized by doctors attempting to please their patients. The lack of technical knowledge meant the doctor's role was that of attending to symptoms and experiences.

Throughout the nineteenth century, doctors were most often in some form of private practice. However, they frequently practised charitable medicine in the newly created public or voluntary hospitals. Their patients were often their social inferiors and more passive in accepting medical advice. Hospital patients were often sicker and frequently died. The biomedical model emerged in the eighteenth and nineteenth centuries as hospital doctors were able to conduct autopsies on dead patients and relate the post-mortem findings to signs and symptoms during life. The biomedical model set up the doctor as the expert on disease, and left little room for the patient's opinion, especially if the patient was socially inferior to the doctor. It became normal for the doctor to occupy the dominant role within the doctor–patient consultation.

The 1950s were characterized by the paternalistic doctor-centred approach, typified by Parsons' 'sick-role'.

From the 1960s onwards there has been a general trend towards a relationship involving greater patient participation. In sociological terms, this has been described by relationships of *mutuality* rather than paternalism. In ethical terms, this has been discussed in terms of patient *autonomy* (see Chs 1 and 3).

In 1992 (updated in 1997), the Patient's Charter was introduced in the UK. This formally gave patients a number of rights and affirmed what standards the public can expect from the NHS. The rights patients are entitled to include:

- A clear explanation of treatment, its alternatives and associated risks
- A full investigation of any complaints

- Waiting lists of a maximum of 18 months.

Patients can also expect the following standards:

- To be seen within 30 minutes of an appointment time
- To be seen immediately at A&E or have need for treatment assessed
- To have their privacy, dignity, religious and cultural beliefs respected.

All the current changes seem to be increasing the *consumer* power of the patient. This is partly reflected by the increase in litigation.

Models of the doctor–patient relationship

As mentioned above, Parsons (1951) was the first sociologist to deal with the relationship between doctors and patients. Parsons believed that social functioning was achieved in part by the fulfilment of social roles – each of which had certain prescribed or expected behaviours. This meant that we know what to expect when interacting with mothers, teachers and doctors, and how we in turn are expected to behave in the role of children, pupils and patients. Just as Parsons held that the 'sick role' had certain rights and responsibilities, he believed the 'doctor role' had a number of rights and obligations as well. These are summarized in Figure 7.4.

Parsons viewed the sick role as both *temporary* – only for as long as it takes to get better; and *universal* – the obligations and rights apply to all regardless of gender, race or socioeconomic class. Parsons thought of the doctor's role as complementary – but not equal – to the sick role. The asymmetry in the relationship was not thought to be problematic due to the expectations or obliged attitudes of the doctor, namely:

- *Affective neutrality* – to remain emotionally detached and objective in the diagnosis and treatment of disease
- *Universalism* – to treat patients equally
- *Functional specificity* – the doctor should be concerned only with those matters that are of direct medical relevance to the patient.

This is of course an 'ideal' model of the doctor–patient relationship. Everyday, reality departs from this ideal.

Armstrong (2003) outlines three different types of doctor–patient relationship models:

1. *Consensual models:* such as the Parsons model – where both the doctor and the patient have the same goals framed within the perspective of the biomedical model. That is, even if the doctor and patient don't agree on how best to produce a cure, they have agreed on their aims – specifically to produce a cure.
2. *Conflict models:* where the patient and the doctor have different agendas and perspectives that may often be in conflict – and are often not addressed.
3. *Negotiation models:* where it is recognized within the consultation that the doctor has a biomedical agenda and the patient a psychosocial agenda, and attempts are made to understand the patient's view and integrate their lay beliefs into a workable plan for treatment.

These models represent different types of relationship between doctor and patient. The Parsons' model is *a paternalistic* one; ultimately, the patient in the 'sick role' is obliged to cooperate with the doctor (Fig. 7.5). Other types of relationship occur when different levels of power and control are exercised by doctors and patients (Fig. 7.6).

In the *paternalistic* relationship, the doctor is authoritative, acting in much the same way as a parent deciding

Fig. 7.4 The role of doctor and patient.	
Patient: sick role	**Doctor: professional role**
Rights	Expectations
1. Allowed to shed normal social role	1. Apply a high degree of skill and knowledge to the problem of illness
2. Regarded as not being responsible for illness	2. Act for the welfare of patient and community
	3. Be objective and emotionally detached
	4. Be guided by professional practice
Obligations	Rights
1. Must want to get well	1. Granted right to examine patients and enquire into intimate areas of physical and personal life
2. Should seek medical help and cooperate with doctor	2. Granted considerable autonomy in professional practice
	3. Occupies position of authority in relation to patient
Adapted from Parsons 1951.	

Fig. 7.5 A comparison of Parsons' doctor–patient relationship and the GMC's Duties of a Doctor.

Parsons (1951)

Apply a high level of knowledge
Be guided by professional practice
Act for the welfare of patient and community rather than self-interest
Be objective and emotionally detached (not judge patient's behaviour in terms of personal value system or become emotionally involved with them).

GMC (2006)

Keep your professional knowledge and skills up-to-date
Make the care of your patient your first concern
Make sure that your personal beliefs do not prejudice your patients' care

Fig. 7.6 Types of doctor–patient relationships.

Patient control	Physician control	
	Low	**High**
Low	Default	Paternalism
Goals and agenda	Unclear	Physician set
Patient values	Unclear	Assumed
Physician's role	Unclear	Guardian
High	Consumerist	Mutuality
Goals and agenda	Patient set	Negotiated
Patient values	Unexamined	Jointly examined
Physician's role	Technical consultant	Advisor

Adapted from Roter 2000.

what is best for their child. The agenda for the consultation is determined by the doctor, who assumes patient values without enquiring after them. For example, a doctor may assume all patients who have a sore throat desire antibiotics, when in fact they may simply want reassurance or vice versa. Recognition of patient autonomy means that consultations are leaning away from this paternalistic approach, although it may still be the most prevalent style of consultation. However, some sections of the population such as the elderly may prefer a paternalistic approach. Paternalism may also be more prevalent in other cultures (e.g. Japan is reported to have a more paternalistic medical profession).

A relationship of *mutuality* sees doctors and patients in a 'meeting of experts'; the doctor with clinical skills and knowledge, and the patient with experience and expectations of the illness and possibly complex ideas about its causation. This is the sort of relationship that is encouraged in the Western practice of modern medicine.

A *consumerist* relationship may develop if the patient becomes demanding, and the doctor acquiesces to their demands, e.g. for antibiotics for a viral infection or an unnecessary referral. This type of relationship is more prevalent where patients are paying to see the doctor. This type of consultation is characterized by the patient setting the agenda, and the doctor acting as little more than a facilitator. The patient's values are unexamined by the physician, which may lead to the patient having an ongoing false impression of his or her condition.

A *default* relationship occurs when neither the doctor nor the patient takes an active role in the consultation. The danger here is that the consultation is undirected and the appropriate decisions may not be made.

Of course, these types of consultation represent extremes; a single consultation may contain a mixture of styles, the doctor being paternalistic with an issue she considers important, and the patient being more demanding with others.

The patient-centred consultation

A 'patient-centred' consultation style is increasingly advocated in all settings, but especially in primary care, where there is a high degree of psychological and social aspects to the consultation. What then is 'patient-centredness'?

Mead and Bower (2002) describe the following five dimensions of 'patient-centred care':

1. *The biopsychosocial perspective*: this takes into account the biomedical, psychological and social factors that lead to a patient consulting
2. *The 'patient-as-person'*: this dimension invites the doctor to consider the personal meaning of the illness for that individual patient
3. *Sharing power and responsibility*: the aim of this perspective is to remind doctors to be sensitive to patient preferences, and understand the reasons and values that guide their actions
4. *The therapeutic alliance*: this aims to develop common goals and agendas that take into account both the patient's and the doctor's preferences. The idea of developing a mutual goal is that it is more likely to be achieved than one that is simply dictated by the doctor.
5. *The 'doctor-as-person'*: this aspect reflects a need for doctors to be introspective to a degree – being aware of how their own personal qualities and their subjectivity affect their practice of medicine. Doctors' assumptions of patients' preferences may have more

influence than the actual preferences of patients – resulting in actions deemed unnecessary by the doctor and unwanted by the patient.

The term 'patient-centred consultation' is used to draw attention to the importance of the patient in the consultation. However, it is characterized by *mutuality* as described above – where both patient and doctor are partners in the process treating the patient – rather than a consumerist relationship, which the term 'patient-centred consultation' might suggest. Some authors prefer to describe this as '*relationship-centred care*' in order to avoid this problem and to recognize the importance of the reciprocal relationship between the doctor and the patient, and the integration of the biomedical and real-life or personal perspective of the patient. Such consultations (whatever we choose to call them) are characterized by being:

- medically functional – the consultation must work within the framework of a healthcare system. History-taking, examination, diagnosis and treatment are expected of the consultation
- informative for the patient – in general, patients want to know as much information as possible about their conditions. Some studies have shown that when patients are better informed (e.g. what the symptoms of a heart attack are) they are more likely to seek appropriate medical care
- facilitative – that is the doctor should aim to elicit the full concerns of the patient and their pre-consultation agenda. The majority of patients do not discuss their full agenda during a single consultation, the consequences of which can be a number of misunderstandings
- responsive – in addition to being experts in health, doctors need to respond to patients at a human level – offering 'support, empathy, concern and legitimation' (Roter 2000) to patients. This helps to build a rapport with the patient, and make them feel that they are being listened to and understood
- participatory – this implies that patients should take a responsible and active role in medical decision-making. The degree to which they are able to do this will be dependent on the patient's desire to be involved in their health care and the encouragement they receive from their doctor to do so.

Patients' agendas

The patients' agendas are their ideas, concerns and expectations. Agendas may include:

- Symptoms – the patient may have multiple symptoms, but through embarrassment or uncertainty about the significance of symptoms, may not mention all of them
- A request for a prescription/or a desire not to have a prescription – some patients may feel that a

prescription represents a positive step towards treating illness, others may feel a prescription treats the symptoms without addressing the cause of illness
- Previous self-treatment
- A request for diagnosis
- Theories about diagnosis
- Reporting of side-effects
- Worries about diagnosis or prognosis – patients often have questions about their health, or need clarifications, but feel unable to ask
- Social concerns.

Conflict in the doctor–patient relationship

As mentioned above, conflict may arise in a consultation due to different expectations – the doctor wishing to pursue biomedical goals, and the patient seeking the resolution of a social problem and a degree of reassurance. However, conflict may also be imposed on the relationship by a number of other factors:

- Competing demands of many patients for limited resources such as doctors' time
- The problem of uncertainty about diagnosis and treatment
- The knowledge that some diagnoses are unhelpful, and some treatments ineffective
- The conflict between the present and future interests of the patient, e.g. when should the doctor reveal a poor prognosis?
- The conflict between the patient's interests and those of his/her family or the state, e.g. whether to inform the DVLA about a newly diagnosed epileptic
- The inability to resolve social problems, such as damp housing, or problem neighbours, which lead to stress and the somatic symptoms
- The conflict with the doctor's other roles, e.g. the doctor's role as a mother and her responsibility to collect her children from nursery.

Resolving conflict in the doctor–patient relationship

- *Doctor's practice style*: The doctor's practice style can be described as doctor-centred or patient-centred. The doctor-centred style is paternalistic and is characterized by the use of closed questions, and active information gathering (e.g. 'do you have any pain?' and 'is the pain burning or stabbing?'). The patient may be interrupted and is expected to be passive. The consultation is limited to the medical problem the patient has and may not address any psychosocial concerns of the patient. By contrast, the patient-centred approach is characterized by open-ended questions (e.g. 'how do you feel?' and 'tell me about the pain'). The process requires greater patient participation and reflects a relationship of *mutuality*.
- *Influence of time*: Lack of time is often cited by doctors as hindering their attendance to the psychosocial

concerns of patients, and 'feeling hurried' is a reason given by patients for not mentioning all their symptoms (or sometimes their major complaint). However, a doctor's practice style may have more important influence on the content of consultations. By adopting a patient-centred approach (which does tend to take longer) doctors are more likely to fully understand the patient's perspective and provide a treatment that is acceptable to both parties. The suggestion has been made that by initially spending extra time with the patient, the doctor may reduce subsequent visits and increase compliance, so saving time in the long run, and benefiting the patient's health. It has also been suggested that a doctor's practice style, rather than length of consultation, is a better predictor of patient satisfaction and the eliciting of complete patient agendas.

- *Influence of structural context*: Consultations with the same patient may vary between the primary and secondary care settings. Patients may adopt a more passive role when seeing a specialist or in an acute setting, but prefer a more active role when consulting the GP. Private patients may be more demanding in their consultations, and their doctors, who are more reliant on the goodwill of the patient, may be more passive.
- *Patients' expectations and participation*: the role the patient takes may change as the consultation process goes on. It has been reported that patients who were passive in their first consultation had increased participation and were more critical by the third.
- *Communications skills*: Communications skills are important in eliciting information from patients in order to get a good history, discovering the patient's concerns, and in conveying information back to the patient about the cause of their illness and its proposed management. The following considerations may be of use in improving these aspects and in avoiding any misunderstanding (see also Fig. 7.7):
  - Removing physical barriers (such as desks) between the doctor and patient

---

Fig. 7.7 Categories of misunderstanding in relation to prescribing.

Britten et al. (2000) studied the sorts of misunderstandings in prescribing that occurred in general practice. Of 35 consultations, 28 had some degree of misunderstanding. The common reasons are outlined below:

1. Patient information remains unknown to the doctor, e.g.:
   a. The patient doesn't mention previous medical history (e.g. side-effects from a previously tried medication) wrongly believing the doctor is already aware of it
   b. The doctor has an inaccurate perception of what the patient wants (e.g. the doctor assumes the patient wants antibiotics, when in fact they merely want reassurance)
   c. The doctor is unaware that the patient is taking over-the-counter medication (either due to failure to ask, or active concealment)

2. Doctor information remains unknown to the patient, e.g.:
   a. Patient does not understand why they have been prescribed a certain medication and therefore takes it incorrectly or not at all
   b. Patient is unaware of the correct dose or is confused about the correct dose

3. Conflicting information given, e.g.:
   a. The patient is confused by receiving different information from the doctor and other sources, e.g. the hospital specialist or the pharmacist

4. Failure of communication about the doctor's diagnosis:
   a. The patient may not understand, remember or accept a diagnosis (e.g. a patient who was receiving two sorts of injections stops taking the wrong one, because he/she misunderstood which one the doctor had advised him/her to stop)
   b. The patient may not understand how treatment can be prescribed in the absence of a diagnosis

5. Relationship factors:
   a. The doctor may write a prescription, not because he thinks it is necessary, but in order to preserve a relationship (e.g. either because it is a repeat prescription by a partner in the practice the doctor does not wish to challenge, or in order to maintain a good relationship with the patient who desires a prescription)

The misunderstandings in prescribing tended to be associated with a patient's lack of participation in the consultation, and in many cases were based on inaccurate assumptions by both doctors and patients

From Britten N, Stevenson FA, Barry CA et al 2000 Misunderstandings in prescribing decisions in general practice. British Medical Journal 320: 485 (Box 1), with permission.

- Use of body language (maintaining eye contact, adopting a relaxed, but not too relaxed posture, appropriate facial expressions)
- Use of appropriate sounds, e.g. 'uh-huh'
- Using 'open-ended' questions
- Giving instructions and advice before other information – this is known as primary effect – people are more likely to remember the first bits of information they are given
- Use of simple, clear, specific instructions
- Repetition – this can be used to clarify parts of the history, or to ensure the patient is confident about how to take their medication
- Providing written information – booklets or leaflets that are relevant
- Asking if the patient has any questions.

Compliance and concordance

Alongside the shift in attitudes about the doctor–patient relationship, from doctor-centred to patient-centred, there has been a shift in the attitude towards those patients with differing agendas to those of their doctors.

Compliance has been described as 'following doctor's orders', and thus, non-compliance has been used to describe any behaviour that is seen as disobedient, for example not taking prescribed medication. Other terms such as adherence and cooperation have been used, but were also criticized for not being far away enough in meaning from compliance.

Qualitative studies have shown that the three main reasons for non-compliance are:

- lack of knowledge or understanding
- unpleasant side-effects from medication
- perceived or real stigma: feeling that taking the medicine isn't 'normal', so patient keeps testing out whether they can stop taking drug and become 'normal'.

In 1997, a report published by the Royal Pharmaceutical Society of Great Britain's working party on medicine-taking, recommended that 'concordance' should replace the term 'compliance'. Concordance is 'a process of prescribing and medicine-taking based on partnership' (Medicines Partnership 2003) between the doctor and the patient.

The need for this sort of approach has arisen subsequent to research showing that many people, especially those with chronic conditions, do not take their medicines as prescribed. Two-thirds of older patients prescribed statin for coronary artery disease will have given up treatment within 2 years, and half of people diagnosed with hypertension do not take the drugs that, as prescribed, may benefit their health. However, Misselbrook and Armstrong (2001) point out that the Medical Research Council trial of treatment of mild hypertension found that 850 patients had to be treated for 1 year for one patient to avoid a non-fatal stroke.

They ask whether mild hypertension should be treated, and who should decide? Heath (2003) points out that a concordance model does not necessarily mean that patients will follow medical advice, or indeed that they should be compelled by the weight of medical evidence.

COMMUNICATION

Compliance and concordance

- *Compliance* refers to a specific patient behaviour, namely did the patient do what was requested by the doctor?
- *Concordance* refers to a consultation process between a healthcare professional and a patient and is based on the ethos of a shared approach to decision-making rather than paternalism.

The advocates of concordance suggest that it is different from compliance, adherence and cooperation, in that it promotes a sharing of power in the doctor–patient relationship. Concordance recognizes the patient's expertise in their experience of illness and response to treatment. While this expertise is different from that of the clinician's, it is of equal relevance and value in terms of deciding on best management. The idea is that doctor and patient will embark on joint decision-making processes to reach a clinically effective treatment that is acceptable to the patient's beliefs, values and ideas about their disease. It is hoped that the ethos of concordance will lead to less drug wastage and fewer hospital admissions due to the iatrogenic effects of drugs.

HINTS AND TIPS

Establishing whether a patient is taking medications as prescribed, exploring their beliefs about their medication, and formulating a plan based on shared decision-making has been a regular theme in both undergraduate and postgraduate clinical examinations. Think about why the patient might want or not want to take a particular medicine, as well as why you want them to be on a particular treatment.

Joint decision-making of this sort requires certain competencies of both doctors and patients (Fig. 7.8). Joint decision-making of this kind is considered to be important (Cox et al. 2003) because it leads to:

- improved satisfaction with care
- increased knowledge of the condition and treatment
- increased adherence

Fig. 7.8 Competencies for doctors and patients to facilitate joint decision-making.

Competencies for doctors	Competencies for patients
1. Develop a partnership with the patient	1. Define (for oneself) the preferred doctor–patient relationship
2. Establish the patient's preferences for information (amount and format)	2. Find a doctor and establish, develop and adapt a partnership
3. Establish the patient's preference for the role in decision-making and any uncertainty	3. Articulate (for oneself) health problems, feelings, beliefs, and expectations in an objective and systematic manner
4. Ascertain and respond to patient's ideas, concerns and expectations	4. Communicate with the physician in order to understand and share relevant information clearly and at the appropriate time in the medical interview
5. Identify choices and evaluate the research evidence in relation to the individual patient	5. Access information
6. Present (or direct patient to) evidence, taking into account (2) and (3). Help patient to reflect on and assess the impact of alternative decisions with regard to his/her lifestyle and values	6. Evaluate information
7. Make or negotiate a decision in partnership with the patient and resolve any conflict	7. Negotiate decisions, give feedback, resolve conflict, agree on an action plan
8. Agree an action plan and complete arrangements for follow-up	

Towle A, Godolphin W 1999 Framework for teaching and learning informed shared decision making. British Medical Journal 319: 766–771, with permission.

- improved health outcomes
- fewer medication-related problems.

However, it has also been suggested that concordance may not be as successful as anticipated. It is reported that leaflets and other aids may increase satisfaction and knowledge but rarely improve physical outcome; even if patients are well informed, doctors may consider patients' decisions to be irrational. Patients tend to overestimate the risks of common complications; patients could not assess the meaning of outcome statistics and some patients have little interest in choice while others are too emotionally compromised.

Morgan (2008) comments that concordance is least problematic when there are several equally appropriate or effective treatments available from which the patient may choose according to personal preference, such as for treatment of menopausal or prostatic symptoms. Problems can arise when a patient demands a new and expensive or ineffective treatment where treatment is being allocated on the basis of cost-effectiveness. Problems may also arise when patients refuse potentially life-saving therapy, such as immunosuppressant medication following a transplant.

HOSPITALS AND PATIENTS

Over the last 30 years, the rates of hospital admission have increased, despite the reduction in the number of beds. This has been achieved by decreasing the length of stay in hospital of each patient, e.g. in 1984, repair of a groin hernia necessitated a stay of 5 days. It is now commonly done as day surgery. When patients are admitted to hospital, they may find themselves disempowered by the experience. Medical staff, by virtue of their technical expertise, good health and familiarity with the practices on the wards, are in a considerable position of power and authority over the patients. The experience is commonly a source of anxiety and stress, due to:

1. the fact that there is 'something wrong' with them that has necessitated their admission
2. a lack of familiarity and privacy on the wards
3. being disturbed (by other patients and staff)
4. lack of sleep
5. lack of information about their health
6. uncertainty about the process of care, procedures on the ward and which investigations will be necessary
7. uncertainty about the pain and risk involved in investigations and treatment
8. what to expect post-surgery – how long they will have to stay in hospital
9. concern about those at home
10. concern about employment and when they can get back to work.

Attempts to combat this negative experience include providing information about what to expect in hospital prior to admission. However, the experience of inpatient care gives rise not only to anxiety, but also to feelings of a *de-personalization* or loss of self-identity. This is due to:

- a loss of normal social roles
- the sense of being part of a 'batch' of patients being treated
- the general impersonal nature of medical procedures
- an institutionalized schedule – being told when to eat, when to get up, when visitors are allowed
- a lack of privacy and personal possessions.

Patients who remain in hospital for long periods of time may be at risk of 'institutionalization'. *Institutionalization* refers to the process by which patients in 'total institutions' (those where individuals are wholly separated from social interaction with the outside world, e.g. old-style psychiatric hospitals, monasteries and prisons) become apathetic and unable to make simple decisions for themselves. This was relatively common in long-stay psychiatric hospitals – and was one of the reasons for the development of 'care in the community' for people with mental disorders.

The psychological well-being of patients also impacts on their physical illness. If patients become anxious, stressed or depersonalized while in hospital, there is a risk that their recovery from their physical illness will be delayed. Patients' beliefs about their illness seem to influence recovery and rehabilitation on discharge from hospital: one study showed that the early identification of illness perception could improve patient outcome following a myocardial infarction.

HINTS AND TIPS

Remember: Assessing a patient's fitness for discharge home includes an assessment of whether they will cope at home and not just whether they are managing well in the institutional environment of a hospital. This is particularly important with frail and very elderly patients.

CHRONIC DISEASE

Chronic disease has been identified as an increasing problem for modern medicine. This is partly due to the ageing population, but also due to the success of medicine in averting death, but not always avoiding permanent injury. Chronic disease often requires a 'caring' approach rather than a 'curative' one. By its very nature, chronic disease is a long-term affliction, and as such has a profound influence on those who suffer with it. Chronic diseases include arthritis, heart disease, some forms of cancer, ulcerative colitis, psoriasis, dementia, multiple sclerosis, asthma and epilepsy. A chronic disease may or may not eventually be fatal, in fact the severity of many of the diseases mentioned fluctuates greatly,

both between sufferers and between days (or even hours) for the same sufferer.

Chronic disease poses a problem for Parsons' 'sick role' (see above), which expects the sick to want to get better and to only occupy the sick role temporarily. For the chronically ill, the 'sick role' must be modified slightly. Sufferers must maximize their ability to carry out social roles within the confines of their illness, and only be accepted to the 'sick role' when their capabilities drop below what they are usually able to do.

Study of the 'experience' of those living with chronic disease and their families has been undertaken since the 1980s in order to bring about a sound, effective and ethical approach to chronic illness. A few of the common problems experienced by the chronically ill and disabled are mentioned below (adapted from Locker 2008):

- *Uncertainty*: chronic disease can be shrouded in uncertainty. Symptoms may be present for many years before a definitive diagnosis is given (for example in multiple sclerosis). However, being given a diagnosis doesn't end the uncertainty. Patients (and doctors) may be unsure of how a disease will progress and at what speed. In addition symptoms may vary from day to day, with little rhyme or reason. One such disease is rheumatoid arthritis – pain level may vary throughout the day, often without a precipitating factor. The uncertainty means it is difficult to make even short-term plans, and living arrangements may need to be constantly revised.
- *Strained family relations*: often family members become carers for those who are chronically ill. The ability of individuals to cope with their role is varied and the carer (as well as the sufferer) may find themselves being excluded from their wider social contacts. Strain may also be placed on marital relationships. In a study of the effects of having a colostomy post rectal cancer, most individuals reported a loss of sexual capacity and a decline in the marital relationship.
- *Problems relating to self-esteem and identity*: the development of a chronic disease can lead to a fundamental rethinking of a person's biography and self-concept (Lawton 2003). This has been termed 'biographical disruption' by Bury (1982). Bury argues that such disruption can take place on many levels – including physical discomfort as well as a rethinking on one's mortality and existential sense. Charmaz (1983) outlined a similar perspective that describes a profound effect on the sense of self-worth, referred to as a loss of self', where individuals separate off the person they may have become as the disease progresses from a cherished view of how they were prior to the disability. Subsequent to the disruption and loss of an earlier conception of oneself comes the rebuilding of one's identity, which incorporates the chronic disease.

Williams (1984) refers to this as 'narrative reconstruction'. This describes the strategies people employ 'to create a sense of coherence, stability and order in the aftermath of the 'biographically disruptive' event of illness onset'. The view of oneself may become linked almost exclusively with that of the disease – to the exclusion of other social roles – so, a patient with multiple sclerosis views themselves as 'an MS sufferer' rather than a mother, a teacher, a theatre-goer or any other role she plays.

- *Problems relating to medical regimes:* patients with chronic diseases need to manage both their symptoms and their medical treatments on a daily basis. Often the treatment may be complicated, e.g. patients in renal failure who have dialysis, and time-consuming. Everyday life must be centred around the routine of medical treatment. This may prevent spontaneity and flexibility within the lifestyles of the chronically ill.
- *Unemployment and economic problems:* the most vulnerable groups in the face of chronic illness are those from low socioeconomic groups, ethnic minorities and women. Lower amounts of disposable income mean that individuals have fewer resources to support themselves through their disease. However, employment is important for reasons beyond simple economic benefit. Being able to be employed is significant in giving purpose and a focus for individuals and being 'included' in a social role may provide valuable benefits in terms of self-esteem.
- *Information, awareness and sharing:* information is a significant resource for the chronically ill. This may be about the disease from which they suffer, about the benefits they are entitled to, or coping strategies, or potential symptomatic treatments. The arena where such information sharing may occur is often a self-help group. The ability to meet others with the same disorder, and similar experiences, may also be beneficial.
- *Stigma and discrimination:* as discussed above.

Living with chronic illness

The ability to adapt to living with a chronic illness can be divided into three different components:

1. *Coping* – the cognitive processes of learning how to tolerate or put up with the effects of illness

2. *Strategies* – the actions people take, or what people do in the face of illness
3. *Style* – the way people respond to and present important features of their illnesses or treatment regimen.

Factors that may aid individuals with chronic disease include (Verbrugge & Jette 1994):

- Extra-individual factors:
  - Medical care and rehabilitation – surgery, physical therapy, speech therapy, counselling, health education, job retraining, etc.
  - Medication and other therapeutic regimens – drugs, recreational therapy, aquatic exercise, biofeedback meditation, rest/energy conservation, etc.
  - External supports – personal assistance, special equipment and devices, day care, respite care, meals-on-wheels, etc.
  - Build, physical and social environment – structural modifications at home or work, access to buildings and public transport, health insurance and access to medical care, laws and regulations, employment legislation, social attitudes, etc.
- Intra-individual factors:
  - Lifestyle and behaviour changes – overt changes to alter disease activity and impact
  - Psychosocial attributes and coping – positive affect, emotional vigour, locus of control, cognitive adaptation to disability, personal support, peer support groups, etc.
  - Activity accommodations – changes in kinds of activities, ways of doing them, frequency or length of time doing them.

Chronic disease is often associated with a degree of impairment in functioning. How this relates to terms like disability and handicap is set out by the International Classification of Impairments, Disabilities and Handicaps (ICIDH) (Fig. 7.9). Crucial to the ICIDH definitions is the idea that handicaps are disadvantages that are not inherent in the individuals, rather they are imposed by the environment. However, the ICIDH definitions have been criticized for using the term 'handicap', which to many is considered a pejorative term.

Disability campaigners over the past 20 years have advocated a theory known as the 'social model of disability'. This approach stands in contrast to the 'medical model of disability', which sees disabilities and handicaps as directly and inevitably derived from impairments. The social model of disability states that:

- disabled people are an oppressed social group
- there is a difference between the impairments people have and the oppression they experience
- 'disability' can be defined as the social oppression, not the form of impairment

Fig. 7.9 International Classification of Impairments, Disabilities and Handicaps (ICIDH) definitions.

Impairment	Any loss or abnormality of psychological, physiological or anatomical structure or function, e.g. osteoarthritis causing painful, stiff joints
Disability	A restriction or lack (resulting from an impairment) of ability to perform an activity in a manner or within the range considered normal for a human being, e.g. difficulty climbing stairs
Handicap	A disadvantage for a given individual, resulting from an impairment or a disability, that limits or prevents the fulfilment of a role that is normal (depending on age, sex and social and cultural factors) for that individual, e.g. an inability to access certain buildings within the community with steps – thus perhaps being unable to visit certain cinemas, libraries, banks and so on

This model describes disability as something imposed upon those with impairments by unnecessarily isolating and excluding them from full participation in society. Disability is the 'social situation' encountered by people with impairments. The importance of this model is two-fold: 1) it identifies the proper approach to disability as being the removal of those barriers that prevent people with impairments from fully participating in society, rather than the previous medicalized approach, which was to cure and 'normalize' impairments and 2) it liberates and empowers the disabled community by locating fault with society rather than with disabled individuals.

However, the social model of disability has been criticized on the following grounds:

1. The denial of the link between physical impairment and social disability has been overstated – denying that disabled people are not also people with impairments is to ignore a major part of the biographies of disabled people.
2. Emphasis on criticizing the need for a 'cure', as stated by the medical model, has led to some disabled groups opposing measures designed to 'normalize' their conditions or maximize their function. For example, the refusal of artificial limbs for amputees and hearing aids for the hearing impaired. This has led to certain conditions having a greater impact on people's lives than might otherwise have been the case.
3. The social model is too rigid in creating an artificial distinction between disability and impairment – the two can be seen as part of a continuum.
4. Some impairments cannot be helped by the removal of environmental or social barriers (e.g. phantom limb pain and significant intellectual impairment).

Disability legislation

In 1995, the Disability Discrimination Act was passed, which begins to address many of the social issues identified in the social model of disability (see www.disability.gov.uk).

DEATH AND BEREAVEMENT

The way in which death is perceived is determined by personal and cultural factors. In an increasingly secular culture, death is seen as a finality, beyond which there is no existence. However, many religions agree in some sort of afterlife, be it reincarnation or a spiritual paradise. In some traditional societies, it is believed that the dead do not really die, at least not in a social sense, rather they remain as an invisible spirit that is still a member of the family and can help, protect, hinder or punish those who continue to survive in an earthly way.

Our perception of death changes as we age. Young children see death as a sleep or departure, not understanding the finality of death until about the age of 7. Children are at first matter of fact and then fearful of corpses. The perception and understanding of death within Western culture is one that tends to incorporate feelings of loss, separation, pain and punishment.

One hundred years ago, less than 10% of people died in hospitals. It is thought that about 75% of people now die (in the UK) in institutions such as hospitals, hospices and nursing homes. The general trend has been for death and the process of dying to be removed from the public domain. Part of the reason for this is the greater ability of medical technology to prolong life; as a result, the process of dying is more drawn out, leading to 'slow deaths'. Figure 7.10 compares slow dying in the modern era with 'quick deaths' in the pre-modern era.

The stages of dying

The typical stages of dying were described in 1969 by Elizabeth Kubler-Ross, an American psychiatrist:

1. *Denial and isolation*: on being told they are dying, patients may enter a state of shock, expressing feelings like, 'It can't be me'. Denial is usually a temporary defence, although it can be sustained. Patients may 'shop around' for a more positive second opinion. A deep feeling of isolation is 'normal' at this stage.
2. *Anger*: shock may be replaced by feelings of anger, resentment and rage. The medical staff – often the nurses – may be subjected to outbursts of 'Why me?' and Why can't you help me?'

Fig. 7.10 A comparison of death and the process of dying in the 'modern' and 'pre-modern' eras.

Conditions facilitating a 'quick death'	Conditions facilitating a 'slow death'
Low level of medical technology	High level of medical technology
Late detection of disease – or fatality-producing condition	Early detection of disease – or fatality-producing condition
Simple definition of death (e.g. cessation of heart beat)	Complex definition of death (e.g. irreversible cessation of higher brain activity)
High incidence of mortality from acute disease	High incidence of mortality from chronic or degenerative disease
High incidence of fatality-producing injuries	Low incidence of fatality-producing injuries
Customary killing or suicide of, or fatal passivity towards, the person once he or she has entered the 'dying' category	Customary curative and activist orientation toward the dying with a high value placed on the prolongation of life

Lofland L 1978 The Craft of Dying: the Modern Face of Death. Beverly Hills: Sage (as reprinted in Scambler G 2003 Dying, death and bereavement. In: Scambler G (ed.) Sociology as Applied to Medicine, 5th edn. Edinburgh: Saunders, p. 93)

3. *Bargaining*: the terminally ill may attempt to negotiate with caregivers or God. They may endeavour to be a 'good' patient in order that the doctor might extend their lives.
4. *Depression*: as patients confront their fate, their anger or shock may give way to depression; it may be reactive – to the condition, or preparatory – based on the impending loss of life itself.
5. *Acceptance*: dying patients may find a sort of peace, an acknowledgement of the inevitability of death. At this stage, the family may need more help, support and understanding than the patient.

Kubler–Ross' model rapidly gained acceptance, according to some, because it filled a void in healthcare theory and re-awakened the topic of dying that had previously been taboo. However, it was criticized because it assumed too mechanistic an approach, with the dying person moving through all five stages in one direction, while the experience of those caring for the dying suggested an oscillation between periods of calm, fear, hope, depression, anger and withdrawal. It also focussed on the psychological aspects of dying, at the expense of physical and spiritual dimensions.

Subsequent authors have modified the stages model of dying by increasing the mixture of emotions and responses exhibited by a person facing death (Fig. 7.11) and marking a patient's progress by the resolution of these emotions, rather than their change. However, this model still suffers from the criticism that it focusses only on the psychological aspects of dying.

Corr (1992) developed a theory that states that individuals who are dying confront tasks in four dimensions of coping with death. These are:

- *Physical*: satisfying bodily needs – such as thirst and pain
- *Psychological*: this includes maximizing psychological security and autonomy

Fig. 7.11 Three-stage model of dying.

Initial stage facing the threat'	Chronic stage 'being ill'	Final stage 'acceptance'
Fear Anxiety Shock Disbelief Anger Denial Guilt Humour Hope Despair Bargaining	Resolution of those elements of the initial response that are resolvable Diminution of intensity of all emotions Depression	Defined by patient's acceptance of death Not an essential state provided that the patient is not distressed, is communicating normally and is making decisions normally

Buckman R 1993 Communication in palliative care: a practical guide. In: Doyle D, Hanks GWC, McDonald N (eds) Oxford Textbook of Palliative Medicine. Oxford: Oxford Medical.

- *Social*: this includes sustaining and enhancing interpersonal attachments of significance to the person, and addressing the social implications of dying; for example, wanting to know that dependants will be cared for after their death
- *Spiritual*: for many people, identifying and reaffirming a sense of spirituality may foster hope or bring reassurance.

Corr maintained that individuals have unique circumstances leading to unique tasks they must cope with in each of these dimensions. The advantage of this model of dying is that it encompasses different aspects of the process rather than focussing on the psychological aspect alone. However, its generality and lack of empirical data limit its usefulness.

The Debate of the Age Health and Care Study Group (Age Concern 1999) produced the following principles necessary for a 'good death':

- To know when death is coming, and to understand what can be expected
- To be able to retain control of what happens
- To be afforded dignity and privacy
- To have control over pain relief and also symptom control
- To have choice and control over where death occurs (at home or elsewhere)
- To have access to information and expertise of whatever kind is necessary
- To have access to any spiritual or emotional support required
- To have access to hospice care in any location, not only in hospital
- To have control over who is present and who shares the end
- To be able to issue advance directives that ensure wishes are respected
- To have time to say goodbye, and control over other aspects of timing
- To be able to leave when it is time to go, and not to have life prolonged pointlessly.

Place of death

As mentioned earlier, over the past 100 years there has been an increasing trend in dying outside the home. This has led to a situation where most people die in hospitals or other institutions. Each location has certain advantages and disadvantages associated with it.

At home

To many, the home remains the proper and natural place to die. Dying at home may be more costly and physically and emotionally demanding for carers. For this reason it requires good communication between hospital services and the carers. Additional support, in the form of respite care, meals on wheels, and Macmillan nurses may be welcomed.

In a hospice

This accounts for around only 4% of deaths. The hospice philosophy is one that concentrates on promoting quality of life over prolonging life. Dying in a hospice may bring reduced levels of anxiety and depression when compared with similar care in hospitals – this may be due to a culture of frank and honest communication.

In a hospital

Hospitals have not historically been especially quick to have wards dedicated solely to the treatment of the terminally ill, fearing the stigma that may be attached to such 'death wards'. However, this has led to some terminally ill patients dying on busy general wards, which is unsatisfactory for all patients, families and staff. One study has demonstrated that many patients' symptoms are not adequately controlled, and many received inadequate nursing care. Furthermore, terminally ill patients may receive only minimal care from senior medical and nursing staff on general wards.

In retirement villages

In North America, retirement villages have been set up and some have been associated with specialist nursing facilities that are available to those requiring terminal care. This sort of facility has allowed elderly residents to talk among themselves about death, and has enabled a shared perspective and collective concern to develop. Residents feel a greater degree of control over the process of dying. It differs from traditional nursing homes, where the dying person is isolated from other residents.

Awareness of dying

Glaser and Strauss (1965) described four different types of 'awareness context' in the management of dying patients in San Francisco Bay area hospitals in the 1960s. These were:

1. *Closed awareness*: where patients were kept ignorant of their impending death by staff and family alike
2. *Suspicion awareness*: where patients had begun to suspect that they were dying and had tried to obtain confirmation of this suspicion from both staff and relatives
3. *Mutual pretence*: where all parties knew that the patient was dying, but no-one acknowledged this fact
4. *Open awareness*: where all parties knew that the patient was dying and were able to talk about dying.

Since the 1960s, there has been a progressive move away from the closed awareness context towards one of open awareness. Open awareness is now seen as a prerequisite for a 'good death'. There is a general consensus that honesty within the medical consultation is necessary, even when the patient has a terminal disease.

Outcomes of open awareness

For the patient:

- Better information and communication from staff
- Psychological support
- Participation in decisions about care
- Increased self-esteem
- Decreased anxiety
- Preparation for death
- Acceptance.

For relatives/carers:

- More honest relationship with the patient
- Easier communication with patient and staff
- Better bereavement outcomes.

For the doctors and nurses:

- Easier interaction with the patient
- Shared decision-making
- Less anxiety, guilt, stress that accompany deceiving the patient
- Being able to stop inappropriate treatments.

In the past decade or so, the concept of *conditional open awareness* has developed. This stresses that disclosure can take place over a period of time and that full disclosure of terminal prognoses is conditional on what is desirable for particular patients. Some individuals may not wish to discuss their terminal prognosis. Conditional open awareness is characterized by a shared approach to confronting death, or if the patient wishes to do so, denying a terminal prognosis. The aim is to act in such a way as to produce a positive psychological outcome for the patient.

Bereavement and loss

One-quarter of GP consultations have been identified as relating to some type of loss – these include separations, incapacitation, bereavement and job loss. Any loss can lead to a detrimental effect on physical and mental health. A major bereavement, such as the death of a spouse or child, can increase the risk of death from heart disease and suicide as well as increasing the likelihood of anxiety and depression.

Even though mourning can be expressed in a variety of ways, there is still a pattern to grieving, and it can make sense to talk of a 'normal pattern of grief'. Worden (1991) outlines a number of tasks that need to be achieved in the course of mourning if it is to be completed:

- Task I: To accept the reality of the loss – the bereaved is initially shocked, and may experience numbness, disbelief or relief at the death.

COMMUNICATION

Bereavement and patterns of expressed grief

The pattern of mourning varies from community to community. For some Greek-Cypriots, there is a 'socially patterned period of weeping and wailing', followed by a defined period of mourning and wearing black. In Orthodox Jewish communities, there is a prescribed timetable to mourning – in the first 7 days, the bereaved remain at home and are visited by consolers. Mourning dress is worn for 30 days, and recreation and amusement are forbidden for 1 year.

- Task II: To work through the pain of grief – the bereaved may experience anger, sadness, guilt, anxiety, regret, insomnia and even transient auditory or visual hallucinations of the deceased.

Fig. 7.12 Risk factors for poor outcome of bereavement.

Predisposing factors
Ambivalent or dependent relationship with the person who died
Multiple prior bereavements
Previous mental illness, especially depression
Low self-esteem of bereaved person
Age and sex of bereaved person – older widowers are at greater risk than widows and younger individuals. Similarly, the death of a parent is associated with greater risk if the bereaved person is still a child or adolescent, as opposed to an older individual, with their own family
Around the time of death
Sudden and unexpected death
Untimely death of a young person
Deaths due to suicide/murder/manslaughter
Stigmatized death: such as AIDS
After death
Level of perceived social support, e.g. an absent or unhelpful family
Lack of opportunities for new interests
Stress from other life crises

Source: *Based on Sheldon 1998.*

- Task III: To adjust to an environment in which the deceased is missing – this may be characterized by despair and a loss of direction. The bereaved may perceive themselves as helpless, inadequate and childlike.
- Task IV: To emotionally relocate the deceased and move on with life – during this phase, the bereaved may start to develop new relationships and interests. The deceased is no longer central in the bereaved person's emotional life.

There is evidence that losses can help to foster maturity and personal growth; however, there are a number of factors that are associated with a poor outcome (Fig. 7.12).

Key questions

- Define illness, disease, sickness and predicaments.
- What factors are important in the evaluation of symptoms?
- What is the function of self-help groups?
- Why do you think the use of alternative medicine has been increasing?
- What is the 'sick role'?
- What is 'labelling'?

- What characterizes a 'patient-centred consultation'?
- How can communication skills be improved?
- Define compliance and concordance.
- Why is hospital admission associated with anxiety and stress?
- What sorts of problems are experienced by people with chronic illness?
- How do impairment, disability and handicap differ?
- What is the 'social model of disability'?
- What are the 'stages of dying'?

References

Alonzo, A., Reynolds, N., 1995. Stigma, HIV and AIDS: an exploration and elaboration of a stigma strategy. Social Sciences in Medicine 41, 303–315.

Armstrong, D., 1989. An Outline of Sociology as Applied to Medicine, third ed. Wright, London.

Armstrong, D., 2003. Outline of Sociology as Applied to Medicine, fifth ed. Arnold, London.

Banks, M.H., Beresford, S.A., Morrell, D., et al., 1975. Factors influencing demand for primary medical care in women aged 20–44. Int. J. Epidemiol. 4, 189–195 (as reproduced in Armstrong D 2003 Outline of Sociology as Applied to Medicine, fifth ed. London: Arnold).

Blaxter, M., 1990. Health and Lifestyles. Tavistock/Routledge, London.

Boorse, C., 1975. On the distinction between disease and illness. Philos. Public Aff. 5, 49–68.

Boorse, C., 1976. What a theory of mental health should be. J. Theory Social Behav. 6, 61–85.

Britten, N., Stevenson, F.A., Barry, C.A., et al., 2000. Misunderstandings in prescribing decisions in general practice: qualitative study. Br. Med. J. 320, 484–488.

Bury, M., 1982. Chronic illness as biographical disruption. Sociol. Health Illn. 4, 167–182.

Charmaz, K., 1983. Loss of self: a fundamental form of suffering in the chronically ill. Sociol. Health Illn. 5, 168–195 (as reported by Nettleton S 1995 The Sociology of Health and Illness. Cambridge: Polity Press, p. 87).

Corr, C.A., 1992. A task based approach to coping with dying. Omega 24 (2), 81–94 (as reproduced in Copp G 1998 A review of current theories of death and dying. J. Adv. Nurs. 28(2): 382–390).

Cox, K., et al., 2003. A systematic review of communication between patients and health care professionals about medicine-taking and prescribing. GKT Concordance Unit, King's College, London (as quoted in Weiss M, Britten N 2003 What is concordance? Pharma. J. 271: 493).

Damen, S., Mortelmans, D., Hove, E., 2000. Self-help groups in Belgium: their place in the care network. Sociol. Health Illn. 22 (3), 331–348.

Age Concern, 1999. Debate of the Age Health and Care Study Group 1999. The Future of Health and Care of Older People: The Best is Yet to Come. Age Concern, London.

Glaser, B., Strauss, A., 1965. Awareness of Dying. Aldine, Chicago.

Goffman, E., 1963. Stigma: Notes on the Management of Spoiled Identity. Penguin, London.

Hannay, D., 1988. Lecture Notes on Medical Sociology. Blackwell Scientific, Oxford.

Heath, I., 2003. A wolf in sheep's clothing: a critical look at the ethics of drug-taking. BMJ 327, 856.

Kubler-Ross, E., 1969. On Death and Dying. Macmillan, New York.

Lawton, J., 2003. Lay experiences of health and illness: past research and future agendas. Sociol. Health Illn. 25, 26–27.

Locker, D., 2008. Living with chronic illness. In: Scambler, G. (Ed.), Sociology as Applied to Medicine, sixth ed. Saunders Elsevier, Edinburgh.

Mead, N., Bower, P., 2002. Patient-centred consultations and outcomes in primary care: a review of the literature. Patient Educ. Couns. 48, 51–61.

Mechanic, D., 1978. Medical Sociology. The Free Press, New York.

Mechanic, D., Volkart, E.H., 1960. Illness behaviour and medical diagnosis. J. Health Hum. Behav. 1, 86–94.

Medicines Partnership, What is concordance? Online. Available at: http://www.medicines-partnership.org/aboutus/concordance (accessed 20th October 2003).

Misselbrook, D., Armstrong, D., 2001. Patients' response to risk information about the benefits of treating hypertension. Br. J. Gen. Pract. 51, 276–279.

Morgan, M., 2008. The doctor-patient relationship. In: Scambler, G. (Ed.), Sociology as Applied to Medicine. sixth ed. Saunders Elsevier, Edinburgh, p. 55.

Parsons, T., 1951. The Social System. Free Press, Glencoe, IL (as quoted by Morgan M, In: Scambler G (ed.) 2003 Sociology as Applied to Medicine, fifth ed. Edinburgh: Saunders).

Roter, D., 2000. The enduring and evolving nature of the patient-physician relationship. Patient Educ. Couns. 39 (5–15), 8.

Royal Pharmaceutical Society of Great Britain, 1997. From compliance to concordance: towards shared goals in medicine taking. RPS, London.

Scambler, G., 2003. Deviance, sick role and stigma. In: Scambler, G. (Ed.), Sociology as Applied to Medicine, sixth ed. Saunders Elsevier, Edinburgh, pp. 205–220.

Scambler, G., Hopkins, A., 1986. Being epileptic: coming to terms with stigma. Sociol. Health Illn. 8, 26–43 (as reported in Scambler G 2003 Deviance, sick role and stigma. In: Scambler G (ed.) Sociology as Applied to Medicine, fifth ed. Edinburgh: Saunders, p. 196).

Sheldon, 1998. ABC of palliative care: bereavement. Br. Med. J. 316, 456–458.

Toon, P.D., 1981. Defining 'disease' – classification must be distinguished from evaluation. J. Med. Ethics 7, 197–201.

Towle, A., Godolphin, W., 1999. Framework for teaching and learning informed shared decision making. Br. Med. J. 319, 766–771.

Verbrugge, L.M., Jette, A.M., 1994. The disablement process. Soc. Sci. Med. 38, 1–14 (as reproduced in Locker D 2008

Living with chronic illness. In: Scambler D (ed.) An Outline of Sociology as Applied to Medicine, sixth ed. Edinburgh: Saunders Elsevier).

Williams, G., 1984. The genesis of chronic illness: narrative reconstruction. Sociol. Health Illn. 6, 175–200.

Worden, J.W., 1991. Grief Counselling and Grief Therapy. Routledge, London.

Zborowski, M., 1952. Cultural components in response to pain. Journal of Social Issues 8, 16–30.

Zola, I., 1973. Pathways to the doctor: from person to patient. Soc. Sci. Med. 7, 677–889 (as reported in Scambler G 2003

Health and illness behaviour. In: Scambler G (ed.) Sociology as Applied to Medicine, fifth ed. Edinburgh: Saunders).

Further reading

Barry, C., et al., 2000. Patients' unvoiced agendas in general practice consultations: qualitative study. Br. Med. J. 320, 1246–1250.

Scambler, G. (Ed.), 2008. Sociology as Applied to Medicine, sixth ed. Saunders Elsevier, Edinburgh.

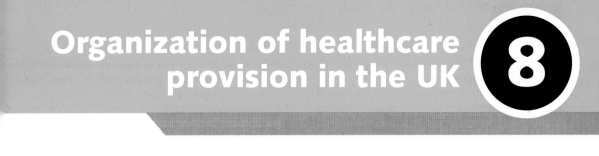
This chapter considers the strengths and weaknesses of the UK National Health Service. Beyond passing exams, it is important for medical students and doctors to understand how health care is provided. This understanding is improved by considering how health care was provided in the UK prior to the NHS, as well as alternatives to a UK-style NHS.

BEFORE THE NHS

Prior to the National Health Service (NHS) there were several elements to healthcare provision in the UK:

- General practitioners (GPs) – mainly for those who could afford them, were also part of insurance schemes, e.g. the Friendly Societies (non-profit-making, mutual benefit organizations) or were affiliated with trade unions.
- Hospitals – primarily used by the poor. They were either *voluntary* (run by charitable foundations) or *municipal* (local authority) hospitals. The latter provided services for the more chronic illnesses.
- Public health and community health services (CHS) – aimed to improve the water supplies and sewerage. Eventually, they attempted to control and treat infectious diseases. Public health and CHS (and housing) were under the control of the local authorities, not health services, and this continued until the early 1970s.

Another crucial aspect to remember is that, in the nineteenth century, hospitals were considered very dangerous places owing to the lack of anaesthesia and aseptic techniques. For those who could afford it, a fee-for-service consultation with a qualified practitioner in the surgery or at home was possible. Friendly Societies (see above) and trade unions allowed other groups, e.g. skilled workers, to use GPs.

The same period also saw the *Poor Law* system being practised. The 'poor laws' were enacted at the time of Queen Elizabeth I and represented the oldest form of government intervention in welfare. The poor laws catered for the needs of the very poorest people and the unemployed. However, patients had to be 'deservingly poor' to qualify for treatment. Even though the standards of these hospitals rose in the 1930s when they were taken on by local authority health departments, their status always remained low, owing to their origins.

NATIONAL HEALTH INSURANCE

In 1911, the UK government took over and extended the role of the Friendly Societies by introducing a 'National Health Insurance' (NHI) scheme for GP services. Insurance premiums were paid to the government in the form of deductions from pay packets; these premiums then funded general practice cover for that person. Workers who earned under £160/year had to insure themselves by paying fourpence; the employer paid threepence; and general taxation paid twopence (The Prime Minister at the time called it the 'ninepence for fourpence'). The NHI scheme covered manual workers between the ages of 16 and 65 years and also provided funds for sickness, accident and disability benefits in cash. Hospital and specialist care were not included. National healthcare services were extended to all the population in 1948 when the NHS came into being. With the inception of the NHS, the government moved from being the organizer of the insurance system to being the provider of healthcare services to all citizens as a civic right.

THE BIRTH OF THE NHS

During the Second World War, it emerged that the state could have a positive impact on the lives of its people by intervening in many areas of public life. All hospitals had been brought under state control as part of the Emergency Medical Service. The landmark Beveridge Report (1942) established the principles for a postwar 'welfare state'. In 1944, the Ministry of Health set out its plans for a comprehensive health service. After a series of negotiations between the government and the

> **Fig. 8.1** Key features of the NHS.
>
> Free at the point of use
> Open to the whole population purely on the basis of healthcare need
> Equality in provision of health services irrespective of means, age, sex and occupation
> Funded almost entirely by general taxation revenues collected by the government

British Medical Association (BMA), the National Health Service Act 1946, created the NHS in 1948 (Fig. 8.1).

Interestingly, the financial estimates that were put to Parliament along with the White Paper setting up the NHS anticipated a fall in the cost of the NHS, based on the assumptions of effective health promotion and improved public health leading to improved health of the population.

Evolution

The NHS has proved to be a fairly dynamic system undergoing continuous reform, particularly since the 1970s. Its ultimate goal has always been to improve the quality of patient care.

Its changes can be divided into *three* phases:

1. *Hierarchical (1948–1979)* – totalitarian control by officials and politicians (and, some would argue, senior doctors) at a national level. A classic example of 'top-down' regulation
2. *Market (1979–1997)* – introduction of market mechanism, dividing purchasers from providers and encouraging the competitive tendering of support services, e.g. cleaning
3. *Network (1997–present)* – amalgamating the pros and cons of (a) and (b) above. Encouraging collaborations and partnerships within the system (Fig. 8.2).

Current organization

This chapter is based on the organization of the NHS in England. There are variations in other areas of the UK. The organization of the NHS is based on giving the primary care organizations (PCOs) greater freedom to make the purchasing decisions for local health services. All GPs are members of PCOs. It also strives to streamline the system overall, while being user-friendly for the patient (Fig. 8.3).

The NHS has several strengths and weaknesses. These need to be understood so that as decision-makers of the future, we know what areas to tackle (Fig. 8.4).

Fig. 8.2 Chronological list of landmark events in the shaping of the NHS.

Period	Problems	Solutions
1948–1974	Divisions between GPs, local authority health services and teaching hospitals	More integrated structure with regional health authorities overseeing area health authorities so correct dispatch of finances to hospitals and community health services
	Inequalities in the geographical distribution of hospital beds and staff requirements	GPs remained independent
	Rising expenditure relative to conservative estimates	*Hospital plan for England and Wales* proposed the creation of a modern district general hospital (DGH) that could treat 250 000 people
		Charges introduced for spectacles, dentures and prescriptions
1982–1987	Difficult for central government to set policy, oversee expenditure and monitor performance	Single general manager appointed at every level in the NHS with power to undertake executive decisions over the resources they managed
		Quantitative performance indicators (PIs) introduced
1988	Demand greater than supply	Increased general taxation
	Inadequate funding resulting in poor maintenance of infrastructure, low staff pay and lowering standard of care	
	Increasing waiting lists	
1989–1990	Funding crisis continues	*Community Care Act* 1990 became law
		Internal market introduced to separate the roles of purchaser and provider
		New GP contract giving autonomy to larger GP practices
		Medical audit made compulsory for both hospitals and GPs
		Health authorities streamlined
		Increase in the number of managers to increase efficiency

Fig. 8.2 Chronological list of landmark events in the shaping of the NHS—cont'd.

Period	Problems	Solutions
1991–1997	Poor implementation of internal market Too much control by central government	'New Labour' elected in 1997 – tried to find an intermediate ground between market forces and socialism
1997–2000	Too much emphasis on *quantity* rather than *quality* of health care Internal market getting chaotic	A new system based on 'partnership' and 'collaboration' Regional autonomy – separate White Papers introduced for England, Ireland, Wales and Scotland Individual funding for GP practices abolished, instead they got their funding from their local Primary Care Group (PCG) or Primary Care Trust (PCT) National Institute for Clinical Excellence (NICE) set up in 1999 to assess the best available evidence on the effectiveness and cost-effectiveness of treatments, drugs and technologies (old and new) and to produce official guidance on whether they should be funded as part of the NHS Commission for Health Improvement (CHI) set up in 2000 to monitor and improve the quality of NHS services
2000–2012	Lack of modernization Waiting lists increasing Varying public confidence	Making the NHS more receptive to the needs of its users Establishment of NHS Direct and NHS walk-in centres Setting NHS plan performance targets Public–private partnerships encouraged 'Choose and book' system allows patients to choose (within limits which hospital they are referred to (this includes a number of non-NHS facilities)
2012	An economic depression in the UK, Europe and the USA Lack of access to GPs Lack of choice over long-term treatment and residential care	The Heath and Social Care Act 2012 aims to reduce costs by reducing a layer of management (abolishing PCTs) and making groups of GPs (commissioning consortia) responsible for local funding decisions Government plans to remove geographical boundaries for access to a GP. Access to most types of health care based on which GP patients are registered with rather than where they live Proposed personal budgets for patients, who might be allowed to choose how their personal allocation is spent

A major issue that continues to confront the NHS is the imbalance that occurs between healthcare funding and usage. This has possibly been exaggerated by what Heath (2008) called the 'credibility gap', where governments promise services and quality standards without considering the context or providing additional resources. The result, according to Heath, is that patients are ever more demanding while healthcare professionals become less vocational and more business-orientated.

One of the main demands on the NHS, which appears to be increasing, relates to an ageing population in the UK. It is estimated that one-third of all men aged between 50 and 65 years old do not work. This is due partly to early retirement and pension incentives or to employer-based age discrimination. Furthermore, the all-cause death rates have decreased in the last 20 years. People are living longer. According to the government's own estimates, the number of people aged 65 years or older will double by the year 2036. NHS services to people in this age group account for a large proportion of NHS resources.

Inevitably, there will be increased spending by the government. However, the birth-rate has also been declining, meaning that there will be fewer young people entering the job market. If current trends continue, there will be a shortage of future taxpayers relative to the elderly. Other sources of finance will have to be sought apart from possible increases in general taxation.

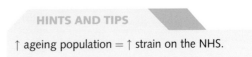

HINTS AND TIPS

↑ ageing population = ↑ strain on the NHS.

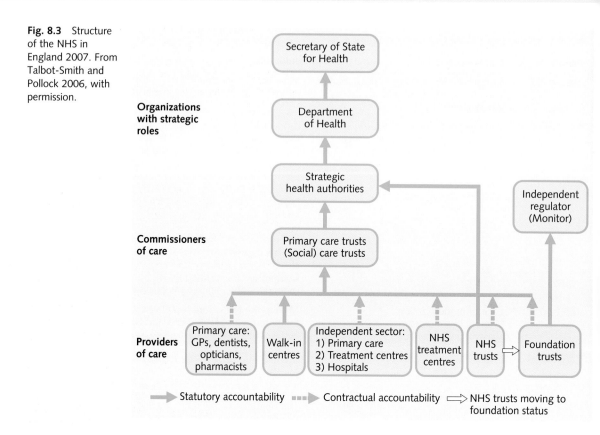

Fig. 8.3 Structure of the NHS in England 2007. From Talbot-Smith and Pollock 2006, with permission.

Fig. 8.4 Positives and negatives of the NHS today.

Positives	Negatives
Wide public support	Lack of receptiveness to the needs of the patient coupled with lack of choice
Control of general spending while providing beneficial social programmes	Professionals still regulate the service
Good value for money	Increased demand for greater spending budget has not increased proportionately to demand or in line with other European countries
Many services available with few user charges	Fewer healthcare professionals – doctors, nurses, etc.
Services based on demand	Restricted access to latest drugs and technology
General taxation provides finance	Large discrepancy between quality and availability of specific services
Fair allocation of resources to different parts of the country	Parallel privately financed companies may compromise the fairness of the NHS in providing health care
Excellent primary care via GPs	Interference by ministers in the fine details of healthcare management
Competent staff because of high-quality? clinical training	Less easy to access specialists
High degree of coordination	Variability of experience among GPs
	Initial assessment in hospitals often conducted by junior and inexperienced doctors
	Relative lack of responsiveness

OTHER SYSTEMS FOR ORGANIZING AND FUNDING HEALTH CARE

Funding and provision of health care varies greatly in different countries. Over the course of the twentieth century, governments have taken an active role in trying to provide the best possible health services. Patients also have individual rights and expectations of their healthcare system.

According to Fitzpatrick (2003) and Field (1973), healthcare systems can be divided into four categories (Fig. 8.5):

1. The pluralistic health system, e.g. USA
   a. several non-integrated methods of providing funds, e.g. insurance, fee-for-service, etc.
   b. healthcare facilities owned by private groups or the state.
2. The health insurance system, e.g. Canada, USA and Japan
   a. third party gathers resources in the form of compulsory insurance.
3. The health service system, e.g. UK and Sweden
   a. the state owns *most* facilities
   b. independence of doctors, despite the fact that they receive most of their income from the government.
4. The socialized health system, e.g. the former USSR
   a. the state owns *all* facilities
   b. nearly all healthcare professionals are employed by the government.

HEALTH PROFESSIONS

A vast number of professional groups provide health care in modern Britain. These include hospital doctors, nurses, radiographers, GPs, community nurses, care assistants, pharmacists and social workers, to name but a few. With so many professionals looking after the patient, there are bound to be problems, such as misunderstandings, poor communication, mistrust and sometimes conflict.

Health professions and multidisciplinary working

The medical profession as we currently know it in the UK, historically began as three different types of practitioner: physicians, surgeons and apothecaries. Physicians needed to have a university degree in medicine and had to be members of the Royal College of Physicians. A physician was not allowed to cut into the body, but had to direct a surgeon to do so. Surgeons were trained by apprenticeship, and had to be members of the Royal College of Surgeons (for a discussion of what the Royal Colleges do today, see Chapter 2). Apothecaries made the medicines which the physicians prescribed but were not allowed to give medical advice. From 1815, apothecaries were obliged to obtain a licence from the Worshipful Society of Apothecaries (this involved 6 months of hospital experience as well as courses in pharmacy and medicine). During the eighteenth century, 22 different licensing bodies allowed individuals to practise medicine. Conflict arose between the different groups of practitioners, all of whom wanted the right to practice independently and to regulate 'official' healthcare provision. In 1858, the *Medical Registration Act* created the General Medical Council (GMC), and united doctors into a single professional group. Even towards the end of the twentieth century, however, doctors could qualify for practice in three ways: a medical degree, a conjoint diploma from the Royal Colleges of Physicians and

Fig. 8.5 The advantages and disadvantages of different healthcare systems.

System	Advantages	Disadvantages
Pluralistic	Closest to a market-driven system	Lack of access – many people cannot afford it Medical monopoly resulting in increased cost Individual access and lack of public-health initiatives
Health insurance	Easier access to private medical care Reduced waiting time Access to leading specialists	Insurance policies favour the use of cheaper medical procedures Premiums may vary according to age Not all medical procedures are covered by the policy
Health service	Universal access *Free* at point of use	Priority issues – continuous planning and changing of healthcare provision Rationing – waiting lists bound to increase
Socialized	Everyone is equal and no other option, e.g. no private care for patients	Difficult to maintain quality and keep up with latest technologies Rationing Lack of responsiveness Risk of bribery as everyone is employed by the state

Surgeons, or a licence in medicine and surgery from the Society of Apothecaries.

The boundaries between doctors and nurses have changed. Nurses now take on prescribing and treatment roles. Also in the UK, the reduction in the number of working hours for junior doctors means that nurse practitioners have assumed some of the roles previously undertaken by doctors. Many types of healthcare professional look after patients. There has been strong appreciation for the roles played by social workers, pharmacists, physiotherapists and nutritionists. Medical students' knowledge of the roles of other healthcare professionals can be tested in both written and clinical examinations.

Carr-Saunders and Wilson (1933) defined 'professionals' according to their characteristics or traits:

- Possession of altruistic values – these are integral for functioning and performance is valued more than financial reward
- High ethical standards
- Discrete body of knowledge over which members have complete control
- High social status
- Monopoly position in market
- Able to regulate their own working conditions independent of the state
- Lengthy period of training, the quality and content of which is determined by the profession itself
- Striving to serve others.

While the 'trait-approach' has received criticism, it does serve to highlight the independence and power of some professional groups, particularly doctors. Larson (1977) introduces the idea of a 'professional project', which entails developing claims to a privileged social position and the ability to sustain this over time. MacDonald (1995) argues that professionals attempt to build up assets or capital in three ways:

1. *Economic assets* – including prestigious properties owned by The Royal Colleges
2. *Organizational status* – healthcare professionals are given power by the state to control large-scale organizations, e.g. the NHS
3. *Cultural assets* – adequate scientific knowledge, reputation and credentials supported by the activities of the professional bodies, e.g. the Royal Colleges allow members to be key advisors to the government.

In general, the medical profession accumulated a lot of power up to the middle of the twentieth century. Professional groups are under continuous scrutiny by the government, the public and the media. The entire medical profession has been shaken by high-profile cases of medical negligence and malpractice.

HINTS AND TIPS

Remember: Medical students' knowledge of the roles of other healthcare professionals can be tested in both written and clinical examinations. For example, do you know the respective roles of the occupational therapist, physiotherapist and district nurse in facilitating the discharge from hospital of an elderly patient?

THE HOLISTIC MODEL

A holistic model of care involves all aspects of patient needs being addressed. The services provided by social workers, physiotherapists, pharmacists, nutritionists and occupational therapists are all important in providing a 'holistic' model of care for the patient. Some of the roles of the doctor are now performed by nurses. These include prescribing and treatment roles.

In the UK and elsewhere, some operations can be performed by surgical care practitioners (SCPs). SCPs are experienced nurses who have undergone further training to perform specific procedures, thereby giving the surgeons time to deal with more complicated cases.

CARE IN THE COMMUNITY

The term 'community care' describes how society should meet the health and social needs of dependent people – specifically, care in the community (i.e. not in hospital) by the community (i.e. by carers/community healthcare practitioners). It also refers to the services that are currently provided to dependent groups.

Dependent groups include:

- The elderly
- The chronically ill
- People with disabilities.

Since the 1980s, informal care from family, friends, relatives and voluntary organizations has become more significant and public, as the shift from institutional care to community care has been enacted. The key obstacles to implementation of effective community care are a lack of resources, managerial difficulties and coordination between social and health services. All healthcare professionals should acknowledge the rise of carers and provide them with sufficient information and support to both help the person they care for and help themselves.

The *NHS and Community Care Act 1990* dictated the working together of local authority social services and the NHS, so as to harmonize packages of care with other agencies and users. Subsequent legislation requires these services also take account of the needs of informal carers.

The fundamental driving forces for community care are:

- Reduction in hospital beds – their number has been diminishing for a long time, partly due to improvement in techniques and policies that allow short stays in hospital, and also to reduce costs. There has also been an increase in the use of day surgery and reduced stay for acute medical conditions
- Patient and client groups – all patients can benefit from good community care. In particular, dependent groups can be treated more effectively in this manner and reduce the time spent at institutions, e.g. hospitals (Fig. 8.6).

Community care can, to a certain extent, be funded by the reduced costs brought about by the closure of bigger institutions, but sufficient bridging funding must be established so that appropriate community care is set up prior to discharging people from bigger institutions.

Setting up effective community healthcare initiatives has several hurdles:

- *Political accountability* – the government determines the healthcare system that a nation adopts and as such decides how much funding it gets
- *Diversity* – how many services can the organization provide, e.g. podiatry, psychiatry, community nursing, etc.
- *Complex and rapidly changing external environment* – economic, sociological, technological and political

factors will determine which health policies are rapidly initiated

- *Changing technologies* – unlike hospitals, which have the latest technology, human skills in community-care settings have been taken for granted and it is only recently that the latter has benefited from advances in information technology
- *Working conditions* – stakeholders in community care need to recognize the factors that motivate their health professionals and support staff.

Basing more health care in the community has been one of the arguments behind the 2012 Health and Social Care Bill, as well as putting GPs in charge of much of the NHS's £106 billion annual budget (at time of writing).

GOVERNMENT DEPARTMENTS

A range of government departments – apart from the Department of Health (DoH) – have responsibilities that impinge on health, and work in partnership with the NHS. They include:

- *Communities and Local Government*: responsible for housing, regional and local government. See: www.communities.gov.uk
- *Home Office*: lead responsibility for progress on the drug strategy; the Home Secretary chairs the cross-government Cabinet ministerial subcommittee on drugs policy, local crime and disorder reduction partnerships. See: www.homeoffice.gov.uk/drugs
- *Department for Education*: responsible for children's social care policy, child safeguarding and initiatives to improve health, education and emotional development for young children in disadvantaged areas. The Healthy Schools programme is run jointly with the DoH. See: www.education.gov.uk
- *Department for Environment, Food and Rural Affairs*: responsibilities include: water, farming, fisheries, horticulture, and some aspects of rural health and well-being. Protection from the effects of pollution or toxic chemicals is a particular concern. See: www.defra.gov.uk.

Factor	Explanation
Demographic	An ageing population is safer under community care
Economic	Value for money, flexibility of community services and minimal fixed costs
Technological	More can be done at home by the GP and community nurses
Consumer choice	The general feeling is that it is user-friendly

Fig. 8.6 Why move to community care?

Key questions

- Describe the evolution of the NHS since its birth in 1948, including the major reforms undertaken.
- Briefly discuss the organization of the NHS.
- Outline the strengths and weaknesses of the NHS system in the twenty-first century.

- Compare the different systems for organizing healthcare delivery.
- How did the medical profession develop in the UK?
- Outline some characteristics of a profession.
- Show how the boundaries between medical, nursing and other healthcare professions have changed since the early twentieth century.
- What government departments besides the Department of Health have health-related responsibilities?
- Outline the importance of care in the community.

References

Carr-Saunders, A.M., Wilson, P.A., 1933. The Professions. Clarendon Press, Oxford.

Field, M., 1973. The concept of the 'health system' at the macrosociological level. Soc. Sci. Med. 7, 763–785.

Fitzpatrick, R., 2003. Organizing and funding health care. In: Scambler, G. (Ed.), Sociology as Applied to Medicine, fifth ed. Saunders, Edinburgh, pp. 292–307.

Heath, I., 2008. The mystery of general practice. In: Matters of Life and Death: Key Writings. Radcliffe, Oxford, pp. 87–123.

Larson, M.S., 1977. The Rise of Professionalism: A Sociological Analysis. University of California Press, Berkeley, CA.

MacDonald, K.M., 1995. The Sociology of Professions. Sage, London.

Talbot-Smith, A., Pollock, A.M., 2006. The NHS: a guide to its funding, organization and accountability. Routledge, London.

Further reading

Armstrong, D., 2003. Organizing health care. In: Outline of Sociology as Applied to Medicine, fifth ed. Arnold, London.

Jones, I.R., 2003. Health professions. In: Scambler, G. (Ed.), Sociology as Applied to Medicine, fifth ed. Saunders, Edinburgh, pp. 235–247.

Langmuir, A.D., 1963. The surveillance of communicable diseases of national importance. N. Engl. J. Med. 268, 182–192.

Mays, N., 2008. Origins and development of the national health service. In: Scambler, G. (Ed.), Sociology as Applied to Medicine, sixth ed. Saunders Elsevier, Edinburgh.

Scambler, G. (Ed.), Sociology as Applied to Medicine, sixth ed. Saunders Elsevier, Edinburgh.

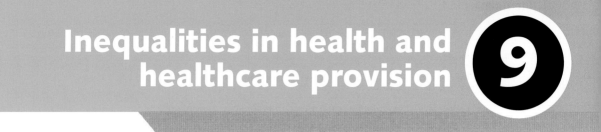

Inequalities in health and healthcare provision

9

This chapter is co-authored with Elizabeth Morrow, PhD Student, Dept of Political Economy, King's College London.

This chapter considers inequalities in health and healthcare provision by social class, gender, ethnicity and age.

IMPACT OF SOCIAL CLASS

There is a long tradition in Britain of analysing national statistics to shed light on the nature and causes of social inequalities in health (Figs 9.1, 9.2). In 1837, William Farr set up the General Register Office. Farr, as the first Superintendent of Statistics, clearly believed that it was the responsibility of the national office not just to record deaths, but to uncover underlying linkages which might help to prevent future disease and suffering.

In the nineteenth century, the associations between various occupations and health were put down to: specific work-related hazards and variation of income – which affected the provision of nutrition and housing.

In 1942, the Beveridge Report set out a national programme of policies to combat the 'five giants of Want, Disease, Ignorance, Squalor and Idleness'. In 1977, the Research Working Group on Inequalities in Health, chaired by Sir Douglas Black, was established. The resulting 'Black Report' presented in 1980 attempted to explain trends in inequalities in health. It argued that inequalities in health were a result of inequalities in society. While the recommendations of this report had a significant effect in academic circles, it arguably failed to produce meaningful change in political policies (health inequalities grew throughout the 1980s).

In 1997, the recently elected 'New Labour' government set up an independent inquiry chaired by Sir Donald Acheson. The Acheson Inquiry, published in 1998, identified the following as areas where policy could redress health inequalities by tackling socio-economic factors:

1. Poverty, income, tax and benefits
2. Education
3. Employment
4. Housing and environment
5. Mobility, transport and pollution
6. Nutrition.

The Acheson Inquiry, which published its Report in November 1998, confirmed that for many aspects of health, inequality had worsened throughout the 1980s and early 1990s. The Report recommended that many government departments – not just the Department of Health – should collaborate in order to reduce health inequalities (see Chapter 8 for a list of departments which have an impact on health in the UK).

In 1999, the government outlined its strategy for addressing health inequalities in the document 'Saving Lives: Our Healthier Nation' (DoH 1999). The strategy aimed to improve the health of everyone generally and of the worst-off in particular. More specifically, the strategy set targets to be achieved by 2010 in four major areas of health. These were:

- cancer – to reduce the death rate in people under 75 by at least 20%
- coronary heart disease and stroke – to reduce the death rate in people under 75 by at least 40%
- accidents – to reduce the death rate by at least 20% and serious injury by at least 10%
- mental illness – to reduce the death rate from suicide and undetermined injury by at least 20%.

Social stratification

Social stratification refers to the way in which an individual who is disadvantaged in one area of life tends to be disadvantaged in others as well. Thus, an individual with a low income probably also has a reduced access to quality housing, education and healthcare services. The concept of 'social class' has been used to describe social stratification within British society. The stratification most widely used in current official UK statistics is the National statistics: socioeconomic classification (NS-SEC, Fig. 9.3). Although the NS-SEC is an occupationally based classification, it can also be applied to the adult population at large (ONS 2010).

Classically, discussions of social stratification in the general population refer to:

- 'working-class' – characterized by earning weekly wages in manual jobs; renting homes, mainly from a local authority; and the aspiration of getting their children in a good job as soon as they are allowed to leave school

Fig. 9.1 Health inequality by 'class' measures.

A boy born to one of the two lowest social classes has a life expectancy of 70 years in the UK – 5 years less than a boy born to one of the highest two classes.

Each of the main disease groups shows a wide health gap among men, with those in the highest two social classes experiencing lower mortality than men in the lowest two.

Men aged between 20 and 64 years from the bottom social class are three times more likely to die from coronary heart disease and stroke than those in the top social class.

Mortality from *all major causes* has been found to be consistently higher than average among unemployed men; unemployed women have higher mortality from coronary heart disease and suicide than employed women.

Children from the households of manual workers are more likely to suffer from chronic sickness and tooth decay than children from the households of non-manual workers.

Men in manual classes are about 40% more likely to report a longstanding illness that limits their activities than those in non-manual classes.

Fig. 9.2 Registrar General's classification of social classes.

Social class	Description	Examples
I	Professional	Accountant
		Doctor
		Lawyer
II	Intermediate	Manager
		School teacher
		Nurse
IIIN	Skilled non-manual	Clerical worker
		Secretary
		Shop assistant
IIIM	Skilled manual	Bus driver
		Coal-face worker
		Carpenter
IV	Semi-skilled manual	Agricultural worker
		Bus conductor
		Postman
V	Unskilled manual	Labourer
		Cleaner
		Dock worker

Fig. 9.3 The five-class 'National Statistics: Socio-Economic Classification' (NS-SEC).

Class	Label
1	Managerial and professional occupations
2	Intermediate occupations
3	Small employers and own account workers
4	Lower supervisory and technical occupations
5	Semi-routine and routine occupations

Adapted from ONS 2010.

- men are allocated a social class according to their occupation
- married women are allocated a social class according to their husband's occupation
- single women are allocated a social class according to their own occupation
- children are allocated a social class according to that of their father
- the unemployed/retired are allocated a social class according to that of the last significant period of employment.

Criticisms of the Registrar General's classification include (Bartley & Blane 2008, p. 121):

1. The classification is a measure of social status rather than income.
2. Each class is not internally homogeneous, e.g. for example, 'manager' in social class II includes the owner of a corner-shop and the managing directors of multinational companies.
3. The classification is inadequate in the way it deals with women. A married woman is classified according to the class of her husband, even though her income may be decisive in determining the standard of living of the family.

- 'middle-class' – characterized by earning monthly salaries in non-manual jobs; borrowing money to buy their own homes; and encouraging their children to gain as much formal education as possible.

Because the use of the NS-SEC is relatively new, many examples of social stratification in teaching still use the older Registrar General's classification. This divides the population into five social classes based on occupation according to skill level and general social standing (Fig. 9.2). Within this classification:

4. The classification is increasingly irrelevant given the flexible nature of labour markets, job insecurity and unemployment rates.

Variations in health according to social class

Even though overall death rates have fallen considerably over the past 200 years, the difference between 'rich' and 'poor' has persisted. The Acheson Inquiry observed that:

Inequalities in health exist, whether measured in terms of mortality, life expectancy or health status; whether categorised by socioeconomic measures or by ethnic group or gender. Recent efforts to compare the level and nature of health inequalities in international terms indicate that Britain is generally around the middle of comparable western countries, depending on the socioeconomic and inequality indicators used.

The Acheson Inquiry also reported the following:

- Over the previous 20 years, death rates had fallen among both men and women and across all social groups.
- The difference in death-rates between those at the top and bottom of the social scale had widened.
- In the early 1970s, the mortality rate among men of working age was almost twice as high for those in class V (unskilled) as for those in class I (professional). By the early 1990s, it was almost three times higher (Fig. 9.4). This increasing differential is because, although rates fell overall, they fell more among the high social classes than the low social classes. Between the early 1970s and the early 1990s, rates fell by about 40% for classes I and II; about 30% for classes IIIN, IIIM and IV but by only 10% for class V.
- Both class I and class V represent only a small proportion of the population that falls at either extreme of the social scale. Combining class I with class II and class IV with class V allows comparisons of larger sections of the population. Among both men and women aged 35–64 years, overall death rates fell for each group between 1976 and 1981 and 1986–1992 (Fig. 9.5). At the same time, the gap between classes I and II and classes IV and V increased. In the late 1970s, death rates were 53% higher among men in classes IV and V compared with those in classes I and II. In the late 1980s, they were 68% higher. Among women, the differential increased from 50% to 55%.
- These growing differences across the social spectrum were apparent for many of the major causes of death, including coronary heart disease, stroke, lung cancer and suicides among men; and respiratory disease and lung cancer among women.

- Death rates can be summarized into average life expectancy at birth. For men in classes I and II combined, life expectancy increased by 2 years between the late 1970s and the late 1980s. For those in classes IV and V combined, the increase was smaller: 1.4 years. The difference between those at the top and bottom of the social class scale in the late 1980s was 5 years; 75 years compared with 70 years.
- In the 1970s and 1980s there was a 2-year improvement in life-expectancy for women in classes I and II, yet for women in classes IV and V there was only a 1 year improvement in life expectancy.
- A good measure of inequality among older people is life expectancy at age 65 years. Again, in the late 1980s, this was considerably higher among those in higher social classes, and the differential increased over the period from the late 1970s to the late 1980s, particularly for women.

With regards to morbidity, the Acheson Inquiry stated the following:

- There is little evidence that the population is experiencing less morbidity or disability than 10 or 20 years ago. There has been a slight increase in self-reported long-standing illness and limiting long-standing illness.
- Among men, major accidents are more common in the manual classes for those aged under 55 years. Between 55 and 64 years, the non-manual classes have higher major accident rates. For women, there are no differences in accident rates until after the age of 75 years, when those women in the non-manual group have higher rates of major accidents.
- 10% of men in classes IV and V were dependent on alcohol compared with 5% in classes I and II.

In addition, the 1997 Health Inequalities Decennial supplement (ONS 1997) showed the following:

- There is a social class gradient in the prevalence of hypertension (Fig. 9.6).
- The manual classes consult their GP more often than non-manual classes.
- In both sexes, members of social class I had more positive health-related behaviours – such as not smoking, regular dental and ophthalmic check-ups, eating well and exercising regularly – than social class V.

Why do such profound differences in health exist?

The 1977 Black Report (Black et al., 1980) proposed four explanations as to why there was an association between social class and health. These were:

1. *Artefact*: the association is spurious because of the way the concepts involved are measured:
   a. One example of this is numerator-denominator bias: this comes about because

Fig. 9.4 European standardized mortality rates by social class, selected causes, men aged 20–64, England and Wales, selected years.

All causes (rates per 100 000)

Social class	1970–1971	1979–1983	1991–1993
I Professional	500	373	280
II Managerial	526	425	300
III(N) Skilled (non-manual)	637	522	426
III(M) Skilled (manual)	683	580	493
IV Partly skilled	721	639	492
V Unskilled	897	910	806
England and Wales	624	549	419

Lung cancer (rates per 100 000)

Social class	1970–1971	1979–1983	1991–1993
I Professional	41	26	17
II Managerial	52	39	24
III(N) Skilled (non-manual)	63	46	34
III(M) Skilled (manual)	90	72	54
IV Partly skilled	93	76	52
V Unskilled	109	108	82
England and Wales	73	60	39

Coronary heart disease (rates per 100 000)

Social class	1970–1971	1979–1983	1991–1993
I Professional	195	144	81
II Managerial	197	168	92
III(N) Skilled (non-manual)	245	208	136
III(M) Skilled (manual)	232	218	159
IV Partly skilled	232	227	156
V Unskilled	243	287	235
England and Wales	209	201	127

Stroke (rates per 100 000)

Social class	1970–1971	1979–1983	1991–1993
I Professional	35	20	14
II Managerial	37	23	13
III(N) Skilled (non-manual)	41	28	19
III(M) Skilled (manual)	45	34	24
IV Partly skilled	46	37	25
V Unskilled	59	55	45
England and Wales	40	30	20

Accidents, poisonings, violence (rates per 100 000)

Social class	1970–1971	1979–1983	1991–1993
I Professional	23	17	13
II Managerial	25	20	13
III(N) Skilled (non-manual)	25	21	17
III(M) Skilled (manual)	34	27	24
IV Partly skilled	39	35	24
V Unskilled	67	63	52
England and Wales	34	28	22

Suicide and undetermined injury (rates per 100 000)

Social class	1970–1971	1979–1983	1991–1993
I Professional	16	16	13
II Managerial	13	15	14
III(N) Skilled (non-manual)	17	18	20
III(M) Skilled (manual)	12	16	21
IV Partly skilled	18	23	23
V Unskilled	32	44	47
England and Wales	15	20	22

Data source: *Acheson 1998.*

mortality rates (in the Black Report) relied on figures from two different sources. The number of deaths in each social class came from death registration. The number of individuals in each class came from census data. Any attempt to 'promote' oneself in the census would lead to artificially increased rates in social classes IV and V. However, longitudinal study of 1% of the 1971 census population showed this is unlikely.

Fig. 9.5 Age-standardized mortality rates per 100 000 by social class, selected causes, men and women aged 35–64, England and Wales, 1976–1992.

	Women (35–64)			Men (35–64)		
	1976–1981	1981–1985	1986–1992	1976–1981	1981–1985	1986–1992
All causes						
I/II	338	344	270	621	539	455
IIIN	371	387	305	860	658	484
IIIM	467	396	356	802	691	624
IV/V	508	445	418	951	824	764
Ratio IV/V:I/II	1.5	1.29	1.55	1.53	1.53	1.68
Coronary heart disease						
I/II	39	45	29	246	185	160
IIIN	56	57	39	382	267	162
IIIM	85	67	59	309	269	231
IV/V	105	76	78	363	293	266
Ratio IV/V:I/II	2.69	1.69	2.69	1.48	1.58	1.66
Breast cancer						
I/II	52	74	52			
IIIN	75	71	49			
IIIM	61	57	46			
IV/V	47	50	54			
Ratio IV/V:I/II	0.90	0.68	1.04			

Data source: *Acheson 1998.*

Fig. 9.6 Variation in morbidity between social classes.

Condition	Men		Women	
	I	V	I	V
Long-standing illness	31% (in 45–64 year olds)	53% (in 45–64 year olds)	36% (in 45–64 year olds)	50% (in 45–64 year olds)
Obesity (BMI > 30)	10%	13%	12%	21%
Hypertension	16%	24%	22%	26%
Neurotic disorders	–	–	15% (social class I & II)	24% (social class IV & V)

b. Infant mortality and social class: a number of factors were originally used to assign each occupation to a social class, which included housing, behaviour, education and wealth – factors that are known to have an influence on infant mortality. So those factors that cause infant mortality are used to determine a low social class status. To then claim that low social class status itself causes increased infant mortality is artefactual. However, social class grading depends on a number of factors (which are linked to worse infant mortality) – so it is not entirely artefactual.

2. *Social selection*: this explanation argues that rather than social class determining health, health determines social class. The proposed mechanism for this is that if people fall ill, they are unable to secure employment in classes I and II. For example, a schizophrenic with active disease may not be able to work as a doctor or lawyer, but could probably find some semi- or unskilled work. It seems probable that the healthy are socially mobile upwardly, and the unhealthy move downwards. However, this explanation is unlikely to be sufficient to account for the whole of the social class gradient. Scambler and Blane (2003, p. 118) observe that:
   a. the gradient is already present in children before social mobility has had a chance to occur
   b. the gradients are present in retirement after social mobility has occurred
   c. the class differences are roughly the same for acute and chronic diseases – if the gradients were due to social mobility, it would be expected that they would be steeper in chronic diseases where there is more time to move downwards
   d. social mobility tends to occur before serious diseases become prevalent
   e. incapacity does not always lead to downward mobility – it may involve early retirement, unemployment or moving to less-demanding jobs, which might lead to a reduction in income but not a reclassification on the Registrar General's classification.

3. *Behavioural/cultural*: Some consider that the middle and working classes have different cultures. As Armstrong (1989) points out: 'they have different habits, read different newspapers, watch different television programmes, have different leisure activities, have different outlooks on life, and so on'. Therefore different classes may have different health-related behaviours. Relevant health-related behaviours include:
   a. Smoking:
      i. In 1974, 50% of men and 40% of women smoked cigarettes
      ii. In 1996, less than 30% of men and women smoke – this breaks down into: men, 12 % (social class I) and 41% (social class V); women 11 % (social class I) and 36% (social class V)
   b. Alcohol:
      i. The proportion of women who drank more than 14 units of alcohol a week rose from 9% in 1984 to 14% in 1996
      ii. In spite of the major class differences in dependence on alcohol in men, there are very small differences in the reported quantities consumed. The implication is that social harms linked to alcohol are more evident in lower social classes. By contrast, higher class women have been reported in the past to consume more alcohol than lower class women.

   c. Physical exercise:
      i. Women – similar rates in levels of physical activity are reported across the social classes.
      ii. Men – the manual classes report a higher level of physical activity than the non-manual classes. However, the manual classes could be engaging in work-related physical activity, in contrast to the non-manual classes, who are more likely to participate in leisure physical activity.
   d. Diet:
      i. People in lower socioeconomic groups tend to eat less fruit and vegetables, and less food that is rich in dietary fibre.
      ii. One aspect of dietary behaviour that affects the health of infants is the incidence of breast-feeding. Six weeks after birth, almost three-quarters of babies in class I households are still breast-fed. This declines with class to less than one-quarter of babies in class V. The differences between classes in rates of breast-feeding at 6 weeks narrowed slightly between 1985 and 1995.

   The implications of cultural explanations for the health inequalities are twofold:
   • Health inequalities may not be reduced by improved economic equality.
   • Perhaps certain health inequalities *should* not be eradicated – as Armstrong points out: 'If … a working class man smokes because he finds pleasure in the activity, and he is less concerned about the long-term consequences, do middle class health professionals have a right to tell him that his values are mistaken and that he should substitute deferred gratification …? There is evidence that cigarette smoking is an integral component of the lifestyle of many working class people; is it morally right to try and change this for a middle class value?'

4. *Materialist*: this explanation was favoured by the Black Report as being of the greatest significance. The Acheson Inquiry also subscribed to this sort of explanation, barely mentioning artefact and social selection. The materialist argument holds that the association between social class and health is caused by the associated levels of material deprivation. Examples of this include:
   a. Lack of essential material possessions such as clothes and food
   b. Poor (e.g. damp, overcrowded and cold) housing which can (especially for older people) contribute to poor health. Housing may be situated in areas with high levels of atmospheric or environmental pollution and there may not be suitable areas for children to play outside

c. Poor access to education and health care. Housing prices tend to increase in areas with good schools, whereas lower-achieving schools are located in areas of poor housing. The children of poor families are therefore less able to use education as a route out of the cycle of poverty. Tudor Hart (1971) introduced the concept of the 'Inverse Care Law', which claims that health care is least available where it is most needed (i.e. in areas inhabited by the working class) and, therefore, it is under-utilized by the lower social classes. This is somewhat supported by data showing that the lower social classes are less likely to use services such as screening, dental care and postnatal examinations.

Further study has lent support to the materialist explanation. It has been demonstrated that physical and social disadvantage accumulates over the course of a lifetime to produce poor health:

- Low parental social class is associated with health disadvantages *in utero* and in the early years of life, e.g. poor nutrition, increased incidence of chronic illness in childhood, failure to thrive and slow growth that leads to short stature for age and sex.
- Children from low parental class families fare less well at school with poor educational achievement resulting in poorer job prospects and an increased likelihood of long-term unemployment. Childhood disadvantage can thus lead to disadvantaged socioeconomic status in adulthood.
- Low educational achievement is also associated with early parenthood, and lone parenthood (mostly lone mothers), which in turn is associated with increased poverty. The new generation of children born to young or single parents are in turn exposed to significant disadvantages. In the 1970s, 10% of children in the UK lived in poverty, by the late 1990s, the proportion was 35%.
- Government policy, particularly regarding taxation and social security benefits, has played a significant role in this increase in child poverty.

- State benefits have declined in relative value in comparison with the incomes of higher earners. Relative deprivation (rather than absolute deprivation) has been increasing in the UK. That is, the gap between the rich and the poor has been getting bigger.

Relative vs absolute deprivation

Marmot (2003) discusses the importance of social gradients within societies leading to ill-health. He argues there are three ways in which socioeconomic position could be linked to health (Fig. 9.7):

1. Money
2. Status
3. Power.

He argues that although a high income is associated with good health, it is merely an indicator for position within society (status). For Marmot, it is status rather than high income which is the most important predictor of health. He draws a comparison between men in Costa Rica (average income $2000 per annum and life expectancy of 74 years) and Black American men (average income $26 000 per annum and life expectancy of 66 years). Even adjusting for the fact that more can be bought for less in Costa Rica than in the USA ($2000 in Costa Rica could buy the equivalent goods and services of around $6600 spent in the USA), US Black men still have a lower life expectancy, even though they have an income that is almost four times greater. Marmot argues that this is due to the relatively low status occupied by Black American men within US society, rather than due to absolute poverty. The mechanism by which this occurs is the relative disadvantage in terms of income within a society. Marmot suggests that this 'relative inequality ... may correspond to absolute discrimination and social exclusion'.

Marmot describes how health differences occur along a social gradient even within a single socioeconomic group. In his studies of civil servants (known as the 'Whitehall studies'), he demonstrated that an increased mortality and morbidity was associated with progressive loss of power and control over their jobs.

In November 2008, Professor Sir Michael Marmot chaired an independent review to propose the most

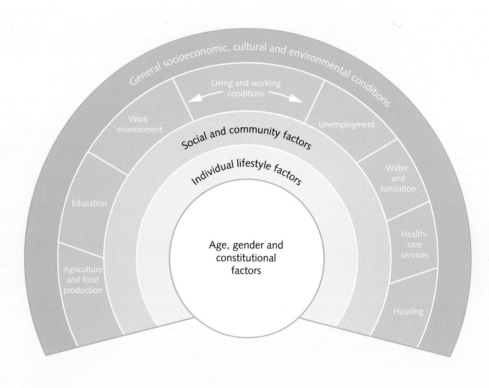

Fig. 9.7 The main determinants of health. (From Acheson 1998, with permission.)

effective evidence-based strategies for reducing health inequalities in England from 2010.

The Marmot Report of health inequalities in England post-2010, 'Fair Society, Healthy Lives', was published in 2010. It highlights six policy recommendations (Marmot 2010):

1. Giving every child the best start in life (highest priority recommendation)
2. Enabling all children, young people and adults to maximize their capabilities and have control over their lives
3. Creating fair employment and good work for all
4. Ensuring a healthy standard of living for all
5. Creating and developing sustainable places and communities
6. Strengthening the role and impact of ill-health prevention.

Reducing inequality between social classes I and V

As mentioned above, the Acheson Inquiry isolated six key areas where policy improvements could help to reduce the health inequalities in this country. In the paper 'Saving Lives: Our Healthier Nation' (DoH 1999), the UK government at the time addressed the Acheson Inquiry's six areas and made policy recommendations as follows:

1. Poverty, income, tax and benefits:
   a. Introduction of the minimum wage
   b. Increased benefits for single mothers and older people
   c. A new system of tax credits for parents.
2. Education:
   a. The 'Healthy Schools' programme, which involves partnerships between local health and education authorities to provide 'healthy' school environments and information for children about health
   b. Establishment of educational resources, such as a health website for children, see: www.wiredforhealth.gov.uk
   c. 'Cooking for kids' – an in-school educational programme, which teaches the basics of healthy eating and cooking.
3. Employment:
   a. the 'New Deal' – to encourage people to leave welfare and enter the workforce

b. 'The Healthy Workplace Initiative' (1999) to encourage healthy practices in the workplace.
4. Housing and environment:
    a. Benefits for fuel
    b. Benefits for making houses energy efficient
    c. The 'New Deal for Communities' provided money to neighbourhoods to be used for developing social cohesion and strong social networks.
5. Mobility, transport and pollution:
    a. Encourage local authorities to prioritize transport improvement in disadvantaged areas
    b. Encourage local service providers, e.g. GP practices, pharmacists, to establish services in disadvantaged areas.
6. Nutrition:
    a. Improve access to affordable healthy foods for people on low incomes
    b. Restrict advertising of food high in salt, fat and sugar targeted at children
    c. 'Five-a-day' advertising campaign to increase the amount of fruit and vegetables people eat
    d. Reduce salt and fat content in processed foods.

Many of these policies are 'upstream' policies designed to have a wide range of consequences – including benefits to health. The Acheson Inquiry recommended both 'upstream' and 'downstream' policies – those that deal with wider (upstream) influences on health inequalities such as income distribution, education, public safety, housing, work environment, employment, social networks, transport and pollution, as well as those which have narrower (downstream) impacts, such as on healthy behaviours.

HINTS AND TIPS

Health inequalities and social class

- The materialist perspective contends that health inequalities are due to inequalities in wealth
- Inequalities in health are associated with a variety of social and environmental factors
- The Acheson Inquiry did not consider artefact and self-selection to be significant causes of inequalities in health between social classes – research in the 1980s and 1990s showed that materialist and behavioural explanations are more useful tools for understanding health inequalities
- Social inequality leads to a life-time accumulation of disadvantages that contribute to poor health outcomes. On this, the Department of Health relevantly concluded that it is likely that cumulative differential exposure to health damaging or health promoting physical and social environments is the main explanation for the observed variations in health and life expectancy.

GENDER DIFFERENCES

Like social class, gender influences long-term health. This is not simply due to the different biological aspects of the two sexes, rather it is due to the combined effects of biological, social and cultural influences.

COMMUNICATION

Definitions of sex and gender
- *Sex*: refers to the classes of 'male' and 'female' as determined by biology.
- *Gender*: refers to the classes of 'masculine' and 'feminine' as socially and culturally constructed.

Levels of gender health differences

Mortality

It has often been said that 'women get sick and men die'. In general, this is true; however, it belies a rather more complex picture of the gender biases in mortality and morbidity (Fig. 9.8). Mortality is the easier of the two to measure – death being a far more objective measure. Men die younger and in greater numbers in all age groups:

- Life expectancy for males: 74.3 years (EU average 74.3)
- Life expectancy for females: 79.5 years (EU average 80.7).

In childhood, the mortality in males is raised due to accidental deaths – especially due to poisoning and injury caused by drowning, road-traffic accidents and fire (Fig. 9.9). The difference between male and female deaths rises to a maximum in the 20–24-year-old group, where male mortality is 2.8 times that of female. The major causes of this disparity are road-traffic accidents, other accidents and suicide (Fig. 9.10). Figure 9.11 outlines the different causes of death in men and women.

In general, the gender differences are greatest in areas of relative deprivation, and least in affluent areas. Remarkably, affluent men still have a greater risk of mortality than deprived women.

Morbidity

Morbidity highlights an apparent paradox: males have higher mortality rates, but females have higher rates of morbidity. However, the broad assumption that females experience more ill-health than males conceals specific gender differences in both directions.

Childhood and adolescence
- Boys are more likely to report long-standing illness (18% M:15% F).

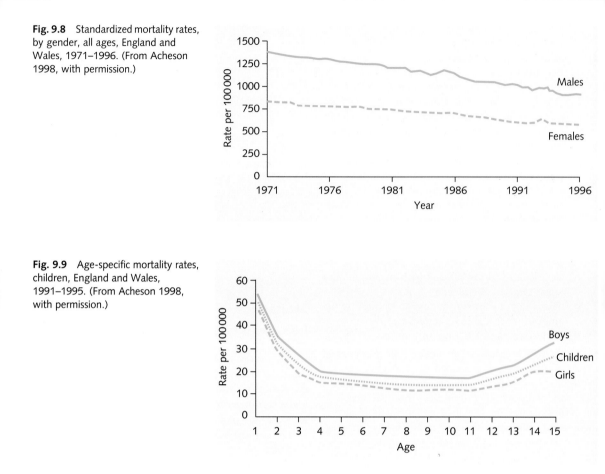

Fig. 9.8 Standardized mortality rates, by gender, all ages, England and Wales, 1971–1996. (From Acheson 1998, with permission.)

Fig. 9.9 Age-specific mortality rates, children, England and Wales, 1991–1995. (From Acheson 1998, with permission.)

- Boys are 30–40% more likely than girls to have consulted at a general practice for serious conditions, but about 10% less likely to have done so for minor conditions.
- While boys have higher rates of chronic physical illness in childhood, this pattern is reversed in early to mid-adolescence, when there are higher rates for girls.

Female longevity

Female longevity has not always been manifest:

- It is thought that there was a substantial male advantage in longevity in the sixteenth and seventeenth centuries.
- In the first half of the nineteenth century, male and female life expectancies were more or less equal.
- By the 1960s, women were living about 6 years longer than men.

The gap in life expectancy may be closing once again:

- The major change in female mortality is due to changing patterns of child-bearing and the reduction in maternal mortality.

- The levels of female mortality in the developing world resemble nineteenth-century mortality rates in the UK.
- For psychological disorders, mostly neurotic, an excess in boys is replaced by an excess in girls by mid-adolescence.

Young people and working adults

- Women have more morbidity than men from poor mental health, particularly from anxiety and depressive disorders.
- Men have higher rates of schizophrenia and alcohol and drug dependence.
- Women are more likely to consult their GP than men (ratio of 6:4 consultations per year).
- GPs see women more frequently for consultations regarding cancer, obesity, anaemia, migraine, osteoarthritis and back pain.
- GPs see men more frequently for consultations regarding diabetes, heart attacks and angina.
- Women are placed at greater iatrogenic risk, e.g. by taking the oral contraceptive pill and undergoing

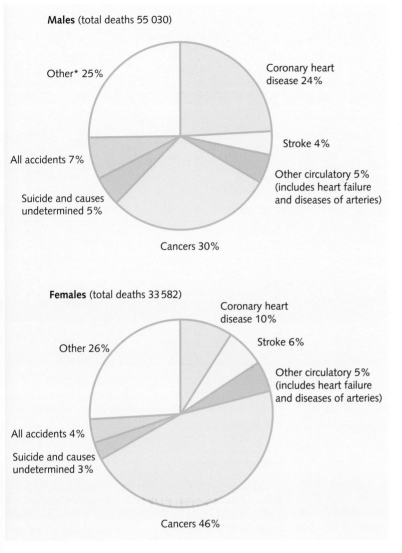

Males (total deaths 55 030)

Other* 25%

Coronary heart disease 24%

Stroke 4%

Other circulatory 5% (includes heart failure and diseases of arteries)

All accidents 7%

Suicide and causes undetermined 5%

Cancers 30%

Females (total deaths 33 582)

Coronary heart disease 10%

Stroke 6%

Other 26%

Other circulatory 5% (includes heart failure and diseases of arteries)

All accidents 4%

Suicide and causes undetermined 3%

Cancers 46%

Fig. 9.10 Major causes of mortality under 65 years, by gender, England 1996. (From Acheson 1998, with permission.) *Deaths occurring under 28 days of age are included, but not allocated to a specific cause, included in 'Other'. The major categories here are those identified as priority areas for 'Our Healthier Nation'. All remaining causes assigned to 'Other' category.

hysterectomies, they may be at greater risk of conditions such as deep venous thrombosis.

Elderly adults

- Osteoporosis is more common in women. The lifetime risk, from the age of 50 years, of fracture of the hip, spine or distal forearm – for which osteoporosis is a major determinant – is 14%, 11% and 13%, respectively, for women compared with 3%, 2% and 2%, respectively for men. The causes of the differences in fracture rates between men and women are not fully understood, but differences in bone density, size and architecture, together with a difference in the rates of falls between the sexes, are likely to be major contributors.
- Women have much higher rates of disability than men, especially at older ages. For instance, 80% of

men over 85 years were able to leave the house and walk down the road, compared with just over 50% of women.
- Of women over the age of 65 years, 14% suffer from functional impairments that require help on a daily basis to remain living in the community, compared with only 7% of men.
- By the age of 85 years and over, these figures have risen to nearly 40% for women and 21% for men.
- Some 64% of women over 65 years of age live in communal homes, compared with 3% of men.

Explaining the gender health differences

There are three different explanatory models for understanding the health differences between men and women:

Fig. 9.11 Causes of death in men and women.

Disease category – male (per 100 000 population)	Death rate	Disease category – female (per 100 000 population)	Death rate
Ischaemic heart disease	227.8	Ischaemic heart disease	175.0
Cerebrovascular disease	88.9	Cerebrovascular disease	134.9
Lung cancer	69.2	Pneumonia	72.4
Bronchitis	51.3	Breast cancer	43.0
Pneumonia	49.4	Lung cancer	41.4
Prostate cancer	34.7	Bronchitis	38.9
Bowel cancer	29.1	Bowel cancer	24.7
All accidents	23.9	All accidents	17.6
Stomach cancer	13.5	Diabetes mellitus	11.8
Chronic liver disease and cirrhosis	12.7	Pancreatic cancer	11.7
Diabetes mellitus	11.4	Chronic liver disease and cirrhosis	7.2
Pancreatic cancer	11.3	Stomach cancer	7.0
Suicide	10.1	Uterine cancer	3.7
		Suicide	2.8

1. That the differences are due to artefact
2. That the differences are due to genes or biology
3. That the differences are due to social causation.

Artefact

The artefact explanation suggests that the differences were created by the method used to collect the data. The implication is that women may self-report more illness because they have a greater awareness of their symptoms and/or less cultural stigma in 'admitting' disease:

- It has, however, *been found by clinical observation*, that men are more likely to overrate their symptoms (of a cold) in comparison to women – this suggests that women in fact underestimate their symptoms.

Genetic/biological explanations

Some of the differences have been put down to solely biological factors, e.g. women have greater resistance to heart disease because of endogenous female sex hormones. Male babies are more likely to die than female babies because their lungs tend to be less developed than those of girls of a similar gestation. Furthermore, conditions such as menstruation, pre-menstrual syndrome, morbidity due to pregnancy and childbirth, diseases of the female reproductive organs and the menopause are specific to women. However, genetic

and biological differences cannot explain the full range of differences in morbidity and mortality between men and women.

Social causation

Social causes reveal that men and women lead very different lives, and social expectations and stereotypes are well established. A few explanations for the observed health differences based on such expectations and stereotypes include:

1. Men lead lives that make them more vulnerable to death from accidents and violence, e.g. men tend to drive faster than women.
2. Women may suffer more illness because they undertake more social roles. Even in couples where both are in full-time employment, women still undertake the majority of domestic work. Women are also more likely to undertake a 'caring' role with regard to their children and spouses.
3. Women are more likely to suffer poverty than men – women tend to be employed in part-time work that pays less and has fewer benefits.
4. Health-related behaviour also differs between the sexes. Historically, men drank and smoked more than women. This has resulted in their higher rates of liver cirrhosis and lung cancer. It is expected that the rates of lung cancer will equalize between the sexes now that levels of smoking have equalized.

Remember: Like social class, gender influences long-term health. This is not simply due to the different biological aspects of the two sexes, rather it is due to the combined effects of biological, social and cultural influences.

ETHNIC MINORITIES

The Patient's Charter codifies the expectation that those receiving treatment from the NHS can expect their privacy, dignity, religious and cultural beliefs to be respected. The GMC issues guidelines that 'personal beliefs' should not prejudice patient care and that doctors 'must never discriminate unfairly' against patients or colleagues. However, there are noticeable differences in the health status of different ethnic groups. Sociological and epidemiological studies have tried to find out whether these differences arise from biological differences, or whether they are the result of social discrimination.

A brief history of immigration to the UK

The idea of 'race' first appeared in the English language in the early seventeenth century. However, the idea of race being used as an 'explanation' for differences in observed behaviour only became popular later on. By the mid-nineteenth century, the idea that there were 'distinct' races, each with a 'biologically *determined* capacity for cultural development' was etched into the collective consciousness.

Eighteenth-century estimates put the African population in England at 0.2% (mostly former slaves), although by the early nineteenth century, this began to decline due to the abolition of slavery. Immigration in England began to increase as a result of the following:

- The earliest large-scale migration was probably the post-famine Irish in the 19th Century
- Jews migrated to the England between the two wars
- Caribbean immigrants began arriving after the Second World War in response to labour shortages, and often ended up working for the transport industry or in other low-paid jobs
- The health service actively recruited from India and Pakistan shortly after its foundation
- Thousands of doctors who had trained overseas immigrated in the 1950s, 60s and 70s
- The 1962 Immigration Act placed restrictions on entry into this country
- East-African Asians expelled from Kenya and Uganda in the 1970s travelled to the UK – many were professional or business families

- Modern-day immigration by refugee populations has occurred from Iraq, the Balkans and Afghanistan.

Characteristics of ethnic minority groups

- Ethnic minorities make up approximately 8% of the UK population – the majority of this number are British-born ethnic minorities
- Ethnic minorities tend to be based in urban environments – often within minority communities. Over half the ethnic population lives in south-east England – forming 20% of Greater London
- The age and gender distribution of minority ethnic groups is different from the majority population:
  - Some minority ethnic groups have more men than women, and all are relatively young
  - Afro-Caribbean and South Asian communities have a higher proportion of households with children than the white population
  - Pakistani and Bangladeshi households are also larger because they are more likely to have three or more adults, while Afro-Caribbean households are more likely to be headed by a lone parent.

The health of ethnic minorities

Generally, the research on ethnic minorities has focussed on ethnicity. Key features about the health of immigrant populations include:

1. A higher rate of mortality than people born in the UK
2. A lower rate of mortality than those from their home country. (Although the Irish are an exception here.)

The reason for this has been described as the 'healthy migrant' factor – which claims that immigrants tend to be healthier than average for their home population but not as healthy as the population they move into. It has been suggested that the mortality rates are higher than for those born in the UK because they bring with them the risks of mortality of their earlier life, and then adopt the risks associated with British society.

Definitions

- *Ethnicity* – refers to social groups who often share a cultural heritage with a common language, values, religion, customs and attitudes. The members are aware of sharing a common past, possibly a homeland, and experience a sense of difference.
- *Culture* – reflects ethnicity, and refers to habits of thought and beliefs, diet, dress, music, art.

- *Race* – is a construct based on phenotypical biological differences (usually skin colour); social assumptions (often negative) are attributed to biological differences.
- *Racism* – deterministically associates inherent biological characteristics with other negatively evaluated features or actions. Racial discrimination is against the law.

Source: Hillier 2003, with permission.

Mortality

- Ischaemic heart disease accounts for the largest proportion of deaths among men regardless of country of birth.
- Men born in East Africa, the Indian subcontinent and Scotland show higher mortality, and those from the Caribbean lower mortality, compared with the UK average.
- Cerebrovascular disease was the next major cause of death for men from the Caribbean, West/South Africa and the Indian subcontinent.
- Lung cancer is the next main cause of death for Scottish and Irish men, among whom mortality was 46% and 57% higher than the average, respectively.
- Irish and Scottish men showed higher mortality from accidents, injuries and suicides. For both of these causes, mortality of Scottish and Irish men in class IV/V was more than twice the national rate.

Morbidity

A nationwide survey, 'The Health Survey for England – The Health of Minority Ethnic Groups 1999' (Erens et al., 2001), looked in depth at the health of minority ethnic groups, including minority individuals born both outside and in England. The survey findings included:

Long-standing and limiting long-standing illness

- Chinese men and women were less likely to report long-standing and limiting long-standing illness than both the general population and all other groups.
- The prevalence of limiting long-standing illness was higher for Pakistani, Bangladeshi and Irish men (35–65% above the general population) and for Afro-Caribbean and South Asian women (20% and 44%, respectively above the general population).

Acute sickness

- Chinese men and women were much less likely to report acute sickness than those in the general population and all other minority ethnic groups.

Cardiovascular disease

The survey looked at a range of cardiovascular disease (CVD) conditions: angina, heart attack, stroke, heart murmur, irregular heart rhythm, 'other heart trouble', reported high blood pressure and diabetes:

- For all the above-mentioned conditions with the exception of diabetes, Chinese men and women had lower rates than the general population, and for diabetes the Chinese rates were not significantly higher than those of the general population.
- All South Asian groups showed higher rates than the general population for most conditions, and both Pakistanis and Bangladeshis showed higher rates than Indians.
- Afro-Caribbean men (but not women) had significantly lower prevalence of angina and heart attack than the general population, and both men and women had higher prevalence of diabetes.
- Irish people did not differ substantially from the general population in the prevalence of CVD conditions.
- For some of the main CVD risk factors examined, the differences between people with and without CVD varied within minority ethnic groups and between these groups and the general population. Risk factors where age-adjusted risk ratios were higher in those with CVD than in those without, included having a raised waist–hip ratio (except Bangladeshi men); being overweight/obese (Indian and Bangladeshi women only); and high blood pressure, while risk ratios for cigarette smoking were higher among those without CVD than among those with CVD.
- When all risk factors (such as high blood pressure, cigarette smoking and obesity) were taken into account simultaneously in logistic regression models, the differences in prevalence between each minority ethnic group and the general population were small, and none was significant.

Hypertension

- Compared with men in the general population, mean systolic blood pressures (SBP) were significantly low for Chinese, Pakistani and, in particular, Bangladeshi men.
- Compared with women in the general population, mean SBP were significantly low for Bangladeshi and Chinese women, and high for Pakistani women.
- Pakistani women (risk ratio 1.25) and Afro-Caribbean women (1.21) were significantly more likely to have high blood pressure than women in the general population.
- Within minority ethnic groups, there was no clear and consistent relationship between high blood pressure and either social class or equivalized household income, for either men or women.

Diabetes

- Pakistanis and Bangladeshis of both sexes showed rates over five times higher than the general population and Indians almost three times higher.
- Mortality is three to four times greater in Caribbean-born individuals, three times greater in Asians, and double in African-born individuals.
- Even though Afro-Caribbeans have higher rates of diabetes and hypertension, they have lower CVD.

Explanations for variation in cardiovascular disease

1. *Insulin resistance hypothesis*: The association of insulin resistance and heart disease is well recognized. Diabetes and heart disease are both raised above the levels of the general population for Bangladeshi, Pakistani and Indian immigrants. Insulin resistance is associated with patterns of fat deposition – specifically abdominal fat. However, it is not clear that most immigrants from South Asia who have heart disease also have diabetes.
2. *Social stress*: This theory claims that the stress associated with any migration and living with ongoing stressors (such as social deprivation and racism) leads to an increased rate of CVD. It is claimed that the prevalence of CVD across social classes within South Asian immigrants is evidence for this theory. *However*, the presence of CVD across social classes is suggestive of a biological reason for increased prevalence. Also, if the stress association with migration was responsible, then *all* immigrants would be expected to show raised levels of CVD, but, Caribbean-born men – who are perhaps subject to even more stress (as a population in terms of social deprivation) than South Asian immigrants – had the lowest rates of CVD.

Mental illness

- Irish immigrants are the most likely to be hospitalized for mental illness, followed by Caribbean-born immigrants.
- South Asian immigrants have a lower rate of hospital admission compared to the general population.
- Women are admitted more frequently than men in all immigrant populations except Caribbean populations.
- Admissions due to schizophrenia and paranoia are three times greater for men and two times greater for women from Caribbean-born populations than the general population. This group is also more likely to present to mental-health professionals via the police, or courts, and as a group are *more* likely to be subjected to compulsory detention, compulsory administration of psychotropic drugs and electro-convulsive therapy. This group is *less* likely to be given psychotherapy (or other 'talking' therapies).

Explanations for variations in mental illness

- *Due to 'real' differences* – some people have argued that the stress caused by migration and by subsequent racism leads to increased schizophrenic episodes in Afro-Caribbean populations.
- *Due to misdiagnosis and exaggeration of minor symptoms* – others have claimed that the higher levels of mental illness are due to cultural misunderstanding. Annandale (1998) notes that schizophrenia in Afro-Caribbeans is thought of in terms of '*threats* to the white community, rather than the *distress* of those who experience mental health problems', and has linked this to a 'predisposition on the part of white people in Britain to interpret Black people's behaviour as signs of insanity and danger'.

Use of health services

- South Asian and Afro-Caribbean men were more likely than the general population to have consulted their GP in the past 2 weeks and to have had more than one consultation over this period.
- Among women, contact rates were significantly higher for South Asian and Irish women.
- Relative to the general population, consultation ratios for psychological distress were significantly higher for Irish men (1.5 times) and lower for Chinese men and women (0.59 and 0.41 times) and for Bangladeshi women (0.64 times).
- Relative to the general population, levels of prescribed medicine use by men were low among Chinese men (0.5 times) and high for South Asian men (1.26–2.04 times). Indian and Bangladeshi men who had been prescribed medicines were also likely to be taking more drugs per person on medication than the general population on medication. Chinese women were low users of medication (0.59 times), while Bangladeshi (1.37 times) and Pakistani women (1.42 times) were relatively high users.
- Afro-Caribbean and South Asian men were two to three times more likely to be on drugs prescribed for endocrine disorders. For example, about one-third of drugs dispensed in this group relate to diabetes control.

General explanations for variations in mortality and morbidity

As mentioned above, the inequalities seen in any population, when compared with the general population, can be due to:

1. artefact
2. biological differences
3. material differences
4. cultural differences.

The inequalities of the ethnic population are probably due to a combination of all of these influences. Artefacts may arise due to the use of census data, which tends to underestimate the size of ethnic populations. Material inequality is common among immigrants; however, with some diseases, such as CVD, there is not as steep a gradient across social classes of South Asian immigrants as there is for the ethnic majority population, which may indicate a biological difference (e.g. increased central obesity and insulin resistance). Finally, cultural differences, such as the 'somatization' of psychological distress in South Asian women, may account for increased GP consultations and reduced diagnosis of mental illness.

THE AGEING POPULATION

Mortality is related to age. This fact seems self-evident: the older you are, the less life you have to live. However, the relationship between mortality and age is not altogether linear, rather it is a lopsided U-shape – a high rate in the first year (i.e. infant mortality) – a rapid decline and a flat area before rising gradually in middle age and then steeply in older people. Diseases that are predominant in the West are also predominantly associated with ageing such as coronary artery disease and cancer.

However, some sociocultural influences are also thought to affect health:

1. Environmental influences – such as diet, degree of physical activity and smoking, contribute to the diseases of old age.
2. Societal treatment of older people may lead to their 'disengagement' from social roles. This withdrawal may be associated with psychological distress such as anxiety and depression, which in turn may lead to physical sequelae.

The changing population

During the 20th century, life expectancy rose, and the birth rate fell. These changes have led to an increase in both the absolute number of older people and the proportion of older people within the general population. Within 20 years, nearly a quarter of the UK population will be aged 65 or over. People are now spending an average of 7 years longer in retirement than in the 1970s, and it is unclear what proportion of these extra years will be healthy (Banner 2011).

HINTS AND TIPS

UK reforms supporting longer working lives (adapted from Banner 2011)

Following the implementation of the Equality Act 2010, the Default Retirement Age (DRA) is being phased out. From 6 April 2011 it was no longer legal to issue notifications of retirement using the DRA procedures, unless the employer can provide objective justifications for compulsory age-based retirement. These measures are intended to prevent age discrimination in the workplace, and to allow capable older workers the right to continue if they so choose. The Pensions Bill 2011 sets out a timetable for increasing the state pension age (SPA). It proposes that women's SPA will be equalized with men's, reaching 65 by November 2018. SPA for both men and women will then increase to 66 between 2018 and 2020.

Older people (i.e. those over 65 years) have been classed as the largest 'dependent' group in society, and they outnumber children. The word 'dependent' is used because the conventional view is that older people do not work and are, therefore, 'dependent' on the proportion of society that does. This classification reveals a generalized view that considers ageing and older people to be a 'problem'. This view has been challenged – a Royal Commission on the long-term care of the elderly in 1999 (Sutherland 1999) stated:

> There is now a clear opportunity to see old age for what it is, a stage of life where we have the gift of time to be able to acquire knowledge and experiences for which there may not have been time during working lives. ... Society should recognise the value inherent in older people, and the value to society in using its ingenuity to help older people to continue to realise their potential more effectively.

There are good reasons to challenge the idea that old age and older people are problems or threats:

• Many people expect to live 20 or 30 years beyond retirement.
• Only 5% of older people either live in a care home or receive care at home from a local authority.
• While acute health problems (e.g. colds and accidents) do increase with age, they still only affect 20% of males and 25% of females in the very oldest age groups.
• Almost 50% of those over 75 years do not have any illnesses or disabilities that impair their activity level.

However, there are some 'medical' problems of old age. These include:

• A progressive inability to undertake 'activities of daily living'. These activities include washing oneself, dressing oneself, feeding oneself, climbing stairs and going to the toilet

- Multiple pathology – elderly people are more likely to have more than one concurrent medical problem than younger people
- Polypharmacy – the oldest 16% of the population receives 40% of the drugs. Many elderly patients take more than one type of medication – this can lead to poor compliance (especially if the patient is confused) and a greater number of drug interactions
- Dementia – only affects 2% of the 65–75 year group, but affects 10–20% of 80+ year olds
- Use of health services – rates of hospital admissions are greater for older people than for other groups and this is also true for most hospital specialties. Older people are also more likely to consult their GP. It has been estimated that the cost of long-term care for older people will rise from £11.1 billion (1995) to £45.3 billion (2051).

Social factors compounding medical problems in older people

In addition to biological factors, social factors may also lead to illness in older people. Such social factors include:

- Poverty:
  - Older people are more likely to be living in poverty compared with the general population. This is especially true of elderly women.
  - State pensions in the UK are not generous in comparison with the rest of the European Union.
  - Older people from social classes IV and V experience more respiratory problems and hypertension compared with older people from social classes I and II.
  - On average, a 65-year-old man from social classes I and II can expect to live 2.6 years longer than a 65-year-old man from social classes IV and V.
  - Poor older people may be less likely to receive some healthcare services, or may have poorer health outcomes after receiving these services than wealthier elderly individuals. For instance, severe visual problems are more likely to remain unrecognized and untreated in older people from low socioeconomic groups.
- Poor housing:
  - Older people tend to live in older housing – this is associated with problems such as increased heating costs and damp. This means that many elderly individuals end up with the dilemma of choosing whether to have adequate heating or adequate food. Hypothermia or malnutrition may result.
- Poor mobility:
  - Degenerative disease, such as osteoarthritis, can lead to restriction of access to:

- *Goods* – an inability to drive may mean that older people are reliant on small local shops. Prices may be higher, and the availability of fresh fruit and vegetables may be reduced.
  - *Services* – such as those provided by their GP, may be difficult to attend. Elderly women as a group commonly require home visits by the GP.
  - *Social contacts* – immobility can hinder the participation of an individual with wider society – this may lead to isolation.
- Fear of crime:
  - Older people may fear crime more than younger people. This fear may cause older people to restrict their activities, which can result in further social isolation.

Ageing and health policy

The ageing population has created a need for specific health policies on how best to provide for older people. One problem that has hindered policy creation is a lack of certainty as to what demands will be made on the state by the ageing population. Moody (1995) has argued that there are four possible scenarios:

1. *Prolongation of morbidity* – the increase in life years is not accompanied by an increase in quality of life – although absolute lifespan has increased, healthy lifespan has not
2. *Compression of morbidity* – good health is experienced almost up to the end of peoples' lives, when a 'terminal drop' of health rapidly leads to death
3. *Lifespan extension* – the healthy lifespan is extended due to advances in medical science and preventative medicine
4. *Voluntary acceptance of limits* – this scenario aims for the development of a shared 'meaning of old age', which informs views on which health interventions are appropriate (in the sense of being beneficial) and which are futile or merely life-extending.

Sociological views and older people

Higgs (2003) outlines three theories that have been used to account for the position of older people within society:

1. *Disengagement theory*: This American theory claims that old people gradually disengage from a range of social activities until they become unable to fulfil the roles they had previously held and ultimately become dependent. Dependence may be:
   a. financial – receiving a state pension
   b. domestic – needing help to wash, dress, cook or shop
   c. medical – receiving treatment for ill-health

d. social – older parents become less central to the lives of their children as the children themselves become parents.

As people disengage from social roles – especially upon retirement – they may experience initial relaxation followed by a period of turmoil, depression and anxiety. This reaction to the loss of status may be similar to the grief of bereavement and has been called *desolation*.

However, questions have arisen as to whether elderly people choose to disengage or are forced to do so by society. Theories that suggest that older people are forced by society to disengage include:

2. *Structured dependency theory*: This theory stresses the importance of social structures in creating the circumstances elderly people find themselves in:

    a. Financial – retirement marks the formal withdrawal from the labour force. In addition, the poverty of older people is a result of poor state pensions.

    b. Labelling and ageism – if older people are seen as 'disengaging' from society and are expected to do so by society, then this becomes a self-fulfilling prophecy. The placement of older people in 'old people's homes' compounds this problem by removing older people from communities. In effect, such elderly people become 'out of sight and out of mind'.

    c. Cultural emphasis on 'youth' almost by definition excludes older people. For example the 'Cool Britannia' movement pioneered by the New Labour Government in the 1990s and early 2000s tailored its approach to 'young, modern Britain', which may be inappropriate in light of population demographics.

3. *Third ageism*: This theory is at odds with the previous two, and holds that in fact older people are able to enjoy relatively good health and affluence. 'Third ageism' observes that retirement is forming an increasingly large part of people's lives. There is a blurring between middle age and old age, and older people are increasingly undertaking activities, such as travelling and learning a new skill, that were once seen as the younger preoccupations.

General explanations for health inequalities in older people

Once again it is useful to consider inequalities through the lenses of artefact, biological and social causation. Clearly, biology has a considerable role to play, with increasing age associated with increasing disease. However, this is not the sole cause of health inequalities between young and older people. The elderly are, through a number of mechanisms, deprived of social benefits that help to prevent worsening of health. Relevant deprivations include a lack of material benefits such as wealth, housing and access to services. Additionally, there may be cultural constraints, which lead to older people being less likely to demand the health care or support services available to them. This might include a dislike of strangers in the house; concerns about modesty; or not wanting to complain, leading (respectively) to refusing home help for housework; refusing assistance with activities of daily living such as washing and dressing; or generally not seeking help when problems arise.

Key questions

- What areas for redress of health inequalities did the Acheson Inquiry highlight?
- What are the aims of the government document 'Saving Lives: Our Healthier Nation'?
- What are the categories of the Registrar General's classification of social classes?
- What explanations for health inequalities between social classes did the Black Report consider?
- What explanations for health inequalities between social classes did the Acheson Inquiry consider?
- In what ways could health inequalities between social classes be reduced?
- What is the difference between sex and gender?
- What types of explanation exist for gender inequalities in health?
- What is the difference between race and ethnicity?
- Why do immigrants in general have a higher mortality than people of similar ethnicity who are born in the UK?
- What is the social stress theory?
- What general explanations can be given for variations in mortality and morbidity in ethnic minorities?
- How might advanced age create health inequalities?

References

Acheson, D. (Chairman), 1998. An Independent Inquiry into Inequalities in Health Report. TSO, London.

Annandale, E., 1998. The Sociology of Health and Medicine: A Critical Introduction. Polity Press, Cambridge.

Armstrong, D., 1989. An Outline of Sociology as Applied to Medicine, third ed. Wright, London.

Banner, N., 2011. An Ageing Workforce. The Parliamentary Office of Science and Technology, London, postnote 391, October 2011. Online. Available at: http://www.parliament. uk/business/publications/research/briefing-papers/POST-PN-391 (accessed 29.04.12.).

Bartley, M., Blane, D., 2008. Inequality and social class. In: Scambler, G. (Ed.), Sociology as Applied to Medicine, sixth ed. Saunders Elsevier, Edinburgh, pp. 116–132.

Beveridge, W., 1942. Social Insurance and Allied Services. HMSO, London.

Black, D., Morris, J., Smith, C., Townsend, P., 1980. Inequalities in Health: Report of a Research Working Group. Department of Health and Social Security, London.

Department of Health, 1999. Saving Lives: Our Healthier Nation. HMSO, London, Cm 4386. Online. Available at: http://www.archive.official-documents.co.uk/document/cm43/4386/4386–uk/document/cm43/4386/4304.htm.

Erens, B., Primatesta, P., Prior, G. (Eds.), 2001. The Health Survey for England – The Health of Minority Ethnic Groups 1999. The Stationery Office, London. Online. Available at: http://www.archive.official-documents.co.uk/document/doh/survey99/hse99.htm.

Higgs, P., 2003. Older people, health care and society. In: Scambler, G. (Ed.), Sociology as Applied to Medicine, fifth ed. Saunders, Edinburgh, p. 167.

Hillier, S., 2003. The health and health care of ethnic minority groups. In: Scambler, G. (Ed.), Sociology as Applied to Medicine, fifth ed. Saunders, Edinburgh, p. 146.

Marmot, M., 2003. Understanding social inequalities in health. Perspect. Biol. Med. 46 (3), S9–S23.

Marmot, M., 2010. Fair Society, Healthy Lives: Strategic review of health inequalities in England post-2010. The Marmot Review, London.

Moody, H., 1995. Ageing, meaning and the allocation of resources. In: Scambler, G. (Ed.), 2003 Sociology as Applied to Medicine, fifth ed. Saunders, Edinburgh, p. 172.

Office for National Statistics (ONS), 1997. Health Inequalities. Office for National Statistics, London, Decennial Supplement. Online. Available at: http://www.statistics.gov.uk/StatBase/Product.asp?vlnk=1382&More=Y.

Office for National Statistics (ONS), 2010. The National Statistics Socio-economic Classification. ONS, London (NS-SEC rebased on the SOC2010).

Scambler, G., Blane, D., 2003. Inequality and social class. In: Scambler, G. (Ed.), Sociology as Applied to Medicine, fifth ed. Saunders, Edinburgh, pp. 107–123.

Sutherland, S. (Chairman), 1999. With Respect to Old Age: Long Term Care – Rights and Responsibilities. A Report by The Royal Commission on Long Term Care. Online. Available at: http://www.archive.official-documents.co.uk/document/cm41/4192/4192.htm.

Tudor Hart, J., 1971. The inverse care law. Lancet i, 405–412 (as described by Armstrong D 1989 An Outline of Sociology as Applied to Medicine, 3rd edn. London: Wright, pp. 112–114).

Further reading

Scambler, G. (Ed.), 2003. Sociology as Applied to Medicine, fifth ed. Saunders, Edinburgh.

Epidemiology and public health ⑩

INTRODUCTION

Epidemiology is the study of the distribution and the determinants of health or ill-health in populations, and its application to modify this distribution. In other words, epidemiologists are concerned with the health of the population as opposed to the health of the individual patient.

Public health is the systematic application of epidemiology, i.e. the promotion of health and disease prevention, thus prolonging life and improving the quality of life through the concerted efforts of society.

Since the 1960s, epidemiology has become important in assessing risk factors for, and reducing the incidence of, multifactorial diseases such as heart disease. The epidemiological approach studies:

- Definitions of disease
- Aetiologies (causes of disease)
- How disease spreads/occurs – the risk factors in individuals both within the population and in the environment
- How to control disease
- How to prevent disease
- How to eliminate disease

Uses for this discipline in planning healthcare provision include:

- Identifying factors that can affect the occurrence of disease
- Assessing the effectiveness of preventive and therapeutic interventions (this is sometimes known as *clinical epidemiology*)
- Assessing the impact of healthcare services
- Predicting future healthcare needs.

Prior to 1968, smallpox disease killed approximately 10 million people worldwide per year. The eradication of this disease in 1979 was heralded as the single greatest achievement of the public health initiatives (Fig. 10.1).

TYPES OF EPIDEMIOLOGICAL RESEARCH

Epidemiological studies, regardless of type, seek to understand the frequency, pattern and causes of disease in populations. They all permit comparing the experience of disease in terms of time, person or place.

The main types of study-design that one will be confronted with as a clinician are:

- ecological
- cross-sectional
- case–control
- cohort
- randomized-controlled trial (RCT)
- meta-analysis.

Another useful way of classifying the various types of studies is shown in Figure 10.2.

Ecological study

Ecological studies use groups or populations rather than individuals as units of observation. They include studies of geographical differences and time trends in disease incidence and prevalence. While ecological studies provide useful information on exposure, disease and modifying factors, they are in most cases inadequate to establish causal relationships. An example of such a study would be one that compares the incidence of skin cancer for people living at different latitudes.

Cross-sectional studies

Describe the distribution of a disease in relation to:

- person (age, sex, race, marital status, occupation, lifestyle)
- place (variation between and within countries)
- time (variation over time and season).

Advantages include:

- Quick and easy
- Relatively cheap and easy to carry out
- Useful for healthcare providers to allocate resources efficiently and plan effective prevention
- Providing clues leading to hypotheses that can be tested in analytical studies
- Status of individuals with respect to absence or presence of both exposure and disease assessed at *the same point in time*.

Disadvantages include:

- Hypothesis is generally poorly defined
- Confounding is high and hence it is difficult to prove causality
- Cannot distinguish whether exposure preceded disease
- Selection and recall bias.

Fig. 10.1 Smallpox eradication plan, illustrating the epidemiological approach.

Step	Answer
Definition	Infectious disease
Cause	*Variola* virus
Risk factors	Overcrowding, excessive mobility of population due to political instability and extreme poverty leading to poor hygiene and poor nutrition
Control	Risk factors could not be altered adequately, so decided to eliminate virus
Prevention	Administer smallpox vaccine en masse Also continuous surveillance and containment of infected patients

An example of a cross-sectional study would be studying the different reasons for people consulting their GPs in three different cities by using a cross-section of the individual populations in the three cities.

Case–control study

A case group with disease is compared with a control group without disease and the proportion of exposure in each group is compared.

Advantages include:

- Quick and inexpensive
- Well-suited for evaluation of diseases with long latent periods
- Optimal for evaluation of rare *diseases*
- Can examine multiple aetiological factors for a single disease.
- Can use expensive tests
- Measurement consistency as exposure and disease collected at the same time.

Disadvantages include:

- Inefficient for evaluation of rare *exposures*
- Cannot compute incidence rates in exposed and unexposed individuals
- The temporal relationship between exposure and disease may be difficult to establish
- Problems with recall and selection bias
- Cannot estimate the incidence of disease.

An example of a case–control study would be the occurrence of eosinophilia-myalgia syndrome (EMS), and the previous use of a specific brand of L-tryptophan.

Cohort studies

Subjects are classified according to presence or absence of exposure to one or more factors and followed for a specific time period to determine the development of

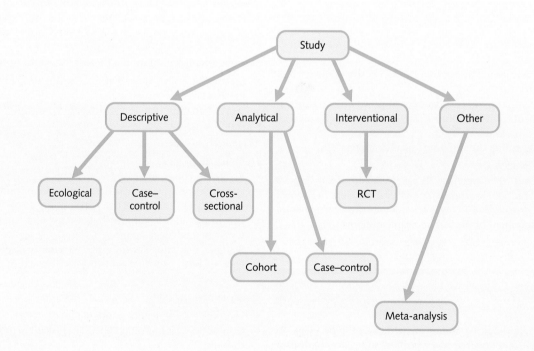

Fig. 10.2 Types of epidemiological study.

disease. There is a follow-up period of several years to allow an adequate number to develop the outcome. *Advantages* include:

- Valuable for rare exposures
- Can examine multiple effects of a single exposure
- Can elucidate temporal relationship between exposure and disease
- Minimize bias in exposure ascertainment
- Allow direct incidence calculation.

Disadvantages include:

- Inefficient for evaluation of rare diseases
- Prospective: expensive and time-consuming
- Retrospective: availability of adequate records
- Losses of follow-up can affect results.

Prospective and retrospective cohort studies

The choice of study type (prospective or retrospective) depends upon whether the outcome of interest has occurred at the time the investigator initiates the study:

- *Prospective* cohort study: exposure may or may not have occurred but disease has not occurred yet
- *Retrospective* cohort study: investigation initiated after both exposure and disease have occurred:
  - A cohort study can start retrospectively by defining cohort and exposures and then follow-up cohort (e.g. congenital malformations and later cancer).
  - Retrospective cohort studies are cheaper and thus better for diseases with a long latency.
  - Retrospective studies require information from pre-existing records (confounder information may be missing).

An example of a cohort study would be dividing 100 000 doctors into four cohorts: non-smoker, light, moderate and heavy smoker, and following them for 10 years to assess their causes of death. The idea is to show that the more you smoke, the greater your chances of acquiring lung cancer.

Trials and meta-analyses

Evidence-based medicine (EBM) has been very successful at identifying and promoting effective treatments (EBM is considered in Chapter 11). The gold standard of evidence-based medicine has historically been the *randomized controlled trial* (RCT). Two important techniques used to collate the information from trials are meta-analyses and systematic reviews. *Meta-analysis* combines the results of many (possibly inconclusive) trials to generate a more precise understanding of the effectiveness of an intervention. Systematic reviews use rigorous selection and analysis of papers to draw the most valid conclusion about whether or not an intervention works.

MEASURES OF HEALTH AND TREATMENT OUTCOMES

Doctors and patients, Armstrong (2003) argues, do not necessarily have the same view of health. This can be a problem when trying to measure health status for the purposes of: research (e.g. is a new drug better than the existing standard?); evaluation (e.g. does this service improve patient health?); or resource allocation (e.g. which group of patients is in most need of care?). In practice, there is a variety of different measures, each with advantages and disadvantages.

Mortality rates

The simplest form of mortality measure is the *crude mortality rate* (CMR):

$$CMR = \frac{\text{No. of deaths in a specified period} \times 100}{\text{Average total population during that period}}$$

The main advantage of using the CMR is that mortality can be expressed as a single figure. This is useful when comparing mortality within an area over a period of time. However, the main disadvantage is that it does not take into account that the chance of dying varies according to age and sex. In fact, standardization is usually aimed at age and sex alone because the effects of these are normally taken as given, whereas possible differences in relation to race and social class are issues for research.

Specific mortality rates refer to the number of deaths occurring in a sub-group of the population. To aid this, there are age-specific and gender-specific mortality rates. These help to detect which parts of the community are most affected by mortality:

$$\text{Age/sex-specific rate} = \frac{\begin{array}{c}\text{No. of deaths in each age/}\\\text{sex group in a period}\end{array}}{\begin{array}{c}\text{Average no. of people in age/}\\\text{sex population in a period}\end{array}}$$

Standardized rates take into account the different age/sex structure of two populations so that their mortality experience can be compared directly. Hence, we eliminate the confounding factors of age and sex.

The most common means of comparison is the *standardized mortality ratio* (SMR), which is the ratio of observed deaths to expected deaths expressed as a percentage:

$$SMR = \frac{\text{Observed deaths} \times 100}{\text{Expected deaths}}$$

An SMR of 100 indicates that observed deaths equals the expected number of deaths (average mortality). An

SMR >100 indicates observed deaths exceed expected deaths, and an SMR <100 indicates observed deaths lower than expected deaths.

It is worth noting that the process of standardizing mortality rates is complex. There are two methods of standardization, *indirect* and *direct*.

Potential years of life lost

- The potential years of life lost (PYLL) is an indicator of premature mortality. It represents the total number of years NOT lived by an individual who died before age 75 years.
- This indicator gives more importance to the causes of death that occurred at younger ages than those that occurred at older ages.
- The upper age limit of 75 years is used to approximate the life expectancy, as that is considered the average life-span for someone in good health.
- Deaths occurring in individuals aged 75 years or older are NOT included in the calculation.
- Infant deaths – deaths among infants under 1 year of age – are not included in the calculation due to their very small numbers. Other methods exclude these deaths since they are often due to causes that have different aetiology from deaths at later ages.

Quality-adjusted life years

Quality-adjusted life years (QALYs) is a single health state measure combining quantity and quality of life (see also Ch. 5). It is a generic measure that sums years spent in different health states using weights (on a scale of 0 (dead) to 1 (perfectly healthy) for each health state). So, 5 years of perfect health = 5 QALYs; 2 years in a state measured as 0.5 of perfect health followed by 3 years of perfect health = 4 QALYs.

Advantages

- Large studies using QALYs have reliable and valid results.
- Used in cost utility analysis – which allows comparison between interventions that nominally differ in terms of outcomes.

Disadvantages

- Theoretical questions: good and bad are qualitative ideas which are assigned a quantitative value.
- Ill people are likely to put values on health that are different from people without illness.
- Calculation is dependent on *who* is asked – patient, doctor – and *how* they are asked.

Morbidity (illness) rates

While death is (generally) a certain and countable event, mortality rates do not tell us much about illness or health in a population. Morbidity, illness and health are, however, considerably more difficult to define, and hence to measure, than death. The following measures are commonly used.

Health service use measures

- Consultation rates, e.g. with GP
- Referral rates, e.g. by GP
- Hospital admission and discharge rates.

These suffer from the problem that access to healthcare providers affects rate of usage.

Illness self-report rates

- General Lifestyle Survey (GLS)
- Sickness-absence rates
- Specific survey studies using a validated questionnaire.

Each of these has its own limitations in terms of coverage. For example, sickness-absence rates do not include people who are not working, such as pensioners or the unemployed. Despite being more difficult to measure, when used carefully, morbidity rates can tell us much about ill-health in specific groups of the population.

MEASURES OF DISEASE OCCURRENCE

Two basic measurements are used to assess the frequency of ill-health events: *incidence* and *prevalence* (Figs 10.3, 10.4).

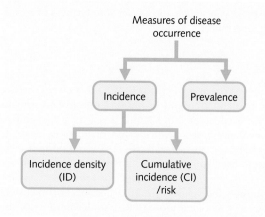

Fig. 10.3 Measures of disease occurrence.

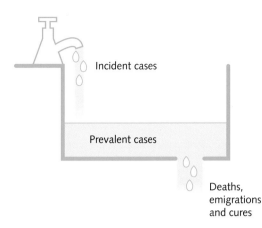
Incident cases

Prevalent cases

Deaths,
emigrations
and cures

Fig. 10.4 Characteristics of incidence and prevalence.

Incidence

Incidence quantifies the number of *new* cases of a disease within a specified time-interval. It measures a change from a healthy state to a diseased state. Hence it can only be assessed using follow-up studies, e.g. cohort studies. There are two categories of incidence rate: cumulative incidence and incidence density.

Cumulative incidence

Cumulative incidence (CI) is the proportion of unaffected individuals who, on average, will contract the disease in question over a period of time:

$$CI = \frac{A \text{ (no. of new cases of disease in a given period of time)}}{N \text{ (no. of disease} - \text{free persons at the beginning of that period of time)}}$$

Incidence density

Cumulative incidence assumes that the entire population at risk at the beginning of the study has been followed-up for the *entire* specified period of time. Often, however, some participants will enter the study years after the start, and some will be lost to follow-up before the study ends. This is a *dynamic* population. In these circumstances, the length of follow-up will not be uniform for all participants.

Incidence density (ID) accounts for these varying time-periods of follow-up and the denominator can be calculated to represent the sum of the individuals' times at risk, i.e. the sum of time that each person remained under observation and was at risk. This is called *the person-time* (PT):

$$PT = \text{average size of population at risk} \times \text{average length of observation}$$

The ID measures the rapidity with which newly diagnosed cases of the disease develop:

$$ID = \frac{A}{PT}$$

Prevalence

This indicates the number of existing cases of the disease of interest in a population. As it is often measured at a particular point in time, it is called *point prevalence* (P):

$$P = \frac{C \text{ (no. of cases in a defined population at one point in time)}}{N \text{ (no. of persons in a defined population of the same size)}}$$

Prevalence is a proportion. It is the only measure of disease occurrence that can be obtained from *cross-sectional studies*. It measures the burden of disease, i.e. the status of a condition in the population.

CAUSAL ASSOCIATION

Association is the statistical dependence between two variables, i.e. the degree to which the rate of disease in persons with a specific exposure is either higher or lower than the rate of disease without that exposure.

Even the best-designed RCTs may contain errors. Even if no errors can be found, it is still necessary to critically evaluate any observed association before reasonably concluding that it is a *causal* one.

Four main areas must be looked at when evaluating a statistical association:

1. *Chance* – we usually draw inferences about the total population from the sample that we have studied. However, it is unlikely that the estimate from our sample is equal to the estimate in the total population and, in fact, different samples from the same population will yield different estimates due to sampling variation, i.e. just as a result of chance. To assess the effect of chance, we perform appropriate statistical significance tests and calculate confidence intervals.
2. *Bias* – leads to an incorrect estimate of the effect of an exposure on the development of a disease or outcome of interest. There are different types of bias:
   a. Selection bias – occurs when there is a systematic difference between the characteristics of the people selected for a study and the characteristics of those who were not, e.g. all patients who enrol for an exercise ECG experiment will probably be health conscious.

Fig. 10.5   Bradford-Hill Criteria (Bradford-Hill 1965).

Criteria	Details
Temporal relationship	Exposure must precede the disease
Plausibility	Results must be consistent with other knowledge, e.g. animal experiments, biological mechanisms, etc.
Consistency	There should be other studies that replicate the results of the study in question
Strength	Measured by the magnitude of the relative risk. Stronger associations are more likely to be causal
Dose–response relationship	If increasing levels of exposure lead to increasing risks of disease, the higher the chance of causality
Specificity	If a particular exposure increases the risk of a certain disease but not the risk of other diseases, then this is strong evidence in favour of a cause–effect relationship
Reversibility	When the removal of a possible cause results in a reduced disease risk, the likelihood of the association being causal is strengthened

b. Measurement or information bias – occurs when measurements or classifications of disease or exposure are inaccurate and do not measure correctly what they are supposed to measure. Errors in measurement may be introduced by the *observer* (observer bias), by the *study individual* (responder bias) or by the *instruments* (e.g. questionnaire or sphygmomanometer) used to make the measurements. Observer bias can also occur if a doctor tends to favour a particular treatment. For example, a doctor may judge the outcome for the patients undergoing a new treatment in a more favourable way than for those in a placebo group. *Recall bias* occurs when patients' recall of their past exposure to risk factors differs from the recall of the controls. If patients with breast cancer are more likely to remember having ever used oral contraceptives than healthy controls, a spurious association between oral contraceptives and breast cancer will result.

3. *Confounding* – occurs when an estimate of the association between an exposure and the disease is mixed up with the real effect of another exposure on the same disease – the two exposures being correlated. For example, a report was published that made the claim that coffee consumption is associated with the risk of cancer of the pancreas. The importance of this association was disputed because it was pointed out that coffee consumption was correlated with cigarette smoking, and cigarette smoking was known to be a risk factor for pancreatic cancer. Therefore, smoking confounded the association between coffee and cancer of the pancreas. For a variable to be a confounder, it must be associated with the exposure under study and it must also be independently associated with disease risk in its own right.

4. *Cause – The Bradford-Hill Criteria, (Bradford-Hill 1965)* are pivotal in identifying a causal relationship between two variables (Fig. 10.5).

> **HINTS AND TIPS**
>
> *Remember*: In epidemiology, it is rare that one study alone will provide sufficient proof that a certain exposure affects the risk of a particular disease. However, the confidence with which you believe in the association between the risk factor and the disease will also depend on whether the correct type of study design is used to demonstrate the association.

MEASURES OF ASSOCIATION BETWEEN EXPOSURE AND DISEASE

The basic aim of epidemiological research is to investigate the association between exposure to a risk factor (e.g. smoking) and the occurrence of disease. This requires that the incidence in a group of persons exposed to the risk factor be compared with a group not exposed. There are two ways of doing this, *relative risk* and *attributable risk*.

Relative risk

$$\text{Relative risk} = \frac{\text{Incidence in the exposed group}}{\text{Incidence in the unexposed group}}$$

The *relative risk* can either be calculated using the *cumulative incidence*, in which case it is sometimes referred to as the *risk ratio*, or calculated using the *incidence rate*, when it may be referred to as the *rate ratio*.

The relative risk is used as a measure of aetiological strength. A value of 1.0 indicates that the incidence of disease in the exposed and the unexposed is identical and thus the data show no association between the exposure and the disease. A value greater than 1.0 indicates a positive association or an increased risk among those exposed to a factor. Similarly, a relative risk less than 1.0 means there is an inverse association or a decreased risk among those exposed, i.e. the exposure is protective.

Attributable risk

Information on the relative risk alone does not provide the full picture of the association between exposure and disease.

The *attributable risk* is a measure of exposure effect that indicates on an absolute scale how much greater the frequency of disease in the exposed group is compared with the frequency in the unexposed group, assuming that the relationship between exposure and disease is causal. It is the *difference* between incidence in the two groups.

It can either be calculated using the *cumulative incidence*, in which case it is sometimes referred to as the *risk difference*, or calculated using the *incidence rate*, when it may be referred to as the *rate, difference*.

The *attributable risk* is especially useful in evaluating the impact of introduction or removal of risk factors. Its value indicates the number of cases of the disease among the exposed group that could be prevented if the exposure were completely eliminated. In RCTs, attributable risk is referred to as 'absolute risk reduction':

Attributable risk = Incidence in the exposed
              − Incidence in the unexposed

Odds ratio

Relative risk can be calculated from cohort studies, since the incidence of disease in the exposed and non-exposed is known. In *case–control studies*, however, the subjects are selected on the basis of their disease status (sample of subjects with a particular disease, i.e. cases and sample of subjects without that disease, i.e. controls), not on the basis of exposure. Therefore, it is not possible to calculate the incidence in the exposed and non-exposed individuals. It is, however, possible to calculate the *odds of exposure*. This is the number of people who have been exposed divided by the number of people who have not been exposed. The *odds ratio of exposure* is the *odds of exposure* in the cases divided by the *odds of exposure* in the controls:

$$\text{Odds ratio} = \frac{\text{Odds of exposure in the diseased group (cases)}}{\text{Odds of exposure in the diseased-free group (controls)}}$$

It can be shown that this *odds ratio* of exposure is generally a good estimate of the relative risk if the disease is rare.

THE CHANGING PATTERN OF DISEASE

As populations change, the pattern of disease within it also changes. This is evident in England from the changing pattern of disease over time, as reflected in mortality rates and life expectancy at birth:

- In 1851 mortality in England: 22.7 per 1000 population
- In 2001 mortality in England: 11.9 per 1000 population
- In 1901 life expectancy: men – 47 years; women – 50 years
- In 2001 life expectancy: men – 75 years; women – 80 years.

These figures show that average life expectancy has increased by around 30 years in the past century. This has been achieved in the main by the reduction of *infant* and *child* mortality. The average life expectancy of a 50-year-old individual in 1850 and a 50-year-old today has not greatly increased.

> **HINTS AND TIPS**
>
> *Life expectancy* helps us to assess the health status of a population. It is defined as the average number of years one can expect an individual of a given age to live if current mortality trends continue.

The mortality rates and life expectancies that the UK experienced 150 years ago are similar to current rates of developing world countries (e.g. Ethiopia – mortality of 23.6 per 1000).

The changing pattern of disease and society

As different types of society have evolved, the major causes of disease have changed.

Pre-agricultural society

Little is known about the health and risks to health of pre-agricultural societies. It is assumed that the major health risks were environmental.

Agricultural society

Agricultural societies produced the bulk of their food by growing crops and through the domestication of animals. As the lifestyle was no longer nomadic, the populations were of a greater density and sanitation was poor. As a result, air-borne (TB), water-borne (cholera), food-borne (dysentery) and vector-borne (malaria) infectious diseases become the major health risk.

Modern industrial societies

Infectious disease has become gradually less important in modern societies. This is probably due to:

- decreased exposure to pathogens, due to changes in domestic housing and reduction in contamination of food and water supplies
- improved nutrition, especially in mothers and children
- increased acquired resistance to infection and the ability to recover from infection – due to improved nutrition
- specific medical intervention, e.g. antibiotics and vaccinations
- economic development and improved standard of living.

However, some populations are still vulnerable to certain infections, e.g. the elderly tend to get pneumonia and certain immigrant populations are at a higher risk of TB. In addition to this, certain infections are now becoming an increasing problem due to antibiotic resistance.

Major causes of death now include:

- Coronary heart disease
- Cancers
- Respiratory disease
- Strokes.

Major causes of morbidity include:

- Arthritis
- Obesity and diabetes
- Mental-health problems.

'Developing world' diseases

The global pattern of disease varies greatly between 'developed' and 'developing' countries. The developed world has a greater burden of non-communicable degenerative disease, e.g. cardiovascular disease, stroke, respiratory disease, cancers and mental illness. In the developing world, the main causes of death are also cardiovascular, stroke and respiratory disease. In addition however, communicable or infectious diseases, e.g. malaria, TB and HIV/AIDS, are major killers and causes of ill-health in the population. The younger population tends to suffer more. About 70% of young children who die from diarrhoeal diseases could be saved if widespread low-cost oral rehydration therapy was available. The problem is compounded by the lack of adequate sanitation, clean water and nutrition; these are commonly exacerbated in conflict zones. Malaria can be prevented by prophylactic measures, e.g. sleeping under mosquito nets, but the cost of implementing these is great. There is also an emerging resistance to the drugs normally used to treat malaria.

The solution to these problems will take roughly the same route as that taken by developed countries. Possible areas of intervention include trying to improve national and local wealth, living standards, clean water supplies and sanitation, nutrition and educational status of the people (see Fig. 10.6).

MEASURING THE HEALTH OF A NATION

Routine data are not often collected for a specific research purpose; however, such data may contain information associated with health and social services. Epidemiologists have access to a multitude of data sources. The accuracy, validity and completeness of such information depends on how regularly it is used and, hence, how much attention is paid to it (Figs 10.7, 10.8). Some different sources of data are outlined below.

Fig. 10.6 Factors affecting health.

Fixed	Social and economic	Environment	Lifestyle	Access to services
Genes	Poverty	Air quality	Diet	Education
Sex	Employment	Housing	Physical activity	NHS
Ageing	Social exclusion	Water quality	Smoking	Social services
		Social environment	Alcohol	Transport
			Sexual behaviour	Leisure
			Drugs	

Fig. 10.7 Sources of routine data.

Demographic and lifestyle data	Census General Lifestyle Survey (GLS) Registrar of births and marriages
Morbidity data	Morbidity statistics from general practice Communicable disease surveillance – infectious disease notification Hospital in-patient enquiry Hospital activity analysis/Hospital Episode System (HES) Cancer registration
Mortality data	Office for National Statistics (ONS) Mortality Statistics Registrar General's Decennial Supplement on Occupational Mortality
Specific datasets	ONS Survey of Disability ONS Longitudinal Study Abortion data Congenital anomalies Workmen's compensation data
Health service data	Immunization levels achieved Uptake of cervical cancer and breast cancer screening District and regional annual reports Chief Medical Officer's annual report Reviews of perioperative mortality and maternal mortality
Other	Social security statistics Private sector and voluntary organization data

Fig. 10.8 Pros and cons of routine data.

Value of routine data	Limitations of routine data
Readily available	Lack of completeness, with potential for bias – may not answer the question
Already collected and available	Incomplete ascertainment, as not every case is captured
Standardized collection procedures	Limited details of determinants such as income and ethnicity
Limited costs	Often poorly presented and analysed – need careful interpretation
Up-to-date and relatively comprehensive; available for past years	Disease labelling may vary over time, e.g. asthma definition has been changing
Wide range of recorded items	Coding changes may create artefactual ↑/↓ in rates
Experience in use and interpretation	Occasionally subject to political influences and manipulation
Useful for identifying hypotheses	Health services' data more geared to process than health status and outcomes
Useful for initial assessment	Public concerns about confidentiality, especially with respect to identifiable data (see Ch. 2)
Provides baseline data on expected levels of health/disease	

Demographic data

This provides us with the denominators necessary to calculate incidence and prevalence. The best example is the *Census* that is conducted every 10 years and gives details on family size, socioeconomic status, highest level of education attained, and the age, sex distribution and geographical location of the population.

The *GHS (General Lifestyle Survey)* collects data from a questionnaire administered to a stratified random sample of households. Data collected relates to population, employment, housing, education, income and family structure and details on many health-related items, such as prevalence of disability, utilization of general practitioners' services, dietary habits, alcohol and tobacco consumption.

Mortality data

This is based upon completion of a standard death certificate, which records the date of death, cause of death, age, sex, date of birth and place of residence. In addition, occupation and other variables may be recorded. Certain causes of death may be poorly recorded. In the UK, for example, it has been shown that deaths from HIV disease and AIDS, which may be stigmatized, are under-recorded in an attempt to maintain confidentiality. Other problems are that data from urban areas may be more complete than data from rural areas, and people belonging to higher social classes are likely to have a more detailed cause of death recorded. The main cause of death in an individual is that pathological process that directly led to the patient's death. The patient may have other co-morbid conditions that worsen the prognosis, but do not directly lead to death, e.g. diabetes or hypertension.

Morbidity data

Morbidity data are often routinely available and provide insights into conditions that may not necessarily result in death. Certain communicable diseases, e.g. meningitis, malaria, need to be reported by law. This information is sent to the Public Health Laboratory Service who surveys and monitors the reported incidence of communicable diseases and detects unusual patterns or epidemics.

DEATH CERTIFICATION

Following the Harold Shipman murders in the 1990s, there remains a general dissatisfaction with the way in which deaths are certified by doctors in the UK. Studies of the accuracy of death certification have found up to one-third of death certificates to contain major errors. A recent English study reported that only 55% of certificates were completed to an acceptable standard. The main explanations for these errors are:

- lack of training of doctors
- inadequate or misunderstood clinical information
- concealment of information that might distress family members
- omissions of information
- coding errors.

Variations between countries in the post-mortem criteria may also lead to differences in diagnostic information and hence the cause of death.

The certificate of death registration (DC) is vital for the funeral to proceed. A doctor may complete this form only if he or she has been in attendance on the deceased during the last illness and has seen the deceased within 14 days of death or after death. There are some cases that have to be reported to the coroner:

- Violent deaths
- Deaths when a doctor has not attended in the previous 14 days
- When the cause of death is unknown or uncertain
- Accidental death
- Doubtful stillbirth
- Deaths related to surgery or anaesthetic
- Deaths within 24 hours of admission to hospital.

When a death is reported to the coroner, he may: certify the death on the basis of the information he has or acquires; certify the death after ordering an autopsy; or certify the death after holding an inquest. The DC must reach the coroner's office in 5 days.

HINTS AND TIPS

There are three categories of death: those certified by a doctor; those certified by a doctor with the coroner's agreement; and those reported to and investigated by the coroner.

PREVENTION

An effective healthcare system aims to provide health services to the sick and public health services to promote health and prevent the spread of disease. *Prevention* refers to actions aimed at *eradicating, eliminating* or *minimizing* the impact of disease and disability. There are three levels of prevention:

1. *Primary* – prevent disease
2. *Secondary* – detect disease
3. *Tertiary* – reduce damage.

Primary prevention

This aims to stop a disease from manifesting itself. It often calls for strategies that aim to remove or destroy agents that cause disease. Other aspects include environmental control and immunization.

Secondary prevention

This proposes to detect a disease at its earliest possible stage followed by initiating measures to cure, or prevent further progression of the condition. The most important example in this category is screening programmes coupled with effective interventions.

Tertiary prevention

This aims to reduce the damage caused by the disease, e.g. encouraging smokers with lung cancer to quit smoking (a modifiable risk-factor that can retard progression of the disease).

Targeting a high-risk group will benefit individuals in this group, but will do little to decrease the overall burden of the disease in the population.

A population-based approach, on the other hand, which yields a smaller benefit in a larger number of individuals, may give better results. Also, there is no need to identify a high-risk group as the strategy targets all.

HEALTH PROMOTION

Health education is empowering individuals through increased knowledge and understanding. Unlike health promotion, there is no political advocacy. *Health promotion* interventions result in only small changes in risk factors and mortality in the general population (Fig. 10.9).

Effective health promotion relies on several factors: Public, Employers, Voluntary groups, Advertising, Media, Primary care, Local authority, Industry, Government, Health services – primary/secondary and Training.

The Quality and Outcomes Framework

In England, health promotion was linked to GP activity by The Quality and Outcomes Framework (QOF) (adapted from the NHS Information centre, at: http://www.qof.ic.nhs.uk/).

The QOF is an annual reward and incentive programme for all GP surgeries in England. The QOF contains four main components (domains): Clinical domain, Organizational domain, Patient experience domain and Additional services domain. Each domain consists of a set of achievement measures, known as indicators, against which practices score points according to their level of achievement. The 2010/2011 QOF measured achievement against 134 indicators; practices scored points on the basis of achievement against each indicator, up to a maximum of 1000 points:

- *Clinical care*: this domain consists of 86 indicators across 20 clinical areas (e.g. coronary heart disease, heart failure, hypertension) worth up to a maximum of 697 points
- *Organizational*: this domain consists of 36 indicators (worth up to 167.5 points) across five organizational areas – records and information; information for patients; education and training; practice management and medicines management

- *Patient experience*: this domain consists of three indicators (worth up to 91.5 points) that relate to length of consultations and to patient experience of access to GPs
- *Additional services*: this domain consists of nine indicators across four service areas – cervical screening, child health surveillance, maternity service and contraceptive services.

The QOF gives an indication of the overall achievement of a surgery through a points system. Practices aim to deliver high-quality care across a range of areas for which they score points. Put simply, the higher the score, the higher the financial reward for the practice. The final payment is adjusted to take account of surgery workload and the prevalence of chronic conditions in the practice's local area.

NATIONAL STRATEGIES FOR HEALTH IMPROVEMENT

The Health of the Nation was the first national strategy in the UK for health improvement. It was adopted in 1992 and set out long-term objectives and measurable targets for the improvement of health in five important areas (DoH 1992):

1. Coronary heart disease (CHD) and stroke
2. Cancers (breast, lung, cervical and skin)
3. Mental illness
4. HIV/AIDS and sexual health
5. Accidents.

These areas were selected because they were major causes of premature death or avoidable ill-health, and effective interventions were possible.

Saving lives: our Healthier Nation came into being in 1999. It is a comprehensive government-wide public health strategy for England (DoH 1999). Its goals are to improve health and to reduce health inequalities. The target was to reduce the following unnecessary deaths by the year 2010 in the following areas:

- Cancer: to reduce the death rate in people under 75 years by at least one-fifth
- Coronary heart disease and stroke: to reduce the death rate in people under 75 years by at least two-fifths
- Accidents: to reduce the death rate by at least one-fifth and serious injury by at least one-tenth
- Mental illness: to reduce the death rate from suicide and undetermined injury by at least one-fifth.

Key developments in *Saving Lives*, were: the emphasis on tackling inequalities, the emphasis on communities, cooperation between government agencies and multidisciplinary work. The document acknowledged the importance of social, economic and political influences. Rayner (2002) argues that despite being less individualistic than *The Health of the Nation*, *Saving Lives* overemphasized the role of the NHS and focussed on health trends and potential risks rather than local authorities, the role of industry

Fig. 10.9   Five approaches to health promotion.

	Aim	Health promotion activity	Important values	Example: smoking
Medical	Freedom from medically defined disease and disability	Promotion of medical intervention to prevent or ameliorate ill health	Patient compliance with preventative medical procedures	*Aim*: freedom from lung disease, heart disease and other smoking-related disorders *Activity*: encourage people to seek early detection and treatment of smoking-related disorders
Behaviour change	Individual behaviour conducive to freedom from disease	Attitude and behaviour change to encourage adoption of 'healthier' lifestyle	Healthy lifestyle as defined by health promoter	*Aim*: behaviour changes from smoking to non-smoking *Activity*: persuasive education to prevent non-smokers from starting and persuade smokers to stop
Educational	Individuals with knowledge and understanding enabling well-informed decisions to be made and acted upon	Information about cause and effects of health-demoting factors Exploration of values and attitudes Development of skills required for healthy living	Individual right of free choice Health promoter's responsibility to identify educational content	*Aim*: clients will have understanding of the effect of smoking on health; they will make a decision whether or not to smoke and act on that decision *Activity*: giving information to clients about the effects of smoking; helping them to explore their own values and attitudes and come to a decision; helping them to learn how to stop smoking if they want to
Client-centred	Working with clients on the client's own terms	Working with health issues, choices and actions which clients identify Empowering the client	Client as equal Client's right to set agenda Self-empowerment of client	*Aim*: anti-smoking issues are only considered if clients identify them as a concern *Activity*: clients identify what, if anything, they want to know about it
Societal change	Physical and social environment which enables choice of healthier lifestyle	Political/social action to change physical/social environment	Right and need to make environment health-enhancing	*Aim*: make smoking socially unacceptable, so it is easier not to smoke than to smoke *Activity*: no-smoking policy in public places; cigarette sales less accessible, especially to children; promotion of non-smoking as social norm; banning tobacco advertising and sports sponsorship

From Scriven 2010, with permission.

and the press. There has been considerable progress to meeting the targets in *Saving Lives* with the notable exception of accidental deaths, which have increased.

SCREENING

Screening is the practice of investigating apparently healthy individuals with the object of detecting unrecognized disease or its precursors in order that measures can be taken to prevent or delay the development of disease or improve prognosis.

HINTS AND TIPS

Remember: Screening tests are generally not definitive. A screening test is usually cheap and simple, and aims to identify people at high risk of the condition. Further diagnostic tests are then done to confirm diagnosis.

Purpose of screening

Screening acts at all three levels of prevention:

1. Early detection of diseases where prognosis is improved by earlier treatment (e.g. screening for breast cancer and offering surgical and other treatments)
2. Detection of people at increased risk of developing disease where interventions will reduce that risk (e.g. screening for high blood cholesterol levels and offering dietary advice and/or drug therapy)
3. Identification of people with infectious disease, where treatment or other control measures will improve the outcome for the individual and prevent ongoing transmission to others (e.g. screening food handlers for salmonella; health workers for hepatitis B, etc.).

Mass, targeted, systematic or opportunistic screening

Screening can either involve the whole population (mass), or selected groups who are anticipated to have an increased prevalence of the condition (targeted). There may be a systematic programme where people are called for screening (e.g. cervical cancer) or screening may be done opportunistically when a person presents to the doctor for some other reason (e.g. blood pressure). Opportunistic screening or case-finding is advantageous, in that over 90% of people will see their GP over a 2-year period, so it is cost-effective, while picking up a large proportion of cases. The problem is that there is reliance on the GP to regularly test for the condition, even if the patient presents with another problem, and with current workloads, this can sometimes be forgotten (Fig. 10.10).

Fig. 10.10 Criteria for screening based on WHO guidelines.

Parameter	Factor
Disease	Important health problem Well recognized pre-clinical stage Natural history understood Long period between first signs and overt disease
Diagnostic test	Valid (sensitive and specific) Simple and cheap Safe and acceptable Reliable
Diagnosis and treatment	Facilities are adequate Effective, acceptable and safe treatment available Cost-effective Sustainable

There are WHO guidelines for deciding when screening is appropriate (drawn up by Wilson and Jungner 1968):

1. The condition being screened for should be an important health problem
2. The natural history should be well understood
3. There should be a detectable early stage
4. Treatment at an early stage should be of greater benefit than at a later stage
5. There should be a suitable, valid test for the early stage
6. The test should be acceptable
7. Intervals for repeating the test should be determined
8. There should be adequate health service provision for the extra clinical workload resulting from the screen
9. The risks should be less than the benefits
10. The costs should be balanced against the benefits.

The validity of a screening test is measured by its ability to do what it is supposed to do, that is distinguish between subjects with the condition and those without (Fig. 10.11).

Evaluating screening programmes

Even after a disease is determined to be appropriate for screening and a valid test becomes available, it does not necessarily follow that a widespread screening programme should be implemented. Evaluation of a potential screening programme involves consideration of three main issues outlined below.

Feasibility

Feasibility will depend on how easy it is to organize the population to attend for screening, whether the screening test is acceptable, whether facilities and resources exist to carry out the necessary diagnostic tests following screening.

Effectiveness

Effectiveness is evaluated by the extent to which implementing a screening programme affects the subsequent outcomes. This is difficult to measure because of a number of biases that affect most of the study designs used.

Selection bias exists as people who participate in screening programmes often differ from those who do not.

Lead-time bias exists because screening identifies disease that would otherwise be identified at a later stage. This may result in an apparent improvement in the length of survival due to screening, which is really due to the earlier date of diagnosis.

Length bias exists as some conditions may be slower in developing to a health-threatening stage, that is, they have a longer preclinical stage. This means they are more likely to be detected at that stage, but they may also have a more favourable prognosis, leading to the false conclusion that screening is beneficial in lengthening the lives of those found positive.

Fig. 10.11 Validity of a screening test.

	Disease +ve	Disease –ve	
Test +ve	a	b	All test +ve: a+b
Test –ve	c	d	All test –ve: c+d
	All disease +ve: a+c	All disease –ve: b+d	

Sensitivity of screening test=proportion of true positive results detected by the screening test (%)=a/a+c

Specificity of screening test=proportion of true negative results detected by the screening test (%)=d/b+d

Positive predictive value (diagnostic value) of the test=the proportion of test positive results which are true positive results=a/a+b

Negative predictive value (diagnostic value) of the test=the proportion of test negative results which are true negative results=d/c+d

The predictive value thus indicates the likelihood of a positive or negative screening test result meaning the presence or absence of the disease, respectively

Knowledge of sensitivity and specificity of a test will influence the decision whether or not to perform it

Knowledge of the predictive value will influence the view that an individual does or does not have the disease, once the test result is available

Predictive values are dependent on prevalence. Even a test with good sensitivity and specificity, when applied to a population with a low prevalence will have a low positive predictive value

Screening programmes need to be tested by randomized controlled trials, partly to avoid the listed biases.

Cost

The cost of screening programmes is important. Resources for health care will always be scarce relative to competing demands. The relative cost-effectiveness of a screening programme compared with other forms of health care should, therefore, be considered. Costs relate not just to the implementation of the screening programme, but also to the further diagnostic tests and the subsequent cost of treatment. On the other hand, in the absence of screening, costs will be incurred by the treatment of patients in more advanced stages of disease (Fig. 10.12).

Possible harms caused by screening

A screening test is a medical intervention that is done to a person who is not ill and usually to someone who has not initiated the request for the test:

- The screening test can cause harm as well as providing benefits:
  - There may be a risk attached to the screening test or subsequent diagnostic test
  - A false positive result can cause unnecessary anxiety
  - There may be other unplanned effects of a positive test, e.g. the issue of diagnostic labelling that leads to the adoption of the sick role
  - A false negative result will give false reassurance.

Therefore, there may be a need for the patient to undergo some form of pre-test counselling.

Some important screening tests used today

Cervical cancer

The objective of cervical cancer screening is to detect cervical intraepithelial neoplasia. All women aged 20–64 years and whose names appear on GP lists held by health authorities are called. Screening occurs every

Fig. 10.12 Advantages and disadvantages of screening.

Screening	Opportunistic	Universal
Advantages	Cheap	Finds those who do not access healthcare services regularly
Disadvantages	Identifies signs not symptoms May not access high-prevalence groups	Stigma of recall for sexually transmitted disease High administration costs

3–5 years. If borderline/mild dyskaryosis is seen, then the patient undergoes a re-smear. If there is moderate/severe dyskaryosis, a referral for colposcopy, laser or loop diathermy is made. Since organized screening began, the number of invasive cervical cancer cases in England and Wales fell by 42% in 6 years: from 15.4 cases per 100 000 women in 1990 to 8.9 per 100 000 by 1996. Problems include inadequately taken smears, laboratory errors and patient apathy/fear towards recall for abnormal smears.

Breast cancer

Screening programmes aim to detect early breast cancer. The NHS Cancer Plan, published by the Department of Health in September 2000, set out future developments in the NHS Breast Screening Programme. The programme has been extended so that women from the age of 50 years up to and including the age of 70 years receive routine invitations for screening. A double-view mammogram is offered at 3-year intervals. Prior to 2004, the age range was 50–64 years and a single-view mammogram was offered. Some argue that screening needs to be increased to include those under 50 years of age. There also remain issues about the overall benefits and safety of mammography and whether a single-view or double-view mammogram is more useful.

Other screening programmes being researched include those for prostate, ovarian and colorectal cancer.

COMMUNICABLE DISEASES

A communicable disease is an illness caused by the *transmission* of a *specific microbial agent or its toxic products* from a *reservoir* to a susceptible *host*. Some common terms need to be understood:

- *Occurrence* – the frequency of a disease in a population without distinguishing between the incidence and prevalence
- *Reservoir* – the site(s) in which a disease agent normally lives and reproduces
- *Causative agent* – a micro-organism, e.g. viruses, bacteria, whose presence is necessary for the disease to occur
- *Transmission* – any mechanism by which an infectious agent is spread from a source or reservoir to another person. These mechanisms include:
  - *Direct transmission* – via direct contact, e.g. kissing, touching, sexual intercourse. Examples of pathogens are *Staphylococcus* and *HIV*
  - *Indirect transmission* – vertical transmission from mother to fetus (e.g. hepatitis B), air-borne/droplet (e.g. influenza), ingestion of contaminated

food/water (e.g. *Salmonella*) and vector-borne (e.g. malaria).

- *Incubation period* – the time interval between exposure to the infectious agent and the appearance of the first sign or symptom of the disease
- *Susceptibility* – the tendency of an individual to contract a disease. Affected by age, nutrition, gender, immunity and genetics.

Understanding the nature of the disease helps us to establish ways of controlling it. Generally speaking, we can use three methods to control the spread of disease:

1. *Controlling the agent* – involves removing agents before they enter into air, water and soil. For microbial agents, this may include prohibiting the consumption of affected foods or the use of bactericides on preparation surfaces.
2. *Controlling the environment* – controlling the vectors, e.g. mosquito nets to prevent the spread of malaria, or treating polluted air, water and soil. Also restricting access to certain areas may help.
3. *Controlling the host* – protecting high-risk individuals, e.g. young, old, sick or immunosuppressed. This can be achieved by promoting personal hygiene, providing immunizations (Fig. 10.13) or fostering health education.

Fig. 10.13 Primary tuberculosis as an example of communicable disease control.

Communicable disease parameter	Primary tuberculosis
Occurrence	5700 cases/year
Reservoir	Primarily human
Transmission	Mainly droplet nuclei
Incubation period	Often asymptomatic; casual short-term exposure is less likely to transmit the disease
Susceptibility – risk factors	Poor nutrition Poor living conditions Some sections of society, e.g. alcoholics, undernourished, some ethnic minority communities, the elderly, and HIV-positive individuals Farm workers who drink unpasteurized milk Gastrectomy patients
Control	Identifying and treating those who already have the disease, to shorten their infection and to stop it being passed on to other people BCG vaccine

IMMUNIZATION

In developed countries, the most beneficial and cost-effective health intervention for the primary prevention of infectious diseases is immunization. The aim of immunization is to provoke immunological memory to protect individuals against particular diseases. It can be defined as the protection of susceptible individuals from communicable disease by administration of a vaccine. Immunization can be *passive* (short-term, e.g. immunoglobulins or antibodies) or *active* (acquired naturally after recovery from infection with the causal organism or induced artificially via a vaccine).

A vaccine is an immunobiological agent injected into the body to stimulate an immune response. There are four types:

1. *Inactivated/killed vaccines* – made from whole organisms killed during manufacture, e.g. pertussis
2. *Live vaccines* – made from living organisms, which are either the disease-causing organisms whose virulence has been reduced by attenuation, e.g. MMR, or less virulent organisms of a species antigenically related to the causal agent, e.g. BCG
3. *Toxoids* – produced from artificially created, but harmless bacterial toxins, e.g. tetanus
4. *Component/sub-unit vaccines* – contain a component antigen(s) of the target organism required to evoke a suitable immune response, e.g. influenza.

Live vaccines are given in a single dose and have a longer duration of immunity. However, they may be less stable and revert to the virulent strain and cause disease in the immunosuppressed.

Inactivated vaccines are given in multiple doses and need a booster (Fig. 10.14). They confer shorter immunity and are stable.

Herd immunity is the immunity of a group or community. For example, if enough children acquire immunity to measles, owing to vaccination, the measles virus loses the ability to circulate in the community. Effective herd immunity can only be achieved with immunization rates of around 90% of the population. This is important for the protection of those who cannot be immunized, and because no vaccine is 100% effective.

Some of the factors associated with poor vaccine uptake are:

- sociodemographic variables
- deprived, inner-city living
- mobile families
- birth order, large families
- children with chronic illnesses
- ethnicity
- personal variables
- attitudes of parents
- attitudes of professionals
- health service variables – generally good in the UK, but be aware of some limitations
- poor coordination (private and public sectors)
- unclear responses, e.g. questioning the potential harms of the MMR vaccine
- access to guidelines and policies.

In the UK, it is a legal requirement for health authorities to be informed of certain 'notifiable diseases'. The Consultant in Communicable Disease Control (CCDC) is responsible for prevention, control and surveillance of communicable diseases. The Public Health Laboratory Service (PHLS) provides support to these doctors at a national level (Figs 10.15, 10.16). An up to date list of notifiable disease can be obtained from http://www.hpa.org.uk/.

MANAGEMENT OF DISEASE OUTBREAKS

The impact of disease can be described as follows:

- *Outbreak* – an epidemic restricted to a localized increase in the incidence of disease, e.g. in a county

Fig. 10.14 The current immunization schedule in the UK.

Age	Immunizations
2 months	Diphtheria/tetanus/pertussis/poliomyelitis/haemophilus type B (DTaP/IPV/Hib) (one injection) and pneumococcal vaccine (one injection)
3 months	DTaP/IPV/Hib (one injection) and meningococcus group C (MenC) (one injection)
4 months	DTaP/IPV/Hib (one injection), MenC (one injection) and pneumococcal vaccine (one injection)
12 months	Hib/MenC (one injection)
13 months	Measles, mumps and rubella (MMR) (one injection) and pneumococcal vaccine (one injection)
3 years and 4 months to 5 years	DTaP or dTaP (one injection) and MMR (one injection) (reduced dose diphtheria vaccine if aged over 10 or completed primary immunizations in infancy)
13–18 years	Diphtheria, tetanus and polio (Td/IPV) (one injection)

Up-to-date information on immunization and infectious disease may be found at: www.immunisation.nhs.uk

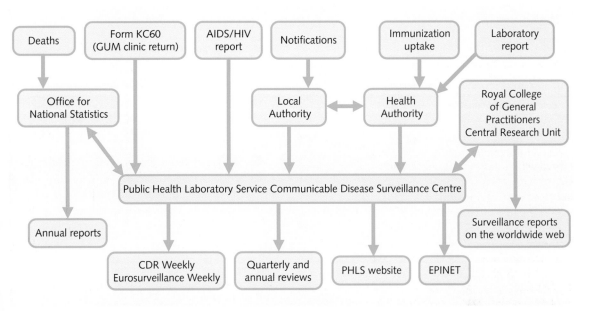

Fig. 10.15 Flow of information about communicable diseases in England and Wales. From Donaldson and Donaldson 2000, with permission.

- *Epidemic* – an increase in the incidence of a disease above that which is ever-present in a population
- *Endemic* – the incidence of a disease that is continuously present in a population
- *Pandemic* – an epidemic occurring across international boundaries and affecting a large number of people.

Surveillance is 'the continued watchfulness over the distribution and trends in the incidence of disease through the systematic collection, consolidation and evaluation of morbidity and mortality reports and other relevant data' (Langmuir 1963).

Sources of surveillance data include:

- Statutory notifications
- Laboratory reports
- Royal College of General Practitioners sentinel reporting system
- Hospital Episode Statistics (HES) data
- Death certificates
- Vaccine use
- Sickness absence
- Special systems: clinical HIV reporting, which is voluntary to the Communicable Disease Surveillance Centre (CDSC), the British Paediatrics Surveillance Unit and the Creutzfeldt–Jakob Disease (CJD) Surveillance Unit (important as cases rise).

Principles of surveillance

- Systematic collection of data
- Analyses of data to produce statistics

- Interpretation of statistics
- Distribution of this information to those who require it for action. Feedback is via Communicable Disease Report (CDR) Weekly, information services, internet information sites, e.g. Public Health Laboratory Service (PHLS)
- Continuing surveillance to evaluate action.

The CDSC publishes reports of notifications of diseases.

Steps in controlling an outbreak

1. Preliminary assessment in outbreak investigation – to confirm the existence of an outbreak. Consult the CDSC. If further investigations are needed, review the literature and survey the data. Form an outbreak control team. Also generate the initial hypothesis and initiate immediate control measures as necessary, e.g. stop symptomatic food handlers from working.
2. Case definition and identification – define 'cases' in terms of time/place/person/symptoms/laboratory results and define the population at risk.
3. Descriptive study – collect and analyse data. Draw the epidemic curve and generate the hypothesis. The aim is to link the cases to a source.
4. Analytical study – can be done using a *cohort study* (population is known, e.g. guests at party) or a *case–control study* for a large population. The aims are to test the generated hypothesis and to attempt to overcome bias.

Fig. 10.16 Notifiable diseases.

Acute encephalitis	Malaria
Acute poliomyelitis	Meningococcal septicaemia (without meningitis)
Acute infectious hepatitis	Measles
Acute meningitis	Mumps
Anthrax	Paratyphoid fever
Botulism	Plague
Brucellosis	Rabies
Cholera	Rubella
Diphtheria	SARS
Dysentery (amoebic or bacillary)	Scarlet fever
Enteric fever (typhoid or paratyphoid fever)	Smallpox
Food poisoning	Tetanus
Haemolytic uraemic syndrome (HUS)	Tuberculosis
Infectious bloody diarrhoea	Typhus
Invasive group A streptococcal disease	Viral haemorrhagic fever
Legionnaires' disease	Whooping cough
Leprosy	Yellow fever
Leptospirosis	

5. Verify hypothesis – by using food and environmental samples sent to the microbiology laboratory.
6. Institute control measures:
   a. Remove source: close outlet, isolate and treat cases, destroy/treat food
   b. Protect persons at risk: improve hygiene and prophylaxis
   c. Prevent recurrence: recommendations and guidelines.
7. Communicate – during the investigation give updated information to the public and professionals. Upon conclusion, publish a report for those involved and interested individuals.

Some of the steps above may be carried out simultaneously, so keep a record of the date and time.

Key questions

- What is epidemiology?
- What is public health?
- Describe the types of studies used in epidemiological research.
- What is the incidence and what is prevalence of a disease?
- What is the Quality and Outcomes Framework (QOF)?
- Which deaths need to be reported to the coroner?
- Can you give an example of an important screening test used today?
- How does immunization prevent disease outbreaks?
- Which diseases are notifiable?
- How are disease outbreaks managed?

References

Armstrong, D., 2003. Measuring health and illness. In: Outline of Sociology As Applied to Medicine, fifth ed. Hodder Arnold, London, pp. 14–23.

Bradford-Hill, A., 1965. The environment and disease: association or causation? Proceedings of the Royal Society of Medicine 58, 295–300.

Department of Health, 1992. The Health of the Nation – A Strategy for Health in England. HMSO, London.

Department of Health, 1999. Saving Lives: Our Healthier Nation. HMSO, London, Cm4386.

Donaldson, L.J., Donaldson, R.J., 2000. Essential Public Health. Petroc Press, Berkshire.

Langmuir, A.D., 1963. The surveillance of communicable diseases of national importance. N. Engl. J. Med. 268, 182–192.

Rayner, G., 2002. Building a UK public health movement. In: Adams, L., Amos, M., Munro, J. (Eds.), Promoting Health: Politics and Practice. Sage, London, pp. 20–25.

Scriven, A., 2010. Promoting Health: a Practical Guide (Ewles & Simnett). Baillière Tindall, Edinburgh.

Wilson, J.M.G., Jungner, G., 1968. Principles and Practice of Screening for Disease. World Health Organization, Geneva.

Further reading

Farmer, R., Lawrenson, R., Miller, D., 2001. Lecture Notes on Epidemiology and Public Health Medicine, fourth ed. Blackwell Science, Oxford.

Saracci, R., 2010. Epidemiology: A very short introduction. Oxford University Press, Oxford.

Vetters, N., Matthews, I., 1999a. Components of health care – preventative health care, health promotion and screening. In: Vetters, N., Matthews, I. (Eds.), Epidemiology and Public Health Medicine. Churchill Livingstone, Edinburgh, pp. 215–220.

Vetters, N., Matthews, I., 1999b. Environmental and occupational health-infectious disease. In: Vetters, N., Matthews, I. (Eds.), Epidemiology and Public Health Medicine. Churchill Livingstone, Edinburgh, pp. 129–136.

Questions about clinical governance and audit have been very popular in interviews for junior medical jobs. As some interviews have been replaced by examinations and extensive application forms, the need for an understanding of these concepts has not gone away – indeed junior doctors may often be asked how they themselves have taken part in clinical governance! This chapter provides a general overview and examines key aspects of clinical governance: evidence-based medicine, audit and risk management.

WHAT IS CLINICAL GOVERNANCE?

Clinical governance has become an increasingly important concept in everyday medical practice. Armstrong (2003) describes this as the tension between institutional control over clinical decisions while allowing individual doctors some freedom to act in the interests of their patients. He explains:

> . . . A hospital might appoint a clinician to lead on clinical governance in that hospital. That person will then discuss with colleagues the sort of actions they should take collectively to ensure that good-quality care is being provided. It may mean stricter adherence to protocols, or expectations that all clinicians will engage in auditing their own work, or arranging for peer review of certain services, or setting up a complaints system, or monitoring of prescribing, etc. The result is a culture of quality control in which all clinicians are aware that they are part of a wider attempt to maintain medical standards through reviewing their own as well as their colleagues' clinical performance. (see Fig. 11.1)

There are major implications for all stakeholders in the NHS, ranging from medical students and junior doctors to consultants. Some of these are:

- development of leadership and knowledge among clinicians
- development of mechanisms to ensure the 'audit loop' is closed, i.e. to ensure that change in clinical practice takes place in the *light of audit, research, evidence, risk management and complaints findings*
- Development of appropriate accountability structures in both primary and secondary care
- Implementation of evidence-based practice across organizations
- Improvement of the clinical information infrastructure of the NHS
- Development of effective multidisciplinary and inter-agency work
- Integration of continuing medical education (CME) and continuing professional development (CPD) into quality-improvement programmes.

The World Health Organization (1988) divides quality into four aspects:

1. Professional performance (technical quality)
2. Resource use (efficiency)
3. Risk management (the risk of injury or illness associated with the service provided)
4. Patients' satisfaction with the service provided.

The 1999 Clinical Governance Framework comprises a number of activities (the seven pillars) that were present before 1999. What Clinical Governance brings is a coordination of these activities, under the umbrella of the 'Seven Pillars of Clinical Governance':

1. Service user, carer and public involvement
2. Clinical effectiveness
3. Clinical risk management
4. Education, training and development

Health gain	Meaningful involvement of patients/public	Evidence-based practice and policy
Confidentiality	Risk management	Audit and evaluation
Accountability and performance	Core requirements	Health promotion

The building blocks of coordinated clinical governance

Coherent team

Managing resources and services	Reliable data	Research and development	Learning culture

Fig. 11.1 The 14 components of clinical governance. (Adapted from Chambers et al. 2007.)

5. Use of information
6. Staffing and staff management
7. Clinical audit.

The main pillars of relevance to medical students and junior doctors, which we will consider further are: clinical effectiveness, clinical audit and clinical risk management.

EVIDENCE-BASED MEDICINE (CLINICAL EFFECTIVENESS)

Evidence-based medicine (EBM) is the conscientious, explicit and judicious use of current best evidence in making decisions about the care of individual patients. It involves much more than just reading research papers. Even the best available external evidence on its own may be inapplicable for an individual patient, while experience, when used in isolation, may result in clinical practice becoming out of date and possibly decreasing delivery of the best possible patient care.

Why practise evidence-based medicine?

Because it:

- provides an efficient and systematic way of reviewing vast amounts of medical literature and translating it into good patient care
- provides a robust way of managing a disease and enhancing the clinical outcome
- serves as a means of modifying current disease-management practices so as to improve the process
- identifies gaps in the current state of knowledge and highlights areas requiring more investigation
- allows one to improve the quality and efficiency of disease-management procedures.

There are some hurdles to practising EBM. These include the following:

- A significant proportion of clinicians lack formal training in EBM and are not able to thoroughly evaluate some research studies
- Clinicians may have the required expertise to analyse the research, but lack the time to do so

- Assuming that all that is required to treat a patient is understanding of the anatomical and pathophysiological changes
- Relying on the fact that it is easier to refer to textbooks, even though they may be out of date
- Lack of EBM guidelines at the point of practice, e.g. the wards
- Bias in terms of what clinical research is funded and what results are published.

Traditionally, EBM has been taught in terms of a hierarchy of evidence. In this hierarchy, systematic reviews and meta-analyses or randomized controlled trials have been seen as the most statistically reliable form of clinical research evidence. By contrast, case reports or personal experience by clinicians has been seen as far less reliable. Increasingly, levels of evidence are matched to the type of research question asked (Fig. 11.2).

HINTS AND TIPS

Traditionally, EBM has been taught in terms of a hierarchy of evidence. The type of evidence should be matched to the type of research question asked and a meta-analysis of RCTs may not always be the best kind of evidence.

Abbreviations and terms

- SR: systematic review
- Homogeneity: a systematic review that is free of worrisome variations (heterogeneity) in the directions and degrees of results between individual studies
- CDR: Clinical decision rule. (These are algorithms or scoring systems that lead to a prognostic estimation or a diagnostic category.)
- RCT: Randomized controlled trial
- SpPin and SnNout: An 'Absolute SpPin' is a diagnostic finding whose Specificity is so high that a Positive result rules-in the diagnosis. An 'Absolute SnNout' is a diagnostic finding whose Sensitivity is so high that a Negative result rules-out the diagnosis.

HINTS AND TIPS

Remember: Evidence-based medicine (EBM) is the conscientious, explicit and judicious use of current best evidence in making decisions about the care of individual patients.

Grades of recommendation

A – consistent level 1 studies
B – consistent level 2 or 3 studies *or* extrapolations from level 1 studies
C – level 4 studies *or* extrapolations from level 2 or 3 studies

D – level 5 evidence *or* troublingly inconsistent or inconclusive studies of any level.

In grades B and C, 'Extrapolations' are where data is used in a situation that has potentially clinically important differences than the original study situation.

How to practise evidence-based medicine

This is a systematic and sequential activity as follows:
1. Define an answerable question(s).
2. Locate the best evidence, which could include guidelines, systematic reviews, primary research or even talking to a senior colleague or doing an internet search using a search engine like Google scholar, PubMed or Medline.
3. Critically appraise the evidence to assess its validity and usefulness for clinical practice.
4. Implement the results of weighing up the evidence in daily practice.
5. Evaluate the implementation of your findings (this is a form of audit).

WHAT IS CLINICAL AUDIT?

All junior doctors are now expected to get involved in clinical audit, and knowledge about audit and the audit cycle can be tested in medical exams.

Start by thinking of the overriding theme:

Audit is the process of reviewing the delivery of health care to identify deficiencies, so that they may be remedied

(Crombie & Davies 1993)

- The principal aim of audit is to improve the quality of medical care.
- Audit looks at how a service ought to be delivered.
- It then compares that to the way it is currently being delivered.

The concept was introduced in the government's White Paper for the NHS *Working for Patients* (DoH 1989), and since the early 1990s, it became a contractual requirement for doctors in the hospital setting.

COMMUNICATION

Audit is a hot topic at interview. Have a two-sentence definition that you could expand on if they push you, e.g. 'Audit is central to clinical governance and is a mechanism for improving patient care. It is a cycle of comparing actual practice with pre-agreed standards or guidelines'.

Fig. 11.2 Matching study type to the question. The Oxford 2011 levels of clinical evidence. (Oxford Centre for Evidence-Based Medicine (OCEBM) 2011; http://www.cebm.net/index.aspx?o=5653).

Question	Step 1 (Level 1*)	Step 2 (Level 2*)	Step 3 (Level 3*)	Step 4 (Level 4*)	Step 5 (Level 5)
How common is the problem?	Local and current random sample surveys (or censuses)	Systematic review of surveys that allow matching to local circumstances**	Local non-random sample**	Case-series**	n/a
Is this diagnostic or monitoring test accurate? (Diagnosis)	Systematic review of cross-sectional studies with consistently applied reference standard and blinding	Individual cross-sectional studies with consistently applied reference standard and blinding	Non-consecutive studies, or studies without consistently applied reference standards**	Case-control studies, or "poor or non-independent reference standard**	Mechanism-based reasoning
What will happen if we do not add a therapy? (Prognosis)	Systematic review of inception cohort studies	Inception cohort studies	Cohort study or control arm of randomized trial*	Case-series or case-control studies, or poor quality prognostic cohort study**	n/a
Does this intervention help? (Treatment Benefits)	Systematic review of randomized trials or n-of-1 trials	Randomized trial or observational study with dramatic effect	Non-randomized controlled cohort/follow-up study**	Case-series, case-control studies, or historically controlled studies**	Mechanism-based reasoning
What are the COMMON harms? (Treatment Harms)	Systematic review of randomized trials, systematic review of nested case-control studies, n-of-1 trial with the patient you are raising the question about, or observational study with dramatic effect	Individual randomized trial or (exceptionally) observational study with dramatic effect	Non-randomized controlled cohort/follow-up study (post-marketing surveillance) provided there are sufficient numbers to rule out a common harm. (For long-term harms the duration of follow-up must be sufficient.)**	Case-series, case-control, or historically controlled studies**	Mechanism-based reasoning
What are the RARE harms? (Treatment Harms)	Systematic review of randomized trials or n-of-1 trial	Randomized trial or (exceptionally) observational study with dramatic effect			
Is this (early detection) test worthwhile? (Screening)	Systematic review of randomized trials	Randomized trial	Non-randomized controlled cohort/follow-up study**	Case-series, case-control, or historically controlled studies**	Mechanism-based reasoning

*Level may be graded down on the basis of study quality, imprecision, indirectness (study PICO does not match questions PICO), because of inconsistency between studies, or because the absolute effect size is very small; Level may be graded up if there is a large or very large effect size;
**As always, a systematic review is generally better than an individual study.
From OCEBM 2011, with permission.

A healthcare professional's aim is to do the best for an individual patient, within the available resources, by addressing the particular needs of that patient.

If there were no agreed standards as to what care the patient with a given illness or condition might expect from the NHS, there would be no reference points against which one could assess and evaluate the quality of clinical care given.

Audit incorporates a structure in which standards are set and then practical solutions are found to bring that service up to a particular standard.

A 'standard' in a clinical audit describes 'what should be done' in a particular clinical situation. It must be up-to-date and be based upon sound research evidence. It is a statement that explicitly lays out (in precise, definite and measurable terms) the quality of care expected.

> **HINTS AND TIPS**
>
> Another way of looking at audit is as:
>
> A cycle of setting standards, monitoring performance, and implementing change to bring performance up to standard
>
> (Healy 1998)

In essence, audit is a review process that *monitors clinical quality* (in a similar way that industries use quality control checks) to ensure that all the energies going into 'intervention X' are as effective as possible, and are not departing from agreed standards of care (Fig. 11.3).

Audit is thus central to all lives as healthcare professionals – it is a powerful tool that helps us to practise medicine to the *best standard*. It is also meant to be a non-threatening exercise for all those involved in it.

However, in order for an audit to be successful, healthcare professionals must be receptive to the possibility that their and the team's clinical practice (and thus the quality of their treatment and care) may in fact be improved.

> **Fig. 11.3**   Key features of an audit.
>
> The aim of audit is to improve quality of care
> Audit involves setting 'standards' and measuring against them
> It examines clinical issues (diagnosis, treatment and patient care)
> Audit involves changing our everyday practice to remedy any deficiencies
> This improves patient outcomes
> The process should be led by clinicians (not academics or management)
> It is a team effort with multidisciplinary involvement

Although patient care is the focus of audit activities, it is also an essential mechanism (as part of clinical governance) for the medical profession and government to move from a 'culture of blame and scapegoating' to achieving an atmosphere where *quality of care* is the focus, i.e. learning from our mistakes – what works well, what does not and making necessary improvements. A 'blame-free' culture has therefore been promoted as the means to encourage the disclosure of information that will improve patient safety and therefore standard of care (Donaldson 2000).

Areas an audit can focus on within the NHS include:

- Regional variations in the delivery of health care ('postcode lottery')
- The use of limited resources (cost-effectiveness)
- Deficiencies in care delivered (improving outcomes)
- Technological advances (how technology is being used)
- Medical education (the process is an educational tool – review and reflection)
- It *can* act as a political tool (e.g. to argue for more resources).

Audit can look at many levels of services, e.g.

- Individual treatments or investigations in a specific hospital
- Departmental performance
- Regional or trust performance compared with national levels.

Society is increasingly scrutinizing the practice of healthcare professionals. This is shown by the rise in demands of pressure groups, press coverage and litigation. Audit helps us to improve our practice of medicine and maintain the respect and appreciation of our patients.

Why should I learn about it?

Clinical audit is a topic that comes up regularly at interview – even if you haven't completed any audits, you are expected to have a working understanding of them.

It is increasingly a mandatory training requirement to conduct audits in the Foundation and Training Years. It is also often a regular feature of in-training appraisals later on in your career. It is thus not only good for the patient, but it is also good for your career!

All specialties hold audit meetings (which include mortality and morbidity meetings) and both as a student and as a junior doctor, it is advisable to understand the basic processes.

Audit is one of the cornerstones of clinical governance. It is also strongly promoted by the National Institute for Health and Clinical Excellence (NICE). Therefore, it is greatly relevant to the future of the NHS and your working environment.

Audit vs research

Confusion often arises between research and audit. Audit is a separate concept from research. Both involve measuring patient outcomes and, although for different purposes, they both have important roles in clinical governance (some differences are considered in Chapter 2).

Figure 11.4 highlights the differences between audit and research. In summary:

- we use research to seek out new information which provides the foundation for agreeing what we should be doing, i.e. it gives us the evidence we need upon which to base our standards
- audit examines current practice to see if we are maintaining the standards we have set for ourselves.

The audit cycle

Audit is a process with discrete stages (Fig. 11.5); however, it is also a continuous exercise, as shown in Figure 11.6.

Fig. 11.4 The differences between research and audit.

Research (What is good care?)	Audit (Is good care being practised?)
Sets standards	Maintains standards
Seeks new knowledge	Tests conformity with tested knowledge
Defines what best practice is	Asks if best practice is being implemented
Aims to increase knowledge	Aims to improve specified outcomes

Fig. 11.6 Medical audit cycle. (Modified from Fowkes 1982.)

Choosing a topic

All aspects of medical care are suited to audit and there are an abundance of topics from all specialties. When considering a topic, you may be responding to an identified problem or to new evidence. Considerations include:

- Is the area of interest of high cost, volume or risk to staff or users?
- Do you have the time and resources to complete the audit cycle?
- Is the project supported by those who have the authority and commitment to put changes into practice?
- Will looking at this area help to improve the quality of patient care?

Ultimately, the only reason for doing audit is to effect change. Without change, it will just become another report or inquiry which gathers dust on the shelves.

> The problem audited should be capable of change and if successful the change should be worthwhile
> (Crombie & Davies 1993)

Fig. 11.5 The essential stages of a clinical audit.

Setting a 'standard of care' (i.e. evidence base)
Assessment by audit (measuring what is currently done)
Comparing current practice with the 'standard of care'
Implement change (alter any deficient practices)
Audit to make sure things have actually improved ('closing the loop')

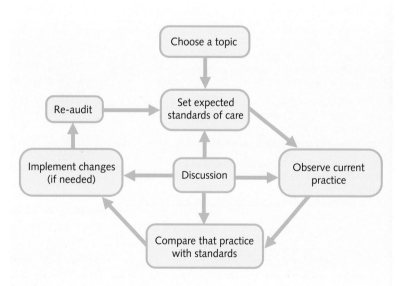

Setting standards

As discussed before, a standard describes 'what should be done' in a particular clinical situation. Standards are the hallmark of audit and the basis of measurement against which we judge a service. However, identifying a standard is arguably the most difficult part of the audit.

The standard should correspond to the specific aims and objectives of your audit; it may come from:

- national standards – such as those set by NICE, a Royal College or a professional body
- regional standards – e.g. agreed levels of care set across an NHS trust
- locally adapted standards – a national standard tailored to your department.

Or:

- there may be no standard – in which case you must set one.

To set your own standards requires considerable effort, but can be ultimately more rewarding. It will be specific to your environment and adaptable to local circumstances. In order to set a new standard, there must be a negotiation both within the audit group and with service deliverers. This will mean that it will be more acceptable to everyone and there will be a sense of ownership.

First, look for evidence and existing standards (such as NICE guidelines):

- A literature search (to see what evidence there is)
- Comparison with other centres (i.e. is there a geographical variation in outcomes between you and another centre)
- Clinical experience (if there is no evidence in that area – an estimation of what level of care should be achieved)
- A consensus to be reached, between all the teams and individuals concerned within that area of patient care.

Second, 'phrasing a standard'. Crombie and Davies (1993) define a standard as having three parts:

1. The setting of 'criteria':
   a. This sets the point at which good care ends and inadequate care begins.
   b. It is a clinically relevant variable, which is easily defined and measured, e.g. an HbA_{1C} of 7% or less for a patient with diabetes mellitus.
2. Outlining a 'target':
   a. The proportion of patients who should meet this criterion.
   b. A target is essential, as some patients will not comply, treatment will fail, etc.
   c. It must be a compromise between clinical importance, attainability (i.e. must be realistic) and acceptability (to all the team).

d. Set too high, the target becomes impossible and you have *created* a healthcare problem. Set too low, and we are not striving for the best medicine, but convenient medicine.
For example – 50% of diabetic patients should have an HbA_{1C} of <7% (this is the current target set for GPs under the *Quality and Outcomes Framework* – see Ch. 10). In our example, the HbA_{1C} is relevant because it indicates good diabetic control over time; it is evidence-based because there is published evidence to suggest that it will decrease the risk of diabetic complications (e.g. nephropathy); it ought to be achievable for the majority of diabetic patients and it is clearly measurable. It is distinct if you are not measuring random or fasting glucose.

3. Defining 'allowable exceptions':
   a. Situations in which the criteria do not apply to certain patients
   For example – If the patient has a concurrent illness at the time of measurement, e.g. a patient with significant educational needs may struggle to take medication or adopt lifestyle changes in a reliable way. In this example, our standard of care is that: 'A good HbA_{1C} measurement is less than 7% mmol/l in a diabetic patient. We aim that 50% of the population will attain this, UNLESS they have a concurrent illness which prevents or alters measurement'.

Irrespective of who set the standard – NICE or John Smith of Any Town Hospital Trust – a standard must convey to everyone (clinicians, auditors and patients) precisely what is expected from the service and what it is being measured against. The standards used should be included in any audit report, as they are what we have measured the service against.

Assessment in audit

This refers to the observation of current practice, and the collection of data. There are different ways of carrying out an audit cycle, and these can vary in complexity from looking at one subset of patients to multicentre analysis of all patients seen.

Data collection is an essential part of the cycle, as without data, we cannot hope to know what to change or how.

It must be broken down into manageable steps:

- Decide where your data are coming from:
  - Is it prospective (collecting new data) or retrospective (getting information from routine sources)?
  - What will be the sources of the data?
  - Who will collect the data?

There are two ways to collect data (retrospectively and prospectively), and the method will depend on which source of information you use:

1. Retrospective audit uses information which is routinely kept by your organization (e.g. waiting times, blood results, patient outcomes). The information should be readily available, accurate and complete (e.g. patients' medical notes, biochemistry results).

2. Prospective audit allows you to set up a reporting system where no such data collection exists (e.g. what time the patient ate or why their discharge was delayed) (Fig. 11.7).
   - Select an audit sample:
     - The important question is: what sample will be sufficient for senior colleagues to agree that they will introduce changes if the audit indicates the need for this?
     - Think about age, aspect of service and time period
     - Ensure the sample is free from selection bias.
   - Create a pro forma (data collection form):
     - The data collected must evaluate every aspect laid out in the standard
     - The questions asked are crucial to successful audit
     - Make sure your data collection sheet is asking the right questions, in a relevant way

- Remember to keep all data confidential (preferably anonymous); though ideally this should be identifiable to the auditors/audit department through use, e.g. of hospital record numbers – this is so that audit results can be checked if necessary
- Use as few words as possible
- Free text is difficult to analyse and should be avoided.
- Trial a pilot audit on a small sample of patients:
  - Sounds boring but can save a lot of later heartache
  - Undertake a mini-audit on a very limited number of patients (e.g. five) to check that: the questions are not ambiguous, the information is answering your questions and that the data are not too difficult to obtain from the record.
- Carry out the audit – you are ready to begin.

Comparing current practice with the standard (data analysis)

At the end of the assessment section of the audit, there will be three sets of data:

1. Those that conformed to the standard
2. Those that didn't conform BUT that fitted the exceptions
3. Those that didn't conform to the standard OR meet the exceptions.

Fig. 11.7 Audit time spans.

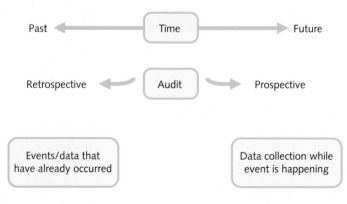

Each should be reported, and you must calculate whether you have met your target or not, for each standard criterion.

At this stage, it is important to have a consensus meeting where you formally present your data to senior colleagues and all the interested members of the healthcare team and patient consumer groups.

Implementing change

This is the final step in the loop, and provides the reason for the whole exercise. By identifying the areas that are not living up to the prescribed level of care, we can start to think of ways to ameliorate the problem.

The aim of audit is to improve the delivery of health care, so there is no point in simply describing a healthcare problem.

Unfortunately, it is usually far easier to identify a deficiency than to solve it overnight. While some problems (such as lack of staff or insufficient training on technique X) may be relatively straightforward to correct, there are many subtle barriers and underlying causes that make effecting change difficult. For example, it may involve more work for the provider of that service with no extra resources or it may be very different from conventional practice and, therefore, seem challenging.

This is a crucial phase, as it offers the possibility for practical solutions to be forged. Therefore, it should be a decision, guideline or change in which all staff involved are consulted for an opinion. Changes must be implemented with care and incrementally, so as not to disrupt the status quo unnecessarily. It should also be explained to staff not directly involved in making the decision why it has been made and it should be stressed that it is hoped that it will lead to improved patient care.

Closing the loop: re-audit

It is too easy to assume that we have effected great change by our efforts. Since audit is intended to improve patient care, we must re-audit ('close the loop') in order to assure ourselves that the solution we have implemented has had an impact upon the original problem.

HINTS AND TIPS

Within management circles and NHS publications, one phrase crops up repeatedly:

The basic principle of audit is that it should be 'complete, accurate, transparent and honest'.

This should be reproduced in any exam question on audit as there is likely to be a mark for saying it!

Other characteristics of audit

Confidentiality

A central part of audit is a duty of confidentiality – not only to those whose care has been reviewed (see Ch. 2) – but also to the clinical staff who managed them. Audit will only blossom where there is confidence that the findings (which may include individual failings) cannot be used for disciplinary actions against individual members of staff. This must be taken into account in the study design.

Multidisciplinary and open discussion

An audit is more likely to be successful if it has the enthusiastic support of all the staff concerned. It will have implications for professions and disciplines other than your own, and so they should be consulted and involved at an early stage. The best way to achieve this is to form an audit group which incorporates representatives from all the teams involved in delivering the service. Involving patients in the process is also considered desirable.

Regular discussion sessions are an important part of audit; the project will benefit and in fact requires input from relevant staff at certain key points.

It is crucial to have a consensus meeting (i.e. a meeting in which all specialties and teams are represented) where agreement is reached that the topic is important (otherwise they are unlikely to help to develop and implement any changes) and on the standards against which you will assess health care (or else they may reject your findings on the grounds that they were inappropriate benchmarks).

For the same reason, another consensus meeting should be held once you have collected your data, so that you can agree that you have identified an important problem, and so you can think about how you are going to change the service and over what timescale you will implement this.

As a general rule, people are far more receptive to change and willing to cooperate in something for which they are responsible and have helped to create, than in something which is imposed from an external source.

The most important points of the cycle are summarized in Figure 11.6. It is worth remembering these for exams and interviews.

Types of audit

Audits can be categorized into the areas of care that they look at:

- *Audits of structure*:
  - What healthcare facilities are there?
  - What buildings, equipment and staff are available?

Typically more of a management issue than a clinician's problem; e.g. looking at staffing levels/bedspaces and how this impacts upon A&E trolley waits.

- *Audits of process*:
  - Did the patient receive the best possible care?

The most common type of audit:

- It considers the investigations, diagnosis and treatment given
  - Was the care given as it was originally intended to be?; e.g. did patients with an acute myocardial infarct receive thrombolysis within 6 hours?
- *Audits of outcome*:
  - What was the end result for the patient?
  - How successful was the intervention for the patient?
  - In other words, did the intervention have the expected benefit, or were there any adverse effects?

Outcome is perhaps the most difficult type of audit because the consequences can be varied and subtle. They can also be extremely subjective. Especially difficult when considering chronic processes – BUT it is the most relevant type of audit, as it asks: 'How did the patient do?', e.g. the Confidential Enquiry into Maternal and Child Health (CEMACH).

There are a number of different measures for patient outcomes. Death is the most extreme outcome; mortality figures are regularly audited for perioperative care (National Confidential Enquiry into Patient Outcome and Deaths), NCEPOD: a continuing national audit programme funded by the National Patient Safety Agency and Department of Health (DoH) but independent of the DoH and professional associations. Other measures include morbidity (how diseased a person is after the intervention), QALYS (quality-adjusted life years) and patient satisfaction. The difficulty with such 'soft' measures is that there is a wide variation in how one interprets them. They rely on subjective values of the doctor or the patient and frequently both.

Why audit does not always work

In an ideal world, there would be no barriers to audit. However, there are both practical and political considerations:

- Set reasonable expectations – you cannot cure the NHS of all its woes overnight!
- Does everyone see it as important a topic as you do? Unless the audit findings are seen as a priority (by senior colleagues or other departments) no change will be effected. This highlights the need for a consensus of opinion and constant discussion.
- There may be different motives behind an audit. Managers may well request an audit because of political pressure on them – if so, the auditors' agenda will be quite different from the managers'.

For example:

- An Emergency Department (ED) physician may want to perform an 'audit of process' for patients presenting with acute myocardial infarcts (e.g. how quickly they were triaged, investigated and definitive care given).
- The management in a hospital may want to have an 'audit of structure' within the ED (e.g. lack of bedspaces, staff shortages and the ensuing trolley waits, meaning that the patient with a myocardial infarct was not taken to CCU).
- Audits can often run into problems when they do not consider this 'ideological mismatch' between the agendas of clinicians, managers and auditors.
- Be aware of other reasons why audit does not effect change – it may be a political rather than practical obstacle.

How to do your own audit

Within each NHS Trust there are Clinical Audit Departments that have staff specifically trained to advise and assist in any of the stages of an audit. They are there to help you get the notes and make sure you perform the audit correctly while maintaining patient confidentiality. Plan your audit carefully and remember that data collection (although the most obvious step) can only happen once you are clear on exactly what information you are trying to find out:

1. Choose a topic
2. Create an audit team (remember – in order to be effective it needs input from all the various disciplines involved in providing the service)
3. Hold a consensus meeting to:
   a. agree on the importance of the topic
   b. set aims and objectives
   c. develop standards
4. Select an audit sample
5. Design a data collection form
6. Pilot the audit
7. Collect the data
8. Analyse the information and write the audit report
9. Present your results and hold another consensus meeting
10. Implement
11. Publish your results
12. Re-audit (after an appropriate length of time).

RISK MANAGEMENT

Risk management is an organizational response to a need to reduce errors and their costs, and is now regarded as an integral component of the management in most NHS Trusts (Hobbs 2001). It places particular emphasis on occasions in which patients are harmed or disturbed by their treatment or care. Errors can involve a complex interplay of human and organizational factors. Dealing with complaints effectively is a key part of risk management (see Ch. 2).

Clinical risk management means having systems to understand, monitor and minimize risks to patients and staff and to learn from mistakes. For example:

- Is there an open and blame-free/reasonable-blame culture?
- How are incidents and near misses reported?
- How does an NHS Trust liaise with other organizations where care is shared?
- What preventative measures are in place?
- What improvements to patient care have resulted from clinical risk management?

THE NHS COMPLAINTS PROCEDURE

The current NHS complaints procedure was instituted in 1996 by the NHS Executive. It was titled: '*Complaints, Listening … Acting … Improving: Guidance on Implementation of the NHS Complaints Procedure*'. The aims of this complaints procedure are to provide a simple, responsive way of tackling complaints, with the goal of improving the level of service provided by the NHS. In essence, it proposed three tiers of response to complaints. The complaints procedure was a method of conflict resolution which patients and next of kin could pursue as an alternative to legal action. Patients may now take complaints to court (in order to seek compensation) as well as pursuing local resolution.

Most complaints should be dealt with at a local level. This would involve the person about whom the complaint was made responding either in writing or in person to the complainant. Hospital Trusts provide a lay conciliator to facilitate such meetings. With honest and open communication, the complainant and the person complained about can see each other's points of view, and resolution to the satisfaction of both parties can be achieved.

A complainant who is not satisfied by attempts at local resolution can request an independent review of the complaint. All Trusts will have a complaints convenor who will decide whether to set up an independent review panel or return the complaint to the local level. There is no automatic right to independent review, and the complainant must state a case for why local resolution has been unsatisfactory.

An independent review panel consists of three lay members advised by clinical specialists. The function of the panel is to investigate the complaint and make a report setting out its conclusions, with appropriate comments and suggestions. It cannot suggest that any person should be subject to disciplinary action or referred to any of the professional regulatory bodies.

The report is sent to the Chief Executive of the Trust, who must then write to the complainant informing them of any action that is being taken as a result of the panel's deliberations and the right of the complainant to take their grievance to the ombudsman (see below) if they remain dissatisfied. It is up to the Chief Executive to decide whether or not to refer the cases to a professional body (e.g. the GMC) or initiate their own disciplinary procedures.

The ombudsman is a civil servant, independent of the NHS, who is responsible for reporting to parliament about the running of the NHS. It is up to the ombudsman whether or not to further investigate any complaints. It is within his power to ask healthcare professionals involved in complaints to appear before a parliamentary select committee in order to give their account of the subject of the complaint. This complaints procedure provides no avenue for the complainant to be compensated. In order to do this, the complainant needs to use the civil justice system (outlined in Ch. 1).

ERRORS AND SIGNIFICANT EVENT AUDIT

In medicine, learning from mistakes can involve sharing and discussing them with patients and colleagues. This requires their accurate reconstruction and description as well as processes to analyse and produce useful outcomes for the future. One such process is significant event audit (or analysis). Not to be confused with clinical audit, this may be conducted for individual cases in which there has been a significant occurrence (not necessarily involving an undesirable outcome for the patient), which are analysed in a systematic and detailed way to ascertain what can be learnt about the overall quality of care and to indicate changes that might lead to future improvements (another process is the clinical incident reporting system).

Fig. 11.8 Reason's Swiss Cheese Model. (Adapted from Reason 2000.)

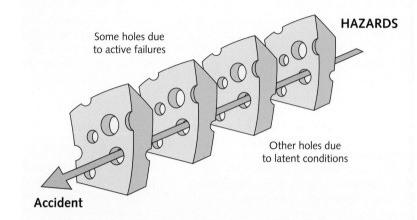

Some holes due to active failures

HAZARDS

Other holes due to latent conditions

Accident

SUCCESSIVE LAYERS OF DEFENCES

Talks on risk management in health care often mention the 'Swiss Cheese' model (Fig. 11.8). Reason (2000) describes the causation of an adverse event as a series of events which must occur in a particular order for the event to occur. He compares this to the holes of several slices of swiss cheese lining up. The slices of cheese are analogous to factors or barriers preventing an accident, and the holes represent flaws or failures in each of the barriers. The holes in the defences arise for two reasons: active failures (e.g. unsafe actions by healthcare staff) and latent conditions (problems within the system such as excess time pressure or understaffing). Nearly all adverse events involve a combination of these two sets of factors. A hole may allow a problem to pass through in one layer but in the next layer the holes are in different places and the problem is stopped. For a catastrophic failure to occur, all the holes in the 'swiss cheese' need to line up.

Violations

Deliberate deviations from rule or policies are known as violations. They generally represent attempts to work around over-complex and undependable systems. They do not necessarily entail a disregard for patient-safety.

Reason (1992) defines violations as deliberate – but not necessarily reprehensible – deviations from practices deemed necessary (by designers, managers and regulatory agencies) to maintain the safe operation of a potentially hazardous system. Hurwitz and Sheikh (2010) outline a number of circumstances that predispose to violations: tiredness, time pressures and rules and procedures that (appear to) lack rationale. They also suggest that violations may not be entirely voluntary on the part of the transgressor. For example, a doctor may decide to allow a relative to translate for an adult patient where there is no available interpreter. This may be a failing of the system but also represents a violation on the part of the doctor who ignores policy in order to allow the patient to consult without delay.

Key questions

- Outline the main components of clinical governance.
- Explain the basic principles of audit.
- Outline the different types of audit.
- Outline the steps involved in carrying out an audit.
- Describe the difficulties involved and the measures taken to tackle them in 'setting standards'.
- What does risk management involve?
- Discuss the difference between a mistake and a violation when thinking about risk management.

References

Armstrong, D., 2003. Clinical governance. In: Outline of Sociology as Applied to Medicine, fifth ed. Hodder Arnold, London, p. 112.

Chambers, R., Booth, E., Rogers, D., 2007. Stage 6: What clinical governance means and how to put it into practise. In: Clinical Effectiveness and Clinical Governance Made Easy, fourth ed. Radcliffe Medical Press, Oxford.

Crombie, I.K., Davies, H.T., 1993. Missing link in the audit cycle. Qual. Health Care 2 (1), 47–48.

Department of Health, 1989. Working for patients. The Stationery Office, London, Cm 555.

Donaldson, L.J., 2000. An organisation with memory: report of an expert group on learning from adverse events in the NHS. HMSO, London.

Healy, K., 1998. Why clinical audit doesn't work. Success depends on type of audit. Br. Med. J. 316 (7148), 1906.

Hobbs, S., 2001. Learning from complaints. In: Lugon, M., Secker-Walker, J. (Eds.), Advancing Clinical Governance. Royal Society of Medicine Press, London.

Hurwitz, B., Sheikh, A. (Eds.), 2010. Health care mistakes, violations and patient safety. In Healthcare Errors and Patient Safety. Wiley-Blackwell, Oxford.

NHS Executive, 1996. Promoting Clinical Effectiveness. A framework for action in and through the NHS. NHS Executive, London.

Reason, J., 2000. Human error: models and management. BMJ 320, 768.

Reason, J., 1992. Human error. Cambridge University Press, Cambridge, MA.

Scally, G., Donaldson, L.J., 1998. Looking forward: clinical governance and the drive for quality improvement in the new NHS in England. BMJ 317, 61–65.

WHO, 1988. Quality Assessment and Assurance in Primary Health Care. World Health Organization, Geneva.

Further reading

Chambers, R., Boath, E., 2000. Clinical Effectiveness and Clinical Governance Made Easy, second ed. Radcliffe Medical Press, Oxford, pp. 1–63, 117–146.

Fowkes, F.G.R., 1982. Medical Audit Cycle. Med. Educ. 16, 228–238.

Oxford Centre for Evidence-Based Medicine (OCEBM) Levels of Evidence Working Group, 2011. The Oxford 2011 Levels of Evidence. OCEBM, Oxford.

Pringle, M., Bradley, C.P., Carmichael, C.M., et al., 1995. Significant event auditing. A study of the feasibility and potential of case-based auditing in primary medical care. Occas. Pap. R. Coll. Gen. Pract. 70, i–viii, 1–71.

WHO, 1983. The Principles of Quality Assurance. (Report on a WHO meeting.) World Health Organization, Copenhagen.

SELF-ASSESSMENT

Single best answer questions (SBAs)

1. Which of the following is NOT an item in the 2010 updated core curriculum for Medical Ethics and Law?
   - (a) Professionalism: 'good medical practice'
   - (b) Justice and public health
   - (c) Medical statistics
   - (d) Towards the end of life
   - (e) Medical research and audit

2. Which of the following options is a framework around which an ethical discussion can be based, regardless of the favourite ethical theory held by the participants?
   - (a) Utilitarianism
   - (b) Deontology
   - (c) Virtue ethics
   - (d) The four principles
   - (e) Socialism

3. Which of the following is NOT required for a clinical negligence case in the civil courts?
   - (a) A duty of care which was not adhered to
   - (b) Proof beyond reasonable doubt that the doctor was guilty
   - (c) Evidence that the patient suffered harm
   - (d) Evidence that the harm was caused by the failure in the duty of care
   - (e) A responsible body of medical opinion which the judge deems reasonable to inform the court

4. The following, which is considered an absolute right, is enshrined in the European Convention on Human Rights:
   - (a) The right to freedom of conscience and religion
   - (b) The right to marry and found a family
   - (c) The right to freedom from torture (inhuman and degrading treatment)
   - (d) The right to privacy
   - (e) The right to freedom from discrimination

5. The following offence would be heard in the civil division of the Courts in the UK:
   - (a) Gross negligence manslaughter
   - (b) Murder
   - (c) Assault
   - (d) Public disorder
   - (e) Negligence

6. The General Medical Council:
   - (a) Supervises standards for postgraduate and undergraduate education
   - (b) Is a trade union
   - (c) Its chief role is to set educational, professional and clinical standards for each specialty
   - (d) Membership is optional for practicing doctors
   - (e) Compensates patients who have suffered as a result of medical negligence

7. The British Medical Association:
   - (a) Provides ethics advice online and on the telephone, but only for its members
   - (b) Provides medical indemnity
   - (c) Supports doctors who are accused of clinical negligence
   - (d) Sets educational, professional and clinical standards for each specialty
   - (e) Enforces professional standards

8. Which is the LEAST likely question which doctors asked of the BMA medical ethics department in 2009–2010?
   - (a) Under what circumstances can confidential health information be disclosed?
   - (b) Who can apply for access to a patient's health records?
   - (c) What is the BMA's position on organ donation?
   - (d) What should a doctor do when they have child protection concerns about a patient?
   - (e) How much information should patients be given in order for consent to treatment to be valid?

9. Therapeutic privilege is:
   - (a) Misleading patients into receiving treatment which they do not need
   - (b) Omitting or lying about information which would affect the choice a patient makes
   - (c) Claiming a qualification or expertise which is not possessed
   - (d) Altering an entry in healthcare records which has been made on a previous occasion
   - (e) Cheating in professional examinations

10. Which of the following statements is true about confidentiality?
    - (a) The Hippocratic Oath holds that confidentiality must be absolute
    - (b) It is an uncommon issue for doctors in the UK
    - (c) Freedom of the press is more important, especially if there is a public interest in knowing which doctors have HIV
    - (d) The use of confidential information in medical research is covered by the Health and Social Care Act 2006 and does not require prior REC approval
    - (e) Confidential information may be disclosed with consent from a person properly authorized to act on the patient's behalf

11. Capacity may be present if a person is:
    - (a) Unable to understand relevant information
    - (b) Unable to retain the relevant information
    - (c) Unable to use the information to come to a decision
    - (d) Unable to communicate the decision
    - (e) Unable to read the relevant information

12. Which of the following best reflects current law on consent?
    (a) Valid consent necessarily requires a signed consent form
    (b) Consent means doing anything a patient wants
    (c) Valid consent requires that the patient knows every detail of a proposed treatment, whether they want it or not
    (d) Information should be withheld if it will cause the patient to refuse treatment
    (e) Consent necessarily requires information about the broad nature and purpose of any proposed treatment

13. The following is NOT one of the five principles of the Mental Capacity Act 2005:
    (a) Every adult must be assumed to have capacity unless it is proved otherwise
    (b) People must be given all appropriate help before they are deemed incapable of making their own decisions
    (c) Individuals retain the right to make what might be seen as eccentric or unwise decisions
    (d) Anything done for or on behalf of people without capacity must be to protect them or others from harm
    (e) Anything done for or on behalf of people without capacity should be the least restrictive of their basic rights and freedoms

14. Do Not Attempt Resuscitation orders should be considered ONLY when:
    (a) Resuscitation is in the best interests of the patient; that is, it is likely to cause a quality of life that is not considered to be worse than death
    (b) There is a decision about whether to commence antibiotics for a pneumonia
    (c) Resuscitation is unlikely to be *futile*
    (d) Resuscitation is in line with the informed wishes of a competent patient
    (e) Resuscitation is contrary to a valid *advance directive*

15. Factors AGAINST a prosecution for aiding and abetting suicide include:
    (a) The victim was under 18 years of age
    (b) The victim did not have the capacity (as defined in the Mental Capacity Act 2005) to reach an informed decision to commit suicide
    (c) The actions of the suspect may be characterized as reluctant encouragement or assistance in the face of a determined wish on the part of the victim to commit suicide
    (d) The suspect gave encouragement or assistance to more than one victim, and these victims were not known to each other
    (e) The suspect was acting in his or her capacity as a medical doctor, nurse, other healthcare professional

16. The Human Fertilization and Embryology Act permits which ONE following activity:
    (a) The creation or use of any embryos outside the human body (however they are created) outside of licensed clinics in the UK
    (b) The creation of 'human admixed embryos' except for research in licensed facilities
    (c) Placing a human embryo in an animal
    (d) Modification of the genetic structure of any cell which is part of an embryo
    (e) Sex-selection of offspring to avoid a having a child with a serious sex-linked disease

17. Which of the following is NOT true about failed sterilization cases:
    (a) They are generally considered as negligence cases in the civil courts
    (b) A court is more likely to award higher damages if a handicapped child is born as a result of negligence
    (c) Courts may consider the discomfort and financial loss resulting from either a subsequent abortion or pregnancy and delivery
    (d) Courts generally award damages for the upkeep of any child born as a result of failed sterilization
    (e) A failed sterilization operation on a man (if negligence is alleged) may result in a case being brought to court by the woman who is his sexual partner

18. Which of the following options correctly pairs a potential source of transplant organs with a relevant ethical issue?
    (a) Cadaveric organ donation – issues relating to the definition of death and ownership of the body
    (b) Organ donation from living people – risk of transfer of diseases from animal to human
    (c) Xenotransplantation – a concern that the poor may be coerced to sell their organs to the rich
    (d) Organ markets – many more people are willing to receive than they are to donate
    (e) Mandated choice – having to discuss organ donation with newly bereaved relatives

19. Which of the following statements is true about challenging resource-allocation decisions in the courts? (Choose the BEST answer):
    (a) A successful Judicial Review case would necessitate compensation for the claimant's loss
    (b) A patient might claim that in not funding a particular service the NHS failed in its statutory duty – this would be a negligence case
    (c) Following the Human Rights Act 1998, Article 3 of the European Convention on Human rights (protections from inhuman or degrading treatment) could be used to challenge refusal of life-saving treatment
    (d) Decisions which are based on a reasonable procedure and relevant grounds are less vulnerable to be challenged in court
    (e) The Human Rights Act 1998 is irrelevant to resource allocation decisions

20. Quality-adjusted life years are:
    (a) Unbiased against any group
    (b) Favour the sick and the elderly because they have greater need
    (c) Derived from interviewing a large number of people to determine what is beneficial and then attempting to quantify it with numerical values
    (d) Biased against the young and the healthy
    (e) Unproblematic because different people all allocate similar values to health and medical treatment

21. Which of the following statements is LEAST accurate about commissioning in healthcare?
    (a) May involve a needs assessment stage
    (b) Involves identifying capacity to meet the need
    (c) Is essentially a resource allocation process
    (d) Involves a procurement stage
    (e) Should include evaluation of the service

22. A healthcare organization's resource allocation committee comes to the conclusion that it will not pay for gender reassignment surgery on the basis that the evidence is unclear whether this is helpful. The committee decides that funding for gender reassignment surgery may be authorized by the Director for Public Health in exceptional circumstances though they do not anticipate this will ever be requested. It does not specify any exceptional circumstances. Which of the following BEST describes the situation?
    (a) A patient with clinically proven gender-dysphoria would not be able to claim that the situation amounts to a blanket ban on gender reassignment surgery
    (b) The likeliest approach with which to challenge the decision in the courts would be as a claim in negligence
    (c) The likeliest approach with which to challenge the decision in the courts would be as a judicial review case
    (d) A judicial review case would award compensation to successful claimants in order to correct any harm caused by the negligent decision process
    (e) A successful negligence action would force the health organization to revisit the decision in a more reasonable manner on more relevant grounds

23. Quality-adjusted life years (choose the BEST answer):
    (a) Are associated with the ethical theory of deontology
    (b) Assign the value of 1 to a year of unhealthy life and more than 1 to different levels of health
    (c) Economists may assign a cost per QALY
    (d) Rest on the assumption that we should measure 'objective function' as the quality part
    (e) Make no claims to introduce evidence into healthcare allocation decisions

24. Which statement about the concept of the epidemiological triangle is CORRECT?
    (a) This deviates from the 'germ theory'
    (b) Disease is seen as an interaction between two entities: the host and the disease agent
    (c) Exposure to the disease agent is sufficient for the disease to manifest
    (d) The disease can be prevented by modifying factors that influence exposure and susceptibility
    (e) More useful in understanding causation of chronic, degenerative diseases than infectious ones

25. Which of the following statements BEST describes the biomedical model?
    (a) The mind and body cannot be treated separately
    (b) The body can be treated as a machine
    (c) Technological interventions are rarely successful in the treatment of disease
    (d) Explanations of disease focus on biological changes in conjunction with social and psychological factors – that is, they are *reductionist* in nature
    (e) It is currently assumed that every disease is caused by a specific identifiable agent

26. Holmes and Rahe (1967) developed the Social Readjustment Rating Scale (SRRS). This consisted of a number of life events that were given a score depending on how life-changing each event was. The LOWEST SCORING life event was:
    (a) Divorce
    (b) Marriage
    (c) Moving house
    (d) Retirement
    (e) Death of wife/husband

27. Which ONE of the following is NOT one of Hannay's (1988) five stages of illness:
    (a) The experience of clinical signs
    (b) 'Lay referral'
    (c) Consultation with a healthcare professional
    (d) Being in the 'sick role'
    (e) Recovery

28. According to Banks et al (1975), which ONE of the following symptoms has to occur MOST frequently to a patient before it results in a consultation with a healthcare professional?
    (a) Backache
    (b) Emotional problem
    (c) Headache
    (d) Sore throat
    (e) Abdominal pain

29. According to Banks et al (1975), which ONE of the following symptoms has to occur LEAST frequently to a patient before it results in a consultation with a healthcare professional?
    (a) Backache
    (b) Chest pain
    (c) Sore throat

(d) Abdominal pain

(e) Headache

30. Which ONE of the following is NOT a common reason given by patients for attending a practitioner of alternative or complementary medicine:
   (a) A greater amount of time and continuity in the consultation
   (b) The attention to personality and personal experience: treatment is 'individualized'
   (c) A comprehensive scientific evidence base
   (d) Hope
   (e) Touch

31. Which ONE of the following statements BEST describes the concept of labelling?
   (a) The pressure that society puts on patients to conform to their idea of what a typical patient looks like
   (b) The expectation that a blind person is quiet and docile
   (c) Labelling causes disease by identifying people as sick or deviant
   (d) Labelling creates disease by identifying people as sick or deviant
   (e) It refers to changes in behaviour as a result of an illness

32. Which of the following statements about the history of the UK National Health Service (NHS) is TRUE?
   (a) During the Second World War, all hospitals had been privatized
   (b) The famous Beveridge Report (1911) established the principles for a post-war 'welfare state'.
   (c) Prior to the NHS there was no healthcare provision for manual labourers
   (d) After a series of negotiations between the government and the General Medical Council (GMC), the National Health Service Act (1946) created the NHS in 1948
   (e) The NHS was originally expected to cost less as the nation became healthier

33. Which ONE of the following statements about healthcare systems is FALSE:
   (a) In a pluralistic health system, healthcare facilities may be owned by private groups or the state
   (b) In a health insurance system, healthcare facilities may be owned by private groups or the state
   (c) In a health service system, the state owns *most* facilities
   (d) In a socialized health system, the state owns *most* facilities
   (e) In a socialized health system, nearly all healthcare professionals are employed by the government

34. Which ONE of the following statements is NOT a characteristic of professions as define by Carr-Saunders and Wilson in 1933?
   (a) Possession of altruistic values
   (b) High ethical standards

(c) Discrete body of knowledge over which members have complete control
(d) Able to regulate their own working conditions independent of the state
(e) A short training period

35. Which of the following is a valid criticism of the Registrar General's classification of social class? (Choose the SINGLE BEST answer):
   (a) The classification is a measure of income rather than social status
   (b) Each class represents similar incomes and responsibilities
   (c) The classification is accurate in the way it deals with women
   (d) The classification is increasingly irrelevant given the flexible nature of labour markets, job insecurity and unemployment rates
   (e) This classification is the stratification most widely used in current UK national statistics

36. Which ONE of the following statements about gender and health inequality is TRUE?
   (a) Men have more morbidity than women from anxiety and depressive disorders
   (b) Women have higher rates of schizophrenia and alcohol and drug dependence
   (c) Women are more likely to consult a GP than men
   (d) GPs see men more frequently for consultations regarding cancer, obesity, anaemia, migraine, osteoarthritis and back pain
   (e) GPs see women more frequently for consultations regarding diabetes, heart attacks and angina

37. Which of the following deaths does NOT necessarily need to be reported to the Coroner in the UK?
   (a) A 90-year-old patient is found dead in a nursing home. A doctor has not attended her in the previous 14 days
   (b) A child has collapsed and died while playing in a sports match. The cause of death is unknown or uncertain
   (c) A piece of masonry has fallen from a building, crushing a man to death
   (d) A patient has died while having a routine laparoscopic hernia repair
   (e) A patient is admitted to hospital with a major stoke. After 3 days in hospital the patient develops a pneumonia and dies 2 days later

38. Which of the following is NOT one of the domains of the Quality and Outcomes Framework for General Practice in England?
   (a) Clinical care
   (b) Emergency services
   (c) Additional services
   (d) Organizational
   (e) Patient experience

39. Which of the following statements best describes screening for disease in a population?
(a) Screening only assists with primary or secondary prevention
(b) Screening may be mass, targeted, systematic or opportunistic
(c) Opportunistic case finding in the UK is more likely to occur in secondary care
(d) Skin and renal cancer screening is routine in the UK
(e) There are no potential harms associated with screening

40. Which ONE of the following is NOT a notifiable disease in the UK?
(a) HIV
(b) Plague
(c) Food poisoning
(d) Ophthalmia neonatorum
(e) Rabies

41. Which of the following statements BEST describes evidence-based medicine?
(a) It provides a way of reviewing very small amounts of medical literature primarily for the pharmaceutical industry
(b) Provides a robust way of managing a disease but does not make a significant difference to clinical outcome
(c) Serves as a means of modifying current disease-management practices
(d) Fails to identify gaps in the current state of knowledge
(e) Is considered separately from the quality and efficiency of disease-management procedures

42. Which of the following statements best describes clinical research?
(a) Defines what best practice is
(b) Maintains standards
(c) Tests conformity with tested knowledge
(d) Asks if best practice is being implemented
(e) Aims to improve specified outcomes

43. Which of the following statements best describes Reason's (2000) model of clinical error?
(a) When several active failures occur in conjunction with latent conditions, a catastrophic failure may occur
(b) Active failures may include problems within the system such as excess time pressure or understaffing
(c) Latent conditions may include unsafe actions by healthcare staff
(d) Hardly any adverse events involve a combination of active failures and latent conditions
(e) The combination of active and latent factors is sometimes described using a metaphor of a game of snakes and ladders

44. A patient dies in intensive care when one of the ventilators fails. It transpires that one of the cleaners has inadvertently unplugged a ventilator in order to use the power socket. According to the principles of risk management, which is the BEST plan to prevent something similar occurring in the future?
(a) The cleaner should be dismissed from his job immediately
(b) A more accessible power socket should be found and all cleaners in the hospital educated about not interfering with medical equipment. An e-mail could be sent to all doctors and nurses to be vigilant for unplugged equipment
(c) A clear warning sticker should be placed above the power sockets of all monitoring or otherwise critical medical equipment, and all the cleaners in the hospital educated about not interfering with medical equipment. The incident could be used as a learning case in staff inductions
(d) A clear warning sticker should be placed above the power socket, and all the cleaners in the hospital educated about not interfering with medical equipment
(e) A clear warning sticker should be placed above the power sockets of all monitoring or otherwise critical medical equipment, and all the cleaners in the hospital educated about not interfering with medical equipment

Extended-matching questions (EMQs)

1. Each of the following is an important concept, theory or framework in Medical Ethics and Law

A. Autonomy

B. A positive right

C. A negative right

D. Act utilitarianism

E. Rule utilitarianism

F. Beneficence

G. The Categorical Imperative

H. Justice

I. Non-maleficence

J. Justice

K. Virtue ethics

Instruction: Select the best option from the list (A–K) to match the descriptions in questions 1–5. Each option may be used once, more than once or not at all.

1. The principle of doing 'good' or improving the welfare of patients.
2. This is illustrated by the 'right to health care,' which imposes a duty on the government to provide hospitals, nurses and doctors for its citizens.
3. This theory is associated with the idea that we should create laws which maximize benefit.
4. The principle of respecting the decisions made by those capable of making decisions.
5. This principle might include the principle (associated with the philosopher Aristotle) of treating equals equally and unequals unequally according to the morally relevant inequality.

2. The following legislation may in some way relate to patient confidentiality and disclosure of information

A. The Children Act 1989/2004

B. Public Health (Infectious Diseases) Regulations 1988

C. Police and Criminal Evidence Act 1984

D. The Health and Social Care Act 2001

E. The Data Protection Act 1998

F. The Mental Health Act 1983 (2007)

G. The Mental Capacity Act 2005

H. The Terrorism Act 2000

Instruction: Select the best option from the list (A–H) to match the descriptions in questions 1–5. Each option may be used one, more than once or not at all.

1. This Act allows the police to access medical records, provided they have a warrant.
2. This Act permits the Secretary of State for Health to allow disclosure of information which is in the public interest.
3. This Act requires all UK citizens to report any information which may be linked to an Act of Terrorism, in the UK or abroad, or face criminal charges if it is subsequently found that they could have done so and did not.
4. This Act allows someone to know what information is held about them (for example by) their GP.
5. This Act maintains that confidentiality is secondary to the prevention of harm to a child.

3. The following is a list of terms associated with consent

A. Written consent

B. Valid consent

C. Invalid consent

D. Implied consent

E. Valid advance directive

F. Invalid advance directive

G. Gillick competence

Instruction: Match the best relevant term from the list (A–G) to the relevant description in questions 1–7. Each term may be used once, more than once or not at all.

1. The doctor tells the patient that she needs a blood test in order to reach a diagnosis and the patient holds out her arm and rolls up her sleeve.
2. An 80-year-old man who has advanced dementia and has lost decision-making capacity (at a close relative's insistence) signs a form stating that in the event that he is gravely ill, he does not wish to receive any medical treatment.
3. An opera singer is told by the surgeon that she needs to have surgery for thyroid cancer. He explains the nature and the purpose of the surgery but neglects to mention a low risk that her voice will be affected as a result of the surgery. She signs a consent form.

4. A patient with special educational needs who is unable to read or write has the nature and purpose of a procedure explained to him in simple terms which he can understand. He agrees to be treated.
5. A doctor is called to see a sick patient in a residential home. She is unconscious but has a signed and witnessed document (which she made at a time when she was assessed to have capacity) which outlines specific treatments she would rather not have and the specific circumstances in which she would refuse them.
6. A 14-year-old boy is brought to hospital with acute appendicitis. The surgical team thinks that he demonstrates sufficient maturity and understanding in order to consent to his operation.
7. A patient signs a consent form for a surgical procedure. When asked immediately after his clinic appointment, he is unable to answer any questions about what operation he is having or why he is having it.

4. The following is a list of terms associated with medically assisted dying

A. Suicide
B. Physician-assisted suicide
C. Murder
D. Attempted murder
E. Voluntary euthanasia
F. Non-voluntary euthanasia
G. Involuntary euthanasia
H. Doctrine of double-effect

Instruction: Match the best relevant term from the list (A–H) to the relevant description in questions 1–5. Each term may be used once, more than once or not at all.

1. Deliberately ending the life of a person who is incapable of expressing any wishes about whether they want to live or die, motivated by a consideration of that person's best interests.
2. Deliberately ending the life of an elderly person who is gravely ill in order to make the bed available to someone who can get more use from it.
3. A competent, able-bodied person has a progressive illness which will render her incapable at a later stage. She seeks medical assistance for medication with which she may end her own life.
4. A competent patient who is in pain and distress but unable to take his own life asks his doctor to administer a lethal injection.
5. A doctor increases the dosage of painkillers or sedation, at appropriate levels to control a patient's symptoms, in the knowledge that this may have a life-shortening side-effect. The doctor is adamant that she only intends the pain-killing and not the patient-killing effect of the medication.

5. The following is a list of terms associated with an approach to resource-allocation

A. Aristotelian justice
B. The Hippocratic Oath
C. Utilitarianism
D. Libertarianism
E. Marxism
F. Communism
G. Rawls theory of justice

Instruction: Match the best relevant term from the list (A–G) to the relevant description in questions 1–5. Each term may be used once, more than once or not at all.

1. Treat equals equally and unequals unequally according to morally relevant inequality.
2. The right not to be killed and to possess property – in simplistic form, each for him/herself.
3. Take from each according to ability and give to each according to need.
4. A rational person who makes a decision behind a veil of ignorance (without knowing who will benefit) will look after the least well-off.
5. Act to maximize welfare for the greatest number (at the least cost).

6. The following is a list of terms associated with sociology and disease

A. Iatrogenesis
B. Clinical iatrogenesis
C. The inverse care law
D. World Health Organization definition of health
E. Social, cultural and structural iatrogenesis
F. General susceptibility
G. Epidemiological triangle
H. The technological imperative
I. Limits to medicine

Instruction: Match the best option from list (A–I) to the relevant description in questions 1–5. Each option may be used once, more than once or not at all.

1. May be caused by medical negligence or error.
2. The idea that the greater availability of healthcare creates increasing dependence on doctors.
3. The notion that technological interventions are generally successful in treating disease.
4. A state of complete physical mental and social well-being.
5. An idea which has developed from the observation that certain groups tend to get certain diseases.

7. The following is a list of the stages of dying from the Kubler–Ross (1969) model

A. Denial and isolation

B. Anger

C. Bargaining

D. Depression

E. Acceptance

Instruction: Match the best relevant stage from the list (A–E) to the relevant scenario in questions 1–5. Each of the following options may be used once, more than once or not at all.

1. After being diagnosed with lung cancer, a patient gives up smoking.
2. A patient with bladder cancer asks about palliative medicine and advance directives.
3. After being diagnosed with end-stage renal failure, a patient seeks a private second opinion.
4. A patient with alcoholic liver cirrhosis swears to his doctors that he will never drink again if his condition can somehow be cured.
5. A patient with ovarian cancer says that she has lost her appetite and is no longer interested in seeing her friends.

8. The following is a list of concepts which have been used to explain the position of older people within society

A. Disengagement theory

B. Structured dependency theory

C. Labelling and ageism

D. Cultural emphasis on youth

E. Third ageism

F. Financial dependence

G. Domestic dependence

Instruction: Match the best relevant concept from the list (A–G) to the relevant description in questions 1–5. Each option may be used once, more than once or not at all.

1. This theory stresses the importance of social structures in creating the circumstances elderly people find themselves in.
2. Old people gradually disengage from a range of social activities until they become unable to fulfil the roles they had previously held and ultimately become dependent.
3. This theory holds that in fact older people are able to enjoy relatively good health and affluence.
4. The placement of older people in 'old people's homes' compounds this problem by removing older people from communities.

5. This theory holds that older people are increasingly undertaking activities, such as travelling and learning a new skill, that were once seen as the younger preoccupations.

9. The following is a list of types of healthcare study

A. Ecological

B. Cross-sectional

C. Case-control

D. Phase I

E. Cohort

F. Randomized-controlled trial (RCT)

G. Meta-analysis

H. Systematic review

Instruction: Match the best option of type of study in the list (A–H) to the relevant description in questions 1–5. Each option may be used once, more than once or not at all.

1. May describe a disease in terms of person, place and time.
2. This combines the results of many (possibly inconclusive) trials to generate a more precise understanding of the effectiveness of an intervention.
3. Subjects are classified according to presence or absence of exposure to one or more factors and followed for a specific time period to determine the development of disease.
4. An example of this type of study might be one that compares the incidence of skin cancer for people living at different latitudes.
5. This uses rigorous selection and analysis of papers to draw the most valid conclusion about whether or not an intervention works.

10. The following is a list of terms associated with public health management

A. Occurrence

B. Transmission

C. Reservoir

D. Incubation period

E. Susceptibility

F. Control

G. Causative agent

Instruction: Match the best relevant term from the list (A–G) to the relevant description in questions 1–5, concerning the public health management of primary tuberculosis. Each term may be used once, more than once or not at all.

1. This may include HIV-positive status, poor housing or malnutrition.
2. This is mainly via droplet nuclei.
3. This is mainly humans.
4. This may include identifying and treating those who already have the disease, to shorten their infection and to stop it being passed on to other people.
5. This may include farm-workers who drink unpasteurized milk.

11. The following is a list of types of research study

A. Case series
B. Systematic review of randomized controlled trials
C. Randomized trial
D. Inception cohort study
E. Systematic review of cross-sectional studies
F. Systematic review of inception cohort studies
G. Mechanism-reasoning
H. Non-randomized cohort follow-up study
I. Local and current random-sample surveys

Instruction: According to the Oxford Centre for Evidence-Based Medicine 2011 guidelines, which type of study from the list (A–I) could be considered to be 'Level 1' evidence for each of the research questions 1–7? Each option may be used once, more than once or not at all.

1. How common is the problem?
2. Is this diagnostic test accurate?
3. Does this intervention help?
4. What will happen if we do not add a therapy?
5. What are the common harms?
6. What are the rare harms?
7. Is this (early detection test) worthwhile?

12. The following is a list of terms associated with the process of improvement in quality of health care

A. Clinical governance
B. Clinical error
C. Clinical audit
D. Significant event audit
E. Evidence-based medicine
F. Risk management

Instruction: Match the best relevant term from the list (A–F) to the relevant description in questions 1–5. Each option may be used once, more than once or not at all.

1. The process of reviewing the delivery of health care to identify deficiencies, so that they may be remedied.
2. The tension between institutional control over clinical decisions while allowing individual doctors some freedom to act in the interests of their patients.
3. A system through which NHS organizations are accountable for continuously improving the quality of their services and safeguarding high standards of care by creating an environment in which excellence in clinical care will flourish.
4. This means having systems to understand, monitor and minimize risks to patients and staff and to learn from mistakes.
5. This may be conducted for individual cases in which there has been an occurrence (with an actual or potential undesirable outcome for the patient). This is analysed in a systematic and detailed way to ascertain what changes might lead to future improvements.

Short-answer questions (SAQs)

Answers for all of these are in the relevant chapter.

Chapter 1

1. Give five examples of ethical issues of particular relevance to medical students.
2. What are the four principles of bioethics? – Give a one-line summary of what each means.
3. What is virtue ethics? – Give an example of a virtue.
4. What are the key differences between a civil case and a criminal case? – Give an example of each relating to health care.
5. Which articles of the European Convention on Human Rights might relate to health care? – Give at least four examples.

Chapter 2

1. Outline the roles of the BMA, the GMC and the Royal Medical Colleges.
2. List the circumstances where a doctor might be required to breach patient confidentiality.
3. Summarize the ethical and professional issues raised by doctors' and medical students' use of social media.
4. What is an intimate examination? – List features of a physical examination that might require a chaperone.
5. List the key ethical considerations when conducting medical research on animals.

Chapter 3

1. What is the difference between explicit and implied consent? – Give examples.
2. What are the criteria of capacity set down in the 2005 Mental Capacity Act?
3. List the components of the Fraser Guidelines for clinicians who give contraceptive advice or treatment to children under the age of consent for sex.
4. List the key types of abuse that frail elderly patients may be vulnerable to.
5. What is the main role of the Mental Capacity Act 2005 and how is this different from the main role of the Mental Health Act?

Chapter 4

1. What is the relevance of defining what counts as a human person? – Give an example of a relevant issue in the healthcare setting.

2. List the key arguments for and against reproductive cloning.
3. Outline the provisions of the 1961 Suicide Act (as amended by the 2009 Coroners and Justice Act) that relate to assisted suicide.
4. List the key arguments for and against euthanasia and other forms of clinician-assisted dying.
5. Outline the ways in which the supply of organs for transplantation might be increased, and summarize the ethical arguments for and against each method.

Chapter 5

1. What is commissioning? – Give examples of each stage of commissioning in the healthcare setting.
2. Give an example of micro-allocation and macro-allocation. Who usually makes these decisions?
3. Outline the different ethical theories which could be used to approach resource allocation.
4. List the advantages and disadvantages of QALYs (quality-adjusted life years).
5. Give a brief summary of the main ethical issues regarding organ transplants and resource allocation.

Chapter 6

1. Summarize 3 ways in which sociology is applied to medicine
2. List 4 assumptions which the biomedical model of disease makes
3. Outline the observations made by the sociologist Emile Durkheim about social integration and suicide
4. Briefly define what is meant by social, cultural and structural iatrogenesis

Chapter 7

1. List the five stages of Illness according to Hannay (1988).
2. Outline two issues which could result from self-management of minor illnesses.
3. What are the five rights and two responsibilities of the 'sick role' according to Parsons (1951)?
4. Summarize the five aspects of patient-centeredness according to Mead and Bower (2002).

Chapter 8

1. Summarize the advantages and disadvantages of the National Health Service in England
2. List the key advantages and disadvantages of a socialised health service, an insurance based health service, and a pluralistic health service
3. What are the characteristics of professionals according to Carr-Saunders and Wilson (1933)?
4. Briefly discuss the challenges to setting up appropriate healthcare in the community

Chapter 9

1. Outline the 'materialist' explanation for the effect of social inequality on health
2. Briefly describe Tudor-Hart's (1971) 'Inverse care law'.
3. Summarize the social causes that might explain some of health inequalities between men and women.
4. Define ethnicity, race and culture.

Chapter 10

1. Outline the epidemiological approach to the eradication of a disease, using an appropriate example.
2. What is the difference between a meta-analysis, and systematic review?
3. What are the Bradford-Hill (1965) criteria for establishing a causal relationship in epidemiology?
4. What are the advantages and disadvantages of studying routine data in healthcare research?

Chapter 11

1. List the key features of an audit.
2. Summarise the key differences between research and clinical audit.
3. What is a significant event audit?
4. Summarize Reason's 'Swiss-cheese' model of risk management

Essay questions

Answers for all of these are in the relevant chapter.

Chapter 1

1. What is medical ethics and why is it an important topic for medical students? – If you think it is not an important topic, please give good reasons why doctors need not have a grounding in medical ethics!
2. 'The Four Principles of Bioethics are the most widely taught approach to medical ethics because they are the best approach for use in the healthcare setting'. Do you agree or disagree? – Discuss this statement, comparing this approach to other ethical theories and frameworks.
3. What is the difference between the civil and criminal division of the law and how might this relate to the healthcare setting?
4. How might the Articles of the European Convention on Human Rights as stated in the Human Rights Act 1998, affect the provision of medical treatment in England and Wales?

Chapter 2

1. What are the main ethical and legal grounds on which a doctor should respect confidentiality? In what circumstances should confidentiality nevertheless be breached? – Provide explanations for your answers.
2. Are there any circumstances where it would be ethical or lawful to lie to or withhold information from a patient? – Discuss the issues involved with examples if possible.
3. You note that one of the doctors in your team has started to make mistakes at work and you suspect he may have a substance misuse problem. What should you do and what issues would you consider before acting?
4. Should doctors have a right to conscientious objection in certain circumstances?
5. What distinguishes ethical from unethical medical research on human subjects? – Your answer should also consider the kinds of things that a research ethics committee might want to know before approving medical research on human subjects.

Chapter 3

1. What are the legal requirements for informed consent? What type of legal case might arise if consent is not present or inadequate?

2. Describe the key provisions of the Mental Capacity Act 2005 in relation to healthcare decisions.
3. 'If a child demonstrates sufficient capacity then he or she should be able to refuse life-saving treatment' – Discuss.
4. Outline how you would approach a case of suspected child abuse. – Your answer should include the main types of abuse described, the legal provisions in such circumstances and any ethical issues you might consider relevant.
5. What are the ethical justifications for compulsory psychiatric treatment?

Chapter 4

1. What are the ways in which ethics and the law define a person? How is this relevant to healthcare decisions?
2. People should be able to exercise autonomy in terms of when how and with whom they have a child. Discuss this statement in the context of reproductive technologies. Explain why you might agree or disagree with this statement.
3. Discuss the ways in which a course of treatment might be considered futile. How is the concept of futility relevant to end-of-life decisions?
4. Should it be a criminal offence for a doctor to assist the suicide of a patient? What ethical reasons do you have for your answer? What are the main counter-arguments to your position and how would you respond to them?
5. How is death defined and how might this be relevant to decision-making in health care?

Chapter 5

1. Are there any particular ethical concerns regarding healthcare commissioning? – Give examples where possible.
2. What considerations might affect the allocation of healthcare resources? – In your answer, include some of the ethical theories which could be applied to rationing decisions.
3. Organ transplantation is a waste of NHS resources – discuss (explain why you agree or disagree with this statement).
4. What are 'Quality-Adjusted Life Years' (QALYs)? – In your answer include the main advantages and disadvantages of using QALYs to guide healthcare resource allocation.
5. How and why might a resource allocation decision be challenged in the courts?

Chapter 6

1. Giving examples from your sociology reading, describe how the study of sociology could improve clinical practice.
2. What are the strengths and weaknesses of the biomedical model of illness? Discuss whether an understanding of social phenomena is helpful or unhelpful.
3. In what ways do social integration, support and life events affect health? Illustrate your essay with examples from your sociological reading.
4. Discuss Illich's (1978) concept of Iatrogenesis. Do you think that this has valid points to make about the effect of healthcare itself on illness? If so why? If not why not?

Chapter 7

1. Discuss the 'Sick Role' as described by Parsons (1951). Is this a relevant concept in modern medicine?
2. What is patient-centeredness and why is it important in healthcare?
3. Using examples from your sociological reading, discuss how conflict may arise in the doctor-patient relationship and how it may be resolved.
4. How can a sociological understanding of death and bereavement improve clinical practice?

Chapter 8

1. How were health services provided in the UK prior to the National Health Service?
2. How has the UK National Health Service changed since 1948?
3. Discuss the advantages and disadvantages of different healthcare systems.
4. Discuss the origins of the medical profession in the UK.

Chapter 9

1. What is the impact of social class on health?
2. "Women get sick but men die." Discuss this statement with reference to gender and health inequalities.
3. How can a sociological understanding of migrant and ethnic minority health improve your clinical practice?
4. What social factors may compound medical problems in older people?

Chapter 10

1. What is the role of epidemiology in healthcare today?
2. What are the advantages and disadvantages of the different types of sociological research?
3. In what ways can we measure health and treatment outcomes?
4. How has the pattern of disease changed over time? How is this relevant in modern medicine?

Chapter 11

1. What is clinical governance and why is it important?
2. Give an example of a clinical audit you could do, identifying each stage of the audit.
3. What is evidence-based medicine?
4. How can we learn from clinical error?

1. C
2. D
3. B
4. C
5. E
6. A
7. A
8. C – Regardless of whether you know this specific fact, the answer could be worked out – all the other issues are regular daily issues for doctors.
9. B – Remember that even if this is done to benefit the patient, it is by definition a form of negligence and may invalidate consent entirely; all are listed by the MPS as dishonest behaviours.
10. E – For example the parent of a young child.
11. E
12. E
13. D
14. E
15. C
16. E
17. D
18. A
19. D
20. C

21. C – It is much more than a resource allocation process.
22. C
23. C
24. D
25. B
26. C
27. A
28. C
29. B
30. C
31. D
32. E
33. D
34. E
35. D
36. C
37. E
38. B
39. B
40. A
41. C
42. A
43. A
44. C

EMQ answers

1. Each of the following is an important concept, theory or framework in Medical Ethics and Law

1. F. Beneficence
2. B. A positive right
3. E. Rule utilitarianism
4. A. Autonomy
5. J. Justice

2. The following legislation may in some way relate to patient confidentiality and disclosure of information

1. C. Police and Criminal Evidence Act 1984
2. D. The Health and Social Care Act 2001
3. H. The Terrorism Act 2000
4. E. The Data Protection Act 1998
5. A. The Children Act 1989/2004

3. The following is a list of terms associated with consent

1. D. Implied consent
2. F. Invalid advance directive. Advance directives must be made by a person with capacity and must be specific. They must not be as a result of coercion.
3. B. Valid consent. Consent is valid to avoid a charge of trespass to the person but is arguably negligent in terms of disclosing risks.
4. B. Valid consent
5. E. Valid advance directive
6. G. Gillick competence
7. C. Invalid consent

4. The following is a list of terms associated with medically assisted dying

1. F. Non-voluntary euthanasia
2. C. Murder
3. B. Physician-assisted suicide
4. E. Voluntary euthanasia
5. H. Doctrine of double-effect

5. The following is a list of terms associated with an approach to resource-allocation

1. A. Aristotelian justice
2. D. Libertarianism
3. E. Marxism
4. G. Rawls theory of justice
5. C. Utilitarianism

6. The following is a list of terms associated with sociology and disease

1. B. Clinical iatrogenesis
2. E. Social, structural and cultural iatrogenesis
3. H. The technological imperative
4. D. World Health Organization definition of health
5. F. General susceptibility

7. The following is a list of the stages of dying from the Kubler–Ross (1969) model

1. C. Bargaining
2. E. Acceptance
3. A. Denial and isolation
4. C. Bargaining
5. D. Depression

8. The following is a list of concepts which have been used to explain the position of older people within society

1. B. Structured dependency theory
2. A. Disengagement theory
3. E. Third ageism
4. C. Labelling and ageism
5. E. Third ageism

9. The following is a list of types of healthcare study

1. B. Cross-sectional
2. G. Meta-analysis

3. E. Cohort
4. A. Ecological
5. H. Systematic review

---

10. The following is a list of terms associated with public health management

1. E. Susceptibility
2. B. Transmission
3. C. Reservoir
4. F. Control
5. E. Susceptibility

---

11. The following is a list of types of research study

1. I. Local and current random-sample surveys
2. E. Systematic review of cross-sectional studies

3. B. Systematic review of randomized controlled trials
4. F. Systematic review of inception cohort studies
5. B. Systematic review of randomized controlled trials
6. B. Systematic review of randomized controlled trials
7. B. Systematic review of randomized controlled trials

---

12. The following is a list of terms associated with the process of improvement in quality of health care

1. C. Clinical audit
2. A. Clinical governance
3. A. Clinical governance
4. F. Risk management
5. D. Significant event audit

Objective structured clinical examination questions (OSCEs)

Many of the concepts in this book can, to a lesser or greater extent, occur in Objective Structured Clinical Examinations (OSCES). It is likely that there will be an ethico-legal or social component to a clinical scenario, though some medical schools have put on OSCE stations that are more overtly testing a knowledge of ethics and the law. OSCEs are a rehearsal for real-life clinical encounters, and are intended to provide some objective evidence to your examiners that you can be a safe and professional doctor. Examiners can usually tell when students have 'learned some words' but do not really know what they mean or are just 'making it up.' The following advice is intended as a way to help you pass OSCES for the right reason – because you have a better understanding- and not as a set of ready answers.

General advice for all OSCEs

- Even OSCEs with a communication-skills theme require a sound medical knowledge
- Remember that you are not usually talking to another doctor, avoid jargon and try and understand what they want to know and what is important to them.
- Always remember to explore the patient's ideas, concerns and expectations (if they are conscious!). And remember that clinical colleagues have ideas, concerns and expectations as well!
- Sometimes the knowledge being tested is less medical and more legal. For example it is entirely fair to expect medical students to know the circumstances in which an autopsy is mandatory. It is also entirely fair to expect students who have done paediatrics to know about Gillick Competence and the Fraser Guidelines. Think about what bits of guidance and the law a doctor might be expected to come across – for example the Data Protection Act, the Mental Capacity Act and the Mental Health Act may well be relevant to doctors in the first two years of practice in the UK. (Students in other countries should think about the equivalent pieces of legislation.)
- Remember that you are usually having a focussed conversation with another person and not just giving and receiving facts. Talking to patients is not a science 'viva' exam.
- The 'clerking' gradually gives way to more flexible discussion with patients as medical students progress towards their final year. (However OSCEs increasingly include communication skills from year 1.)
- Keep an eye out for instructions like, 'Respond to the patient's concerns.' This mirrors real life, as you progress through medical school you will be increasingly be expected to respond to concerns. You cannot respond if you do not know what the concern is!

These are a few examples of ideas that could form the basis of a clinical examination station

1. You witness a doctor behaving in an unprofessional way, or a way which risks harm to patients
2. A patient asks to discuss the care of an adult family member, and asks to see the notes
3. A mother refuses to allow her child to vaccinated
4. A 14-year-old asks for contraception
5. A parent of a teenager would like to know if her daughter is receiving contraception
6. A patient would like the latest and most expensive drug with the fewest side-effects for their condition
7. You have been asked to assess a person who is behaving strangely
8. A patient would like a copy of his notes and a letter outlining his condition so he may obtain assisted suicide abroad
9. A patient would like to discuss having an advance directive
10. You are asked to discuss the need for an autopsy or the possibility of a post mortem with relatives
11. A patient has been newly diagnosed with a chronic disease – what do they want to know?
12. You are asked to talk to an elderly patient about her discharge from the hospital
13. You are asked to talk to a patient whose condition is not improving. You suspect he is not taking his medication
14. A patient has attended with a simple complaint but does not seem to want to discuss it
15. You have just given a patient the wrong vaccination. Discuss this with the patient

Some relevant ideas that may help you improve your OSCE performance in the above scenrarios

1. Look up and read chapter 2 on ethics law and professionalism and the sections on risk management, complaints and errors in chapter 11.
2. Look up and read about confidentiality
3. Look up and read children, parental responsibility
4. Look up and read confidentiality, child protection, Gillick competence and Fraser guidelines
5. Look up and read confidentiality, Gillick competence and Fraser guidelines
6. Look up and read justice, rationing, four principles
7. Look up and read autonomy, mental health, mental health act
8. Look up and read the Data Protection Act, euthanasia

9. Look up and read advance directives
10. Look up and read about the coroner, reasons why an autopsy might be legally required
11. Look up and read chapter 7, experience of health and illness
12. Look up and read the section on older people in the chapter on health inequalities, and on the multi-disciplinary team and care in the community in
13. Look up and read consent, compliance, concordance, patient-centeredness, patient agenda
14. Look up and read sections on patient's agendas, and stigma.
15. Look up and read the sections on risk management, complaints and errors in chapter 11.

Further reading

Papanikitas, A., 2007. We. J. R. Soc. Med. 100, 436–437. Available online at http://jrsm.rsmjournals.com/content/100/9/436.full.
(This short article discusses how medical students and doctors can be more aware of the words that they use in the context of OSCEs and consultations)

Washer, P., 2009, Oxford Core Texts: Clinical Communication Skills. Oxford University Press, Oxford. (This book has links to online audio podcasts as well as numerous examples of helpful and unhelpful language that students and clinicians use).

Index